Discerning Persons

Discerning Persons

Profound Disability, the Early Church Fathers, and the Concept of the Person in Bioethics

Pia Matthews

Franciscan University Press

Franciscan University Press
1235 University Boulevard
Steubenville, OH 43952
740-283-3771

Distributed by:
The Catholic University of America Press
c/o HFS
P.O. Box 50370
Baltimore, MD 21211
800-537-5487

Library of Congress Cataloging-in-Publication Data
Names: Matthews, Pia, author.
Title: Discerning persons : profound disability, the early church fathers, and the concept of the person in bioethics / Pia Matthews.
Description: Steubenville, OH : Franciscan University Press, 2020. | Includes bibliographical references and index. | Summary: "Drawing on rich insights from the early Church Fathers, this book addresses the neglected issue of disablism and how discriminatory attitudes fail to treat people with profound disabilities as persons. This discrimination can be found in the field of bioethics, where the stakes are often high and a matter of life or death. Whereas views that give priority to human beings whatever their capacities are seen as speciesist and so discriminatory, bioethical approaches that are disablist are rarely acknowledged as prejudiced. Many bioethicists do not even realize there is an issue. Current bioethical thinking appears uncritical and unreflective in the way it accepts a separation of the human being from the person and downgrades certain individuals who do not fulfill arbitrarily defined and insubstantial criteria for being persons. Using neglected Patristic thinking and its analogies with the human person, abled and disabled, found in reflection on the image of God and in the Trinitarian and Christological disputes of the early centuries where person language originated, the book makes patristic thinking do important work. It establishes that there are no early historical, philosophical, or theological grounds for calling or treating human beings as anything less than persons. Nor is there foundation for defining the person purely in terms of individuality, rationality, autonomy, or self-consciousness. Patristic insights conclusively call us to be discerning persons: to realize that persons are not so much defined as discerned, and to discern that all human beings, whatever their situations or capacities, are unique and unrepeatable persons"—Provided by publisher.
Identifiers: LCCN 2019044018 | ISBN 9781733988926 (hardcover)
Subjects: LCSH: Human body—Religious aspects—Christianity. | Disabilities—Religious aspects—Christianity. | People with disabilities—Religious aspects—Christianity. | Theological anthropology—Christianity. | Bioethics. | Persons.
Classification: LCC BT741.3 .M36 2020 | DDC 261.8/324—dc23
LC record available at https://lccn.loc.gov/2019044018

Cover Design: Kachergis Book Design
Cover Image: John G. Unnevehr, *Christ Blessing the Children*, ca. 1872. Courtesy of the J. Paul Getty Museum.
Printed in the United States of America.

Contents

Introduction. Discerning or Defining Persons?

Speaking about the Profoundly Disabled Human Being

The words we use matter. Words can build people up or humiliate them; words can influence how people are viewed; words say something about our own attitudes to others. Concern about the power of language has led to movements that encourage respectful language, which applies particularly when speaking about disability. Words like "retard," "moron," "cretin," and "idiot" have rightly been categorized as insulting, and the term "handicapped" is no longer acceptable since it (mistakenly) carries connotations of charity, of coming cap-in-hand.[1] Nevertheless, disability language remains a veritable minefield. Saying someone "suffers" from rather than simply "has" a disability implies a negative understanding of disability. Calling someone wheelchair-bound suggests that the person is tied to the wheelchair. Placing the word "disabled" before "people" puts the focus on disability instead of the person, as if the medical condition is primary. Referring merely to the disabled suggests that people with disabilities are not able to do anything. Moreover, this term does not include any notion of the person. While "people with disabilities" appears to put the person first, it also seems to deny that some people are disabled further by socially constructed barriers. Certainly, words matter. But for people with profound disabilities, it is not merely the arrangement of the words that makes a difference. It is the use of the word "person" itself. While it is no longer acceptable to call a person with profound intellectual disabilities a retard, in some circles it has become acceptable to deny this human being personhood.

The profoundly disabled are first and foremost people. It may seem

1. Hand-in-cap was a game involving exchanges; it then became a term for equalizing a horse race by obliging the stronger horse to carry additional weight.

curious to have to state this at the outset, but when talking about the voiceless profoundly disabled human being, this is the heart of the issue, and there is much at stake. As the brief foray into the minefield of disability language shows, when speaking about disability, many vocal people with disabilities argue that what is significant is not the disability but the person; hence they say that "person" should come first. The term "people" is simply plural for "person." But the sentence "the person with profound disabilities is first and foremost a person" has become a point of issue especially in bioethics, the discipline that concerns itself with the ethics of human life, particularly in the context of health care. This is because two disparate and competing visions of the person—the discerning vision and the defining vision—have gradually unfolded in the recent history of bioethics. According to the now-dominant defining vision, the profoundly disabled human being is not a person.

In the discerning vision, the person is a subject of discernment, or of coming to recognize. Rather than being merely a body to be fixed or cured, every patient is discerned as a person with his or her own story and history. All human beings are persons, and the person as a holistic concept refers to the unity of the material and spiritual aspects of human beings: persons are embodied souls, or ensouled bodies or embodied minds. In the defining vision, the person is the subject of definition, where the individual in question is measured against a set of desired characteristics. Rather than being first and foremost a person, the individual must reach a specific threshold to be considered a person, and only then does the individual qualify for all the privileges that seem to accompany personhood. These two visions underpin notions of human dignity and ultimately how the profoundly disabled human being is treated. As Gilbert Meilaender explains, for those who ground human dignity in certain characteristics that may or may not be present, those lacking these characteristics will also lack personal dignity. When human dignity and personal dignity are compared, there is inequality, and some lives can be judged as having less worth than others. When human dignity and personal dignity are set side by side, however, then "every person, simply by virtue of his or her humanity, is one whose dignity calls for our respect."[2]

2. Meilaender, *Neither Beast nor God*, 6–7.

While Meilaender accepts that dignity means many different things and raises puzzling questions,[3] the term "person" appears to be more clear-cut, even though there are nearly as many definitions of person as there are bioethicists. These definitions tend to have a common foundation in the definition of the person as "a thinking intelligent being, that has reason and reflection, and can consider itself as itself, the same thinking thing, in different times and places, which it does only by that consciousness which is inseparable from thinking,"[4] formulated by the seventeenth-century philosopher John Locke. The Lockean approach has led to a separation of human life into biological life and biographical life. According to this separation, the human being with profound disabilities may have biological life, but without the requisite cognitive capacities, he or she may not have biographical life: some people with disabilities are not persons.

Honoring people with disabilities as first and foremost persons, this book calls for discerning rather than defining persons. Discernment appreciates that no one can fully understand another human being in his or her entirety, and discernment recognizes that the other person is always unique and irreplaceable. This book attempts to speak for the speechless, persons who are not able to cry out when someone more powerful calls them nonpersons, especially when the powerful are those who seek to influence health care decisions. In particular, it is about the person with profound intellectual disabilities, but it is also about other human beings that seem to fall out of some definitions of the person: so-called less good spare embryos, disabled embryos that genetic engineering aims at eliminating, fetuses that are screened out by prenatal diagnosis, fetuses that may or may not have a disability, neonates whose lives are considered to be not worth living, cognitively impaired human beings, frail and demented elderly people, patients in persistent vegetative state. What is at stake is not simply hurt feelings at not being called a person, even if it is someone else's hurt feelings on behalf of those who apparently have no feelings because they cannot express them. What is at stake for the voiceless is something more critical: life itself.

3. Meilaender, *Neither Beast nor God*, 1.
4. Locke, *Essay Concerning Human Understanding*, II.XXVII.9.

Bioethical and Theological Persons

In bioethics, most discussions about the disabled person take place in connection either with beginning-of-life issues or end-of-life issues: the disabled human being merges into one of these issues. This means that disability is often treated as a way of arguing for or against abortion or euthanasia, for instance, rather than being a subject in its own right.

In bioethical discussions on personhood, arguments against speciesism are frequently central. In contrast, disablism is rarely mentioned. As the prominent utilitarian and champion of animal rights Peter Singer explains, "if there is real doubt about whether a being we are thinking of killing is a person, we should give that being the benefit of the doubt. The rule here is the same as that among deer hunters: if you see something moving in the bushes and are not sure if it is a deer or a hunter, don't shoot!"[5] Unfortunately for profoundly disabled human beings, Singer is only speaking of nonhuman animals here. He does not apply this benefit to the profoundly disabled, since there he is in no doubt.

This book examines the personal reality of the profoundly disabled human being. It returns the person to where the concept started, in the theology of the early Church Fathers. Unlike "dignity," which is a relatively new term in bioethics and comes out of classical stoic philosophy rather than theology, "person" appears to be crucial in the early bioethical literature and in later bioethical thinking, and it is rooted in theology as well as philosophy. To return to theology, especially patristic thought, may seem odd for a discipline, even when practiced by Christian bioethicists who lean so heavily toward philosophy. But the opening for such a consideration comes from an unlikely source: bioethicists themselves. Some bioethicists casually refer to theology; in particular, Singer and his coauthor Paola Cavalieri situate the foundations for their view of the person as rational and self-conscious specifically in relation to patristic Trinitarian theology. Singer definitively makes the connection between philosophy and theology when he points out that in the theological writings of Boethius, "Boethius confirmed this by defining 'person' as 'an individual substance of rational nature,' a definition subsequently used

5. Singer, *Practical Ethics*, 119.

by Aquinas and other writers and supplemented by Locke with the element of awareness of one's own existence at different times and places."[6]

Much has been written about Aquinas and the human person.[7] Moreover, Locke himself comes to his definition through theology. Still, apart from a cursory nod to Boethius, patristic thinking has been neglected and, as the subsequent chapters show, misinterpreted by secular bioethicists like Singer. To address this neglect, this book offers a systematic exploration of the thinking of the early Church Fathers on the person. Returning the concept of the person to its beginning in patristic thinking may seem to be merely a telling of its historical story in order to fill in the gaps and avoid ahistoricism. But patristic thinking can also be put to work as a tool to challenge, analyze, expose, and question difficult areas. A return to the early Christian traditions of the Fathers is a worthwhile enterprise precisely because the insights of this tradition can correct mistakes and illumine areas that currently lie forgotten outside the vision of modern bioethics. The early Christian tradition also has something to say to current disability studies. Notably, for disability studies, which challenges discourses of normality versus abnormality or "them versus us," the early Christian tradition treats all human beings as belonging to one family: us. But the claim that patristic thinking can make a significant contribution to a modern debate leads perhaps inevitably on to the vexing question of the relationship between theology and philosophy in bioethics.

Relating Theology, Philosophy, and Bioethics

The conversation about how and if theology and philosophy relate in bioethics is vexing on two main but interrelated accounts: as a matter of the history of the discipline, and as a matter of the contemporary academic understanding of the nature of bioethics.

As a matter of history, long before bioethics emerged as a discipline

6. Singer, *Rethinking Life and Death*, 180.

7. See, e.g., Pasnau, *Thomas Aquinas on Human Nature*; De Young et al., *Aquinas's Ethics*; Ashley, "Anthropological Foundations of the Natural Law," 7–11. For insight into the thinking of Aquinas in connection with the person with disabilities, see Romero, "Aquinas on the *Corporis Infirmitas*," 101–51, and through the lens of Pope John Paul II, see Matthews, *Pope John Paul II*, 41–51.

in its own right, moral theology was the mainstay for medical ethics, and many of the founding fathers of the emerging discipline of bioethics were working in the field of theology. It would appear then that theology is embedded in bioethics. Yet Kevin Wildes notes that religious voices have now receded from the public square, and he charts the shift toward a secular approach to bioethics through the general secularization of contemporary Western societies, the developing focus on law and public policy, and the growing attention to individual patient choice in medical decision making.[8] Moreover, and in reference to analysis by Stanley Hauerwas, Wildes suggests that Christian ethicists also contributed to this shift because they assumed that the Christian vision was commonly shared in society, and so they did not ground their arguments in Christianity, thus opening the way for philosophy to take bioethics in different directions.

John Evans explains the shift toward a secular bioethics in terms of the competition for jurisdiction. Evans charts the first era of bioethics in the 1960s as a competition between scientists and theologians where scientists were seen by theologians as "professional interlopers." In order to capture the ground, theologians used "condensed translation," whereby they abandoned explicitly theological language and used generalized arguments with explicit secular ends. In the second era, Evans says that theology became more and more implicit, allowing the growth of a system of abstract knowledge of the "new profession of bioethics." As the hand of bioethicists grew stronger, the theological challenge receded, and the third era is characterized by bioethicists who wrested jurisdiction from the scientists. Evans concludes that "the bioethics profession did not begin with theological ends and translate to secular language, thus resulting in a debate about various ends. Rather it started with a list of four ends that roughly correspond to the four principles of principlism, portrayed as the values held by all of the citizens, which one could transmute other ends into."[9]

Evans also speaks of the "thinning" of the debate in bioethics, though from a different perspective to Wildes. Evans challenges the claim that

8. Wildes, "Religion in Bioethics," 163–74.

9. Evans, *History and Future of Bioethics*, 4–9. Evans does think, however, that the "bioethics profession" and science and medicine have never been in "serious competition" (104).

this "thin" debate is the result of an acknowledgment of pluralism and its competing notions of the "good life," where the "thick" debate is left within individual traditions themselves, be they Roman Catholic, feminist, or African American. Instead, Evans notes that theology calls for the general public to become more involved in debates, and that this call becomes a challenge not only to the authority of the state but also to those who are pursuing their own interests, whether scientific, economic, or in research. Furthermore, the shift toward thinness in the debate sees the emergence of the "bioethics profession" that has given itself jurisdiction over ethical decision making in both public debate and hospital practice. The creation of expert professional bioethicists is accompanied by specialized knowledge; hence the marginalization of theologians.[10]

Even though theology seems to have been marginalized, however, theology remains a force in the discipline, which has led some writers, like Timothy Murphy, to call for a competing "irreligious outlook" to protect against what he sees as the overreach of religion.[11] Furthermore, and beyond the academic sphere, theology remains relevant for the many health care professionals, patients, and policy makers who identify themselves as religious. As Evans points out, "for a healthy public sphere we must have debate about what our values should be," and both philosophy and theology help us to understand the "big questions" in bioethical debate.[12] Theology, it seems, is here to stay.

In the matter of the contemporary academic understanding, bioethics is multidisciplinary, or at least interdisciplinary, as a result of the migration of theologians, philosophers, sociologists, and lawyers from their own specific disciplines. So, it seems that theology, along with other disciplines, naturally belongs in bioethical discourse. But some have charged theology with particularism, of being significant only for those with a religious outlook. At the same time, some thinkers are beginning to question whether bioethics can be considered *a* field since they find little common agreement within the discipline.[13] As Wildes points out, this claim suggests that philosophy, no less than theology, may be subject

10. Evans, *Playing God*, 5–7, 193.
11. Murphy, "In Defence of Irreligious Bioethics," 3–10.
12. Evans, *History and Future of Bioethics*, 160–61.
13. Engelhardt, "Skeptical Reassessment of Bioethics," 1–28.

to the challenge of particularity: appeals to differing views of reason in philosophy are "as opaque to those who do not share them" as are appeals to views of God.[14] We may also wish to add the complexity of referring to *a* discipline of bioethics in a global world where for instance the dominance of autonomy is perhaps particular to a Western conception of bioethics, and the notion of ubuntu—an understanding of humanity focusing on care, hospitality and a shared life[15]—is beginning to underlie African understandings of bioethics.

Despite these difficulties of particularity, the complex and multidisciplinary nature of bioethics partly acknowledges that a focus on merely practical clinical issues or on issues of policy or on culturally specific questions is not adequate for a discipline that inevitably touches upon deep questions. This need for reflection is reinforced by Helga Kuhse and Peter Singer, editors of *A Companion to Bioethics*, one of many textbooks in the now flourishing field. Kuhse and Singer rightly explain that in contrast to the older medical ethics, bioethics is "a more overtly critical and reflective enterprise." They point out that bioethics has as its goal "a better understanding of the issues," where practitioners are prepared to ask "deep philosophical questions,"[16] and the generally accepted interdisciplinary nature of bioethics advances this goal. Many bioethical textbooks, *Companion to Bioethics* included, accept that, as a branch of applied ethics, bioethics encompasses different ethical approaches that these textbooks identify and describe in their strengths and weaknesses. These textbooks also often acknowledge that there are some serious disagreements on fundamental principles and so admit that there is not necessarily a unique right answer to difficult questions.

Notably for Kuhse and Singer, however, it is only philosophical questioning that appears to be on the table, even though the apparent neutrality of the secular perspective has been challenged.[17] The call for "deep" questioning does not seem to be applied to the notion of person, since the notion is treated as generally accepted or already agreed, and "a better understanding of the issues" does not seem to be relevant to

14. Wildes, "Religion in Bioethics," 170.
15. Tutu, *No Future without Forgiveness*, 34–35.
16. Kuhse and Singer, *Companion to Bioethics*, 4.
17. See, e.g., Iltis, "Failed Search for the Neutral in the Secular," 220–33.

disability even though disability underlies almost all other questions, including resource allocation, where cash is replacing care as the main topic. Instead, issues of disability are framed in terms of deciding whether an individual qualifies as a person. Given the widely recognized interdisciplinary nature of bioethics and the complexity and confusion surrounding the concept of the person, theology surely has a place in the conversation without further justification. Moreover, the very fact that some bioethicists appeal to theology in order to find support for their interpretations from those with whom they do not generally agree seems to support the claim that theology remains relevant. The need for theology is clear, especially when serious mistakes have been made about theology that call out for theologians to correct.

Nevertheless, theology is further singled out, as some ask precisely what the introduction of theology in the now philosophy-saturated field of bioethics is attempting to achieve. Among a range of possible responses, some thinkers, like H. T. Engelhardt, argue that theology and philosophy are entirely separate in bioethics; some, like Charles Camosy, claim that there can be dialogue on the basis of compromise; and some, notably Pope John Paul II, think that theology not only provides a corrective perspective but also offers important insights.

While philosophers like Singer use theology, albeit often in a reductive or dismissive manner, thinkers like Engelhardt point to what Engelhardt sees as the "still widening gulf" between theistic bioethics and secular bioethics, a gulf that has engendered "culture wars" that we must take seriously.[18] According to Engelhardt, bioethics is in chaos, it cannot deliver moral direction, and there is no common ground either within the discipline or between philosophical accounts of bioethics and theology. Engelhardt claims that theological knowledge cannot be adequately understood without distortion outside of a life of right worship and right belief. Indeed, he thinks that it is impossible to give an account of morality grounded in natural law, or the good, or right-making conditions, understandable by all without them becoming Christians. In Engelhardt's understanding, "Orthodox Christians do not have a morality, a moral theology, or a moral philosophy" because true philosophy, "love

18. Engelhardt, "Moral Pluralism," 234–53, at 241.

of the wisdom of God," is directed only to God.[19] Engelhardt seeks to distance Orthodox Christianity from Roman Catholicism in particular, and he claims that Catholicism's alliance of faith and reason is "a much later Christian development born of the second millennium attempt to marry Athens with Jerusalem."[20]

In contrast, in his encyclical *Fides et Ratio,* Pope John Paul II calls faith and reason "two wings on which the human spirit rises to the contemplation of truth." The pope explains that "God has placed in the human heart a desire to know the truth," notably the truth about him or herself as a human being, and philosophy is a way of coming to know the wonder of being a human being in the world, in relationship with others.[21] Certainly, the pope acknowledges that the early Fathers were cautious when it came to philosophy, or in some cases, on their journey to wisdom, they found philosophy disappointing. He explains that this was partly because philosophy was often linked to esoteric speculation such as Gnosticism, and that the Gospel answered all their questions so that philosophy appeared to be remote. Nevertheless, the critical engagement of the Fathers with philosophy demonstrates that "they were not naive thinkers." The pope suggests that for the Fathers of both the East and the West, faith does not preclude philosophy. Instead, "precisely because they were intense in living faith's content, they were able to reach the deepest forms of speculation." Whereas Engelhardt finds little common ground, Pope John Paul II sees the early Christian relationship with philosophy as not only a "meeting of cultures" but also a "meeting of creature with Creator" where reason was opened up to the transcendent.[22]

In about 200 CE, and writing at a time when the "blood of the martyrs" was the "seed of Christians,"[23] Tertullian wrote *De Praescriptione Haereticorum*, a treatise about the practicalities of how Christians should and should not dialogue with heretics. Tertullian, who may have been a Roman lawyer and possibly the first theologian to write in Latin, uses the legal term *praescriptiones* to indicate that the case of one of

19. Engelhardt, "Moral Pluralism," 247.
20. Engelhardt, "Moral Pluralism," 249.
21. Pope John Paul II, *Fides et Ratio*, 4.
22. Pope John Paul II, *Fides et Ratio*, 37–41.
23. Tertullian, *Apology* 50, 12.

the parties, the heretics, was obviously defective and therefore should be ruled out of court. Tertullian's passion for the message of the Gospel led him to make the pithy comment, based on St. Paul's experience in the public arena of the Areopagus, and repeated by Engelhardt, "what indeed has Athens to do with Jerusalem."

In contemporary bioethical thinking, the line seems to have become "What indeed has Jerusalem to do with Athens?" In Tertullian's day, Christianity was the new innovative and provocative thinking, a conversion moment that put a new spin on human existence through Christ and the scandal of the Cross. Today, bioethics is the new thinking, and it is not merely a move away from the paternalistic medical ethic, characterized by the view that the doctor knows best, to the bioethical view summed up by ask the patient—or the philosopher, the sociologist, the lawyer, the politician, the moralist, the media, the celebrity. Evans may take the sociological approach and regard the bioethics profession as defined by a system of abstract knowledge based on the idea that "it is not using the values of the bioethicist, or of a subgroup of citizens, but the values of either those involved in the decision... or the general public."[24] Evans offers just one view of the discipline of bioethics, however. Singer, who sees bioethics as applied ethics and thinks that utilitarianism and its associated values provide the most appropriate method for bioethical decision making, is considered a leading bioethicist, even if he is not a bioethicist according to Evans's definition. In the middle of this academic dispute is the human being with disabilities, and often the life of this human being is at stake.

In a phrase used by Singer, bioethics has begun a "Copernican revolution," an outright rejection of the old fashioned, outmoded Christian ethic that holds back progress.[25] A view that sets store by concepts such as the sanctity of life, that balks at intentionally and directly killing human beings, that genuinely acknowledges that fine distinctions can be made between withdrawing burdensome treatment and deliberately seeking the death of the patient, that fervently believes in the value of all human beings no matter how sick, small, or disabled is, for Singer, a view that clouds the crystal-clear decision making of a practical ethics. Notably, it

24. Evans, *History and Future of Bioethics*, 75.
25. Singer, *Writings on an Ethical Life*, 211.

is the theological view of the human person that is problematic. Now that "we" have rid ourselves of what he sees as the "crumbling" Christian ethic, Singer believes that "we" can question why all human beings—including "infants, mental defectives, psychopaths, Hitler, Stalin and the rest"—should have dignity that no nonhuman animal can achieve.[26] Moreover, the unsanctifying of human life enables "us" to distinguish between human beings and persons and thus solve some of the apparently more intractable bioethical problems: the unwanted fetus, the anencephalic infant, the profoundly disabled, the patient in persistent vegetative state. According to Singer, because not all human beings are persons, it is not wrong to kill certain redundant or inconvenient human beings so long as it is done painlessly.[27] It is the religious view that is obstructive and obviously defective that has lost credibility and therefore should be ruled out of court. Religion risks being relegated to the private and personal sphere, and some would argue that it has no place in the public square.[28]

This move to rule theology out of court does not fully mirror Tertullian's objection to philosophy. Tertullian's view that heretics have "no right to Christian literature" since "this is my property, which I have long possessed"[29] seems to have resonance with Engelhardt's contention that theology outside of worship is a distortion. But Tertullian is not against philosophy itself. According to Tertullian, the problem is that heretics rely on many differing philosophies that are endlessly conflicting, and they rarely examine these philosophies critically. Tertullian himself is keen to explore Pythagorean, Platonic, Epicurean, and Stoic thought, and he uses these philosophies to further his own reflection on human beings, body and soul, and on God. But he rules out of court those who misuse philosophy as well as Scripture because in doing so they distort or lose the truth.[30] For Tertullian, the exclamation "What indeed has Athens to do with Jerusalem?" was a rhetorical device: it was part and parcel of how a rhetorician captured his (and it was usually his) audience. The modern version of this rhetorical question is a more troubling affair because it

26. Singer, *Rethinking Life and Death*, 206; idem, "All Animals Are Equal," 568–77, at 575.
27. Singer, *Practical Ethics*, chap. 7.
28. See Stammers and Bullivant, "Secularism," 83–88.
29. Tertullian, *De Praescriptione Haereticorum* 37,1.
30. Tertullian *De Praescriptione Haereticorum* 7.

suggests that theology has no role to play, and that it cannot even offer a corrective perspective on theology that has been misinterpreted. This is particularly concerning when, as Evans points out, the bioethics profession finds it difficult to say no in public policy bioethics.[31]

There have been attempts to find overlaps in theology and philosophy. Charles Camosy is a significant writer who has shown that there can be fruitful dialogue between Christianity and "Singerite" arguments. In particular, Camosy calls for a reaction to "culture's disproportionate focus on the human person as a consuming, private, supposedly autonomous individual." Camosy thinks that although Singer at times resorts to caricature when critiquing Christian positions, the disagreements between Christianity and Singerites are "actually quite narrow."[32] On the issue of persons, Camosy believes that the severely disabled human being is the same kind of being as other persons, even though disability frustrates the capacity to express this. As part of his project to narrow the gap, however, he does not rule out the possibility that some human beings are nonpersons or that there is a "gray area" between persons and nonpersons.[33] While critical engagement with influential thinkers is an important enterprise, there are always dangers in attempting compromise, and it is no less important to point out when there has been fundamental misinterpretation or misuse rather than mere caricature. The following chapters demonstrate that some bioethicists have not so much presented a caricature of the theological concept of the person. Rather, they have made fundamental mistakes or unwarranted assumptions, and on this basis they have offered what appears to be a clear-cut and uncontentious definition of the human person on which the lives of some people with disabilities depend.

The compromise approach of thinkers like Camosy is certainly appealing, and it may seem to ensure that theology is not dismissed out of hand. Yet there is considerable value in a prophetic approach that has confidence in its own traditions, that is grounded in real life experience, particularly of those who are voiceless and marginalized, and that can offer moral direction. Theologians like Pope John Paul II take up the vi-

31. Evans, *History and Future of Bioethics*, 110–18.

32. Camosy, *Peter Singer and Christian Ethics*, 3, 7, 251.

33. Camosy, *Peter Singer and Christian Ethics*, 23–24; idem, *Beyond the Abortion Wars*, 53–55.

sion of the Second Vatican Council's document *Gaudium et Spes* that faith "throws a new light on all things," and that the Church offers service to human beings who are asking fundamental questions yet are also affected by the "modern dilemma" of being "at once powerful and weak, capable of doing what is noble and base," and in fear of being enslaved by technologies.[34] Theology offers insights and a depth that may be forgotten, neglected, or even misrepresented in the turn toward a more practical bioethic.

Theology: Bridging the Gap

Echoing Tertullian's concern about the misuse of philosophy and Scripture, many contemporary bioethicists, including Singerites, take an ahistorical view of the person and locate its starting point in Locke's definition. By defining the person in terms of a disembodied rational self-conscious entity, Locke cuts the threads that kept the personal and biological aspects of the human being together. While many other philosophers were important in the split between mind and body (notably Descartes), Locke's understanding of the person has been promoted explicitly by prominent utilitarians Singer and Derek Parfit, and it seems to appeal to many bioethicists because it seems "flexible"[35] and compatible with many contemporary views. Locke's definition is taken up uncritically and developed beyond self-consciousness to having desires and interests or a certain level of rational ability.[36] This appeal to the Lockean idea applies across the human life span, from those who comment on the beginning of human life[37] to the end of life,[38] to those who comment in the context of animal rights,[39] and to those who use the Lockean definition in their own broad ethical frameworks.[40] And if a person is defined

34. Second Vatican Council, *Gaudium et Spes*, 3, 9–11.

35. Takala, "Genetic Knowledge and Our Conception of Ourselves as Persons," 92.

36. Gordijn points out that Locke's definition was open to development because his idea of consciousness was not clear. "Troublesome Concept of the Person," 353.

37. See, e.g., Tooley, *Abortion and Infanticide*, 49; Warnock, "In Vitro Fertilisation," 239; Dennett, "Conditions of Personhood," 176; Lizza, "Persons at the Beginning and End of Life," 97–104; Lockwood, "Moral Status of the Human Embryo," 18.

38. See Green and Winkler, "Brain Death and Personal Identity," 105–33.

39. See DeGrazia, *Human Identity and Bioethics*, 6.

40. See Parfit, *Reasons and Persons*, 205–6; Singer, *Rethinking Life and Death*; McMahan, *Ethics of Killing*; Harris, *Enhancing Evolution*, 97.

as a kind of thinking thing, whose material body is "immaterial" to the question of its personal status, then it is clear that some human beings do not qualify, notably, one particular profoundly disabled human being, the cognitively impaired human being. In the clear separation between the human being and the person, biological and biographical life, the human being seems to be nothing more than the animal body, raw material that can be manipulated or acted upon.

As part of this ahistorical approach, on a few occasions reference is made to the Boethian definition of the person as *naturae rationabilis individua substantia*, an individual substance of a rational nature, though this usually occurs without its context.[41] Although it appears that Locke and Boethius make the same connection between rationality and the concept of the person, once the definition by Boethius is returned to its theological Trinitarian context, the gulf between the two thinkers becomes clear. If Boethius means that person equals a rational individual along Lockean lines, then that would suggest that he believes in three gods: the divine Persons appear to be three divine individuals, who can reason about themselves and are self-conscious. Returned to its proper context, this is clearly not what Boethius thinks. Locke arrives at his definition because he does not think that in the afterlife and in judgment before God the body can carry personal identity over time because the body disintegrates, and if it is eaten by cannibals, then this is even more problematic.[42] Nor does he think that the soul can carry personal identity, since in his opinion souls can migrate into other bodies.[43] Instead, he arrives at his definition of person as a "forensic term," one connected to reward and punishment in the afterlife, and he locates person in self-consciousness.[44]

It is deeply concerning that some influential understandings of the concept of the person ignore its true roots and uncritically hold to a definition based on impoverished theological reasoning of eternal reward and punishment. It is also deeply concerning that mistakes are frequently made or that unwarranted extrapolations are drawn from the theological position. Taking an ahistorical approach to the concept of the person

41. Boethius, "Treatise against Eutyches and Nestorius," III.5.
42. Locke, *Essay Concerning Human Understanding*, II.XXVII.3.
43. Locke, *Essay Concerning Human Understanding*, II.XXVII.6.
44. Locke, *Essay Concerning Human Understanding*, II.XXVII.26.

that seems to offer an interpretation that is already tailor-made to some contemporary understandings means that many profound insights are lost. Making misinformed assumptions fails to take theology seriously. As a result, the concept of the person is often considered at a reductive level. To explore the roots of the concept and to point out mistakes is not to expect that all become Christians. Rather, it is to engage critically with this concept, to add depth, and to point to some implications that may at least cause us to pause and reflect more profoundly on what is after all a concept with high stakes that affects us all.

A return to the Fathers reminds us of what the concept really involves, and their reasoned arguments challenge Lockean definitions of the person that focus solely on the actual capacities of reasoning and having future desires. The theology of the early Fathers from both the East and the West can speak across the centuries because what they have to say about persons human and Divine came out of long debate, fine distinctions, and struggles with concepts, language, and silence. And these debates speak not just to theology. They also speak to philosophy, and they contribute to the dialogue on contemporary concerns, particularly to the growing recognition of an opening to the transcendence of the person, whatever his or her situation, through affectivity rather than purely intellectual abilities.

The State of the Question about Persons

From the idea of "person-centered care" to the defense or denial of the person as a central concept in bioethics, the term "person" has been the source of considerable debate, and the stakes are high—literally life and death. Emerging out of the concept of the person, the notion of personhood was developed in the 1980s by Tom Kitwood, a lecturer in psychology, specifically to improve the quality of life of people living with dementia.[45] For Kitwood, personhood is "a standing or status that

45. Rather than being a philosophical enterprise, Kitwood's project in defining personhood was part of a bigger project to improve care, and he took it as understood that all human beings were persons. His ideas, then, are somewhat incomplete and at times inconsistent and ambiguous. Moreover, his definition has been the subject of considerable critique, and personhood remains a hotly contested topic. For a consideration of some of these issues, see Kitwood, *On Dementia*.

is bestowed upon one human being, by others, in the context of relationship and social being. It implies recognition, respect and trust."[46] Rather than take an analytical approach to personhood, Kitwood says that his interpretation of what it means to be a person "gives priority to experience": he sees personhood in relational terms, most notably in terms of the I-Thou relationship of thinkers such as Martin Buber.[47] Kitwood's model of personhood became the underlying condition for delivering person-centered care, an approach to care that looks beyond the merely medical in treating patients.

In academic bioethical discourse, however, the concept of the person seems to have moved from the context of improved care and into the ethics of killing.[48] Writers on bioethics in general[49] and on specific bioethical topics speak of groups of patients who no longer have the right not to be killed,[50] who need not be cared for,[51] who cannot be wronged by being killed,[52] who do not have a "serious right to life,"[53] who do not enjoy a strong "presumption against killing."[54] The term "person" is recognized as value-laden.[55] According to some who write on human life and health care ethics, the human being's moral status changes over a lifetime depending on whether that being exhibits the relevant characteristics for being a person. There are *pre-persons*, beings like the embryo and fetus who, it is claimed, are humans but not yet persons.[56] Pre-persons may also be called *potential persons*.[57] Then there are *former*

46. Kitwood, *Dementia Reconsidered*, 8.

47. Kitwood, *Dementia Reconsidered*, 10–12.

48. See Tooley, "Personhood."

49. Glover, *Causing Death*, 19; Singer, *Practical Ethics*, 83; McMahan, *Ethics of Killing*.

50. Veatch, "Dead Donor Rule," 10–11.

51. Green and Winkler, "Brain Death and Personal Identity," 117.

52. Harris, "Concept of the Person and the Value of Life," 110.

53. Tooley, *Abortion and Infanticide*, 46.

54. DeGrazia, *Taking Animals Seriously*, 265, 267.

55. Merrill, *Defining Personhood*, 4.

56. See, e.g., Harris, *Wonderwoman and Superman*, 66. Harris explains that he is not "seduced" by the potentiality argument, which confers moral status on an individual because of the individual's potential for development (58). It seems that Harris is thinking of potential in terms of mere possibility, whereas the potentiality argument is considerably more nuanced and includes the notion of a power that a thing actually possesses. For a discussion of interpretations of the argument, see Manninen, "Revisiting the Argument from Fetal Potential."

57. Tooley, "Personhood," 132. According to Tooley, although a potential person is not a

persons, human beings with, say, advanced dementia or in persistent vegetative state who, it is claimed, were once persons.[58] Following this outline, most of us begin as pre-persons, become persons at some point in our life story, and if profound disability strikes, cease to be persons, all the while remaining living human beings. But this journey in and out of being a person is just the beginning. There are now other classifications for human beings.

In the human-made new creation, brought about by technological advances in bioethics, there are also what may be termed *un-persons*, those curious entities, human-animal hybrids, who are not one thing or another.[59] In addition, there may be contingent *future persons*, the coming generation to whom we may or may not have duties,[60] and futuristic *post-persons*, genetically enhanced beings whose higher intellectual capacities will supposedly endow them with a moral status superior to that of the rest of us, who will then belong to the new category of *mere persons*.[61] The *person of today* is only the mere person of tomorrow.

Last and ostensibly least in this list of precarious persons is the *non-person*, the human being who has never been and never will be a person.[62] These are those who are conceived or born as profoundly disabled human beings, and they witness in their own lives the living reality of the implications of being, or not being, treated as persons.

Profoundly Disabled People

The profoundly disabled human being can appear within any variety of the so-called human-beings-who-are-not-persons: a pre-person, as an embryo created through in vitro fertilization that is not implanted owing to undesirable genetics or discarded as "spare" and perhaps subjected

---

person, it "contains within itself all the positive factors that are needed in order for it to become a person."

58. See, e.g., Singer, *Practical Ethics*, 191–93. Singer revised his highly influential book in 2011. In the new edition, however, the author is less forthright in his discussion on the person, an indication, perhaps, that he does not take the concept of the person seriously.

59. For an exploration of human-nonhuman combinations, see MacKellar and Jones, *Chimera's Children*.

60. See Fotion and Heller, *Contingent Future Persons*.

61. See, e.g., David DeGrazia, "Genetic Enhancement, Post-Persons and Moral Status," 135–39.

62. See, e.g., Fletcher, *Humanhood*, 16; Tooley, "Personhood," 132.

to destructive research; another kind of pre-person, as a fetus terminated or even a neonate refused life-sustaining treatment simply because of a disability; the former person, as a human being with dementia or diminished cognitive capacities; and the un-person, as an animal-human hybrid where the human element has been deliberately disabled. In the future it may be a post-person, where either the mere person is considered somehow disabled or the post-person is considered no longer fully human. Most obviously, the profoundly disabled human being is a non-person, as a human being that has never had, nor will ever have, the kinds of capacities and abilities that some consider necessary for consideration as a person.

Disablism: The "Last Prejudice"

The elimination of the profoundly disabled from the status of persons in bioethics, and hence from the protection this status brings, seems to run counter to another trend—the criticism of disablism, a new name for a prejudice that is not new.[63] The UK disability charity Scope defines disablism as "discriminatory, oppressive or abusive behaviour arising from the belief that disabled people are inferior to others."[64] This discriminatory behavior fails to treat the disabled human being as a person, and Scope adds that this attitude is rooted not in fear or ignorance but in contempt and prejudice. As Scope points out in its 2008 report *Getting Away with Murder: Disabled People's Experience of Hate Crime in the UK*, people with disabilities are regarded as "less than human," and their lives are judged to be "less valuable."[65] Scope's position demonstrates the

63. See Miller et al., *Disablism*. The eugenics movement of the 1920s and 1930s evidenced a profound disdain for the disabled, although it was largely discredited owing to its adoption by the Nazis. See Jakob Tanner, "Eugenics before 1945," 458–79. Daniel Wikler says that the Nazis followed a program of eugenics and that consequently eugenic ideas became "virtually taboo" ("Can We Learn from Eugenics?," 183). But he argues that eugenics is not inherently wrong and can be done justly. He accepts that there may be some social costs, notably to the well-being of the disabled.

64. "Disablism and Ableism," Scope website, accessed January 11, 2013, http://www.scope.org.uk/disablism/. Dan Goodley explores some other definitions of disablism that are concerned with social oppression or economic and political exclusion in his book *Disability Studies*, 8–9.

65. Scope, *Getting Away with Murder*, 8.

widely held belief that there is something significant about being a human person: human beings are persons, and persons matter; persons are worthy of a level of respect.

The term "disablism" appeared in the 1980s, possibly a consequence of the growth in literature written by disabled people themselves. The rise of disability studies and the identification of disablism are also linked to challenges to the medicalization of disability, to the questioning of notions such as doctors rather than parents knowing best about disabled children, and to the realization that health care professionals tend to overestimate the negative impacts of disability on disabled people and their families.[66] People with disabilities began to identify and articulate the prejudice often leveled against them. But not all disabled people are able to "have a voice." The profoundly intellectually disabled person remains silent. So, even within disability studies, a hierarchy of disability can develop: on the one hand, those who can speak up for themselves—who can demand the rights to independent living, proper support, and the real possibility of choice—can think that they speak for all the disabled in this regard. On the other hand, those who will always be radically dependent, whose choices (if any) are at the most basic level, can make no demands.

Speciesism: The Final Frontier

Whereas disablism is prejudice against some disabled human beings, speciesism appears in direct opposition. Richard Ryder first spoke about speciesism as "a form of injustice . . . hurting others because they are members of another species."[67] Speciesism is defined as "discrimination against or exploitation of certain animal species by human beings, based on an assumption of mankind's superiority."[68] We are urged to ditch the

66. See Goodley, *Dis/Ability Studies*, 5–6; Singer, "People with Mental Retardation," 268 and 280.

67. Ryder, *Political Animal*, 44. Ryder acknowledges that there are different approaches within the campaign against speciesism, and he explains that his approach is based on "painism," that any sort of suffering is the preeminent issue, rather than what he calls the "Rights Theorist" view, that "it is the animal's overall biography that merits respect." He also rejects the utilitarian notion that pains and pleasures can be meaningfully aggregated. See "Speciesism Revisited," 89–90.

68. Peter Singer explains that the term "speciesism" was coined by the psychologist

"arbitrary" speciesist line that has been drawn between humans and other animals[69] and to accept that some lives of nonhuman animals "by any standards" are more valuable than the lives of some humans such that "we must grant these animals a right to life as good as, or better than, such retarded or senile humans."[70] According to anti-speciesists, the term "person" is wrongly limited to the species Homo sapiens.[71] Even though Singer thinks that the root cause of speciesism is theology, since theology bestows a supernatural dignity on human beings such that all human beings regardless of their capacities are considered valuable,[72] Singer also thinks that theology underpins anti-speciesist claims. He points out that because Christianity recognizes as persons "spiritual beings like God and the Holy Ghost," there may be "more tangible persons who are not humans," such as higher primates.[73] But if the intention had been to extend the sphere of moral concern to more creatures, the term "speciesism" soon began to be used to reduce the sphere of the person among human beings.

Theology and the Person

The idea that the Church Fathers have nothing to offer the contemporary ethical debate and the life of persons with profound disabilities assumes that the "modern" Lockean idea of the person is truly new. It also assumes that the two competing bioethical visions are an innovation. Consider the view that human beings "are of the same substance as irrational animals in accordance with the irrational body" and that they are also "of a different substance as rational beings." The author of this view thinks that the human body is merely an animal aspect of the human being: it is simply passive raw material. Loss of the mind, he continues, signifies the destruction of the individual, the end of the person.

The author of these statements is not a contemporary philosopher

---

Richard Ryder in 1970, and Singer links speciesism to racism. See *Rethinking Life and Death*, 173.

69. Singer, *Practical Ethics*, 77–78.
70. Singer, *Writings on an Ethical Life*, 44–45.
71. DeGrazia, "On the Question of Personhood," 40–53.
72. Singer, *Animal Liberation*.
73. Singer, *Rethinking Life and Death*, 181.

or bioethicist, however: it is the fourth-century controversial Christian thinker Apollinarius (ca. 315–92 CE). The view presented by Apollinarius, and other views that offered a fragile and breakable link between the human being and the person or attempted to define human beings by arbitrary characteristics, was the subject of withering critique in the early centuries by patristic theologians. According to the early Fathers, being a person is not simply about the actual possession of rationality: all human beings are persons, and the term "person" involves not only mental characteristics but also the body; human beings are embodied souls.

Person in its Greek and Roman equivalents, προσοπον, *prosopon*, and *persona*, does exist in antiquity. But the word only developed into a deeper concept when it was taken up and forged through the struggles and refinements of early Christian reflection on the Trinity as Three Divine Persons, and on Christology and the Person of Jesus Christ. This theological reflection involved carefully argued disputes, as early Christianity was forced to face problematic views and their consequences. In turn, this led to profound reflection on and rejection or acceptance of differing approaches to what it means to be a person by such thinkers as, on the one hand, Arius (d. 335), Apollinarius, and Nestorius (381–452) and, on the other hand, Athanasius (ca. 295–373), Basil (330–79), Gregory of Nyssa (ca. 331–95), Gregory of Nazianzus (329–90), Augustine (354–430), and Cyril of Alexandria (ca. 378–444). This theological reflection on the person is not only of relevance to ancient theological disputes or to a historical context of the concept of the person. The hard-fought struggles and subtle distinctions made in the past embodied a sustained intellectual effort to formulate, refine, and deepen the understanding of person. Both the confusions, distortions, and myopia and the corrections and insights can enlighten contemporary discussions on the person, particularly since contemporary bioethics often seems to share similar myopic concerns or to make similar confused and distorted moves. Moreover, the enterprise is not purely descriptive. Early theology engages with deep theological and philosophical questions, and it also offers profound reflection, beyond that of the undoubted significance of relationality, on the human condition in its strength and in its weaknesses.

With the advent of Christianity, something new and decisive happens. All human beings, whatever their capacities, share in the dignity of being persons destined for friendship with God. They have this dignity precisely because through his Incarnation the Son assumed human nature, he did not absorb or destroy it, and so he raised humanity to a dignity beyond compare. Moreover, human beings have been promised bodily resurrection through Christ's Resurrection. The human body as well as the soul is the subject of theology.[74]

The Fathers explain this universal human dignity of being a person[75] in ways that can be understood philosophically as well as theologically. The use and misuse of language are common to both disciplines, as are notions of the relationship of human beings to the world and to other nonhuman animals. Both disciplines have an interest in a focus on uniqueness and the reality of the human being rather than simply on rationality or individuality. The significance of dependence and genuine freedom can be explored through a discussion of both philosophical and Christian attitudes.

While the roots of "person" lie in theology, discussion of the person in theology and in bioethics does not lie on strictly parallel lines. Whereas in bioethics the person is often considered in terms of body and mind, biological and biographical life, early theologians developed their anthropology by reference to body and soul, the relations between the Divine persons and the divine and human in Christ. Still, mind as well as body and soul come into theological discourse, notably in the challenges from Apollinarius. Moreover, the traditional Christian and Jewish belief system have influenced some modern secular approaches in its attempts to integrate body and mind, even though mind is not exactly converted to soul or spirit.[76]

Theology has long struggled with trying to do justice to the transcendent aspect of the human person and the aspect that sees him or her as an animal of a specific nature. But theology reminds us that these two aspects are connected: the human person is both material and transcen-

74. Pope John Paul II, *General Audience,* April 2, 1980.

75. Dignity is itself a highly contentious notion and has been (mis)described as confused, vague, or reducible to autonomy (see Rosen, *Dignity*). The early Church Fathers do not make much of the term "dignity," so it does not form part of the discussion in this book.

76. Veatch, "Death of Whole-Brain Death," 22.

dent, a unity, an embodied soul. These struggles, and the reasoning they have produced, can be used to inform and enlighten the current difficulty in which many bioethicists find themselves. Although the theological approach illustrates how difficult it is, it also offers deeper reflection on the human person. In particular, these theological struggles indicate that viewing the concept of person as a problem to be solved or the subject merely of definition according to a level of rationality or a list of intellectual characteristics risks reducing the person to a completely understood physical body or to an arbitrary will unconnected to human nature and human need.

Overview

Chapter 1 begins with a conversation between disability and bioethics. This conversation highlights the logic of some bioethical views that lead directly into disablism, even if the holders of these views do not think that their approaches are discriminatory. The chapter charts the emergence of a clear separation between biological life and biographical life, the erosion of the sanctity of life principle, and how disabled life is not seen as personal life and is therefore without protection. Various competing definitions of what constitutes the concept of the person contribute to the conclusion that bioethical thought on the person is confused. This is further compounded by the fact that some bioethicists use theology to shore up their own specific definitions, yet at the same time their theology itself is inaccurate or confused.

Chapters 2–4 focus on different theological themes identified in chapter 1. Concentrating on texts in Genesis, chapter 2 takes up the theme of human beings made in the image of God. In a challenge to those who think of persons principally in terms of mental capacity, rationality, or possessing interests, early theological reflection on the image of God highlights both the bodily and spiritual aspects of human beings. The image of God provides an underpinning for not only unity in the human being as body and soul, but also unity and solidarity of all human beings in the human family. The chapter also addresses contemporary concerns of speciesism. Chapters 3 and 4 follow more of a historical trajectory because Trinitarian theology and Christology build upon previous theological thinking, and they set the context for chapter 5. Chapter 3 offers more insight through reflection on the image of the Christian God as a personal God, the one impassible God in three Divine Persons of the Trinity. In contrast to mistaken applications of Trinitarian theology that seek to establish a theological basis for a philosophy of consciousness, attention centers on the essentially relational and concrete understanding of person, in the context in which a meaningful language of personhood was first used. Chapter 3 gives serious consideration to equality in the uniqueness of human beings who also exist in relationship with others, themes that are vital for all people with or without disabilities. Chapter 4 turns to Christ and Christological thinking on the God-made-man, for it is in Christ, true God and true man, that the true image of God and thus the true image of the human being, the human person, is found. Patristic reflection on the human and divine in Christ takes place alongside discussion of the reality of human beings, and this descriptive anthropology has many resonances with the problems and mistakes raised by some bioethical approaches to the person. In chapter 4, there are close parallels between the anthropologies of Apollinarianism and Nestorianism and some contemporary thinking. It is a deliberate strategy that chapter 4 makes only passing reference to people with disabilities, because thinking on Christ and human beings is the same for all human beings. Unlike those who are disablist in separating profoundly disabled people from persons, reflection on Jesus Christ applies to all because there is no "them" and "us."

Connections between anthropologies that were rejected or critiqued by the Fathers and some contemporary bioethical approaches are made in chapter 6; however, this is after an analysis of Boethius. The neat definition that Boethius gives of the person figures in many modern discussions. Usually quite briefly, but all too frequently, Boethius is quoted as if his definition can give clear provenance to those who wish to claim that the actual capacity for reasoning is definitive for persons, such that some higher primates can be elevated to the status of personhood and some human beings, notably the profoundly intellectually disabled, fall below the threshold for personhood. In chapter 5, the definition from Boethius is returned to its theological context, which instantly highlights the mistakes made by modern bioethicists who rather casually make passing reference to Boethius without fully appreciating his thinking. Moreover, since Boethius says he depends on Augustine for his understanding of the person, and Augustine is accused of promoting the kind of individualism that fuels modern notions of the person (though notably modern bioethicists do not claim Augustine as one of their own), chapter 5 also looks to Augustine and his view of the self-sufficient person, in connection with Pelagius.

Chapter 6 then illustrates that some theological insights and distinctions have been neglected in secular bioethics, even though they remain relevant and indeed vital. For those thinkers who apparently misunderstand or do not fully appreciate the theological tradition to which they appeal in solving difficult bioethical problems, theology may offer a reflective critique. For those who reject theology as outmoded or as mistaken, theological reflection fruitfully offers a different starting point and approach, perhaps more in tune with the early vision of bioethics. Moreover, because the theological insights and distinctions have significance for the concept of the person even from a philosophical perspective, there is a need to incorporate them into bioethics. It may be true that discernment and reflection have left some problems unresolved, but they have also opened the way for further reflection and a constant deepening. Some bioethical thinking may appeal by its simplicity and its definitive answers; however, theological insights seem to do more justice to the concept of the person that is in fact complex and at times perplexing.

The person with profound disability is not singled out in this book. Reference is at times made to disability, but the point is that people with disabilities are in fact no different from all other human beings: there is no disablism.[77] Definitions of the concept of the person that exclude people with cognitive disabilities by reducing the person to a notion of an insubstantial center of consciousness have simply failed to comprehend the richness of the concept and the depth that it acquired through its formation in theology.

77. This is clearly demonstrated in practical theological terms: all the principles of Catholic social teaching apply equally to all; we all share the same origin and destiny; we are all called to a life of holiness and to cooperate in that call as far as we are able.

1. Defining Persons ➛ *Biographically Speaking*

Introduction

This chapter sets out definitions and accounts of the concept of the person from some influential bioethicists. The aim is not to offer a comprehensive guide to bioethical thinking on persons and nonpersons. Rather, the philosophical logic of these bioethicists leaves them genuinely puzzled by any accusation of discrimination. Put simply, individuals with severe cognitive disabilities or developmentally young individuals are not persons, and there can be no disablism if there is no person there to be harmed or discriminated against. What is chilling is that this logic appears to have been arrived at unreflectively and in the certainty that this is the right answer that can solve most bioethical dilemmas.

Here I explore the way in which the logic of excluding some human beings from the category of the person comes out of the separation of biological life (the life of the individual being) from biographical life (the life of the person). Certainly, there is a conceptual distinction between these two. When the two are polarized instead of kept together, however—that is, when an individual is said to have only biological life—then this allows for the individual to be described as a nonperson. Those bioethicists who support the project to separate biological and biographical life have in their sights one principle in particular: the principle of the sanctity of life. This chapter goes on to examine how this principle has been mischaracterized as both vitalist and purely theological, therefore depriving it of any philosophical merit.

Because the question of biological and biographical life can be found in the first conversations that led to the discipline of bioethics in the 1970s, I also consider the opposing visions of two of the discipline's founding fathers, Paul Ramsey and Joseph Fletcher. Out of these competing visions, Fletcher's view of the person as an autonomous individual and people with severe cognitive disabilities as nonpersons seems to be dominant in academia. Fletcher's view is given added credence by the influential bioethicists Beauchamp and Childress in their textbook *Principles of Biomedical Ethics.* But the many competing accounts of the concept of person have led to confusion and charges of vagueness. This has led to a weakening of the significance of the concept and an approach that defines the person simply in terms of interests or desires.

In this confusion about persons in the secular bioethical conversation, some bioethicists, notably Singer, specifically appeal to theology to shore up their own particular interpretations. But theology is frequently used in an unreflective and often mistaken way, as an overview of the thinking of some bioethicists on the *imago Dei*, Trinitarian theology, and Christology shows. The project of the rest of this book is to disentangle some of these mistakes in order to discover a deeper understanding of the person that can be applied in bioethics.

Disablism and Definitions

To situate the contentious nature and serious consequences of the way in which some bioethicists define the "person" and the relationship of that definition to disability, there is perhaps no better place to start than the frank article written by the lawyer, atheist, and disability activist Harriet McBryde Johnson. "Unspeakable Conversations" was published in the *New York Times* in 2003, some five years before Johnson's premature death. Johnson was born with a degenerative neuromuscular disease, and she had risen to fame as a result of her confrontation with Peter Singer during a question-and-answer session about his book *Rethinking Life and Death.* Singer invited Johnson to speak to his students at Princeton University, where Johnson saw herself as "the token cripple with an opposing view." As Johnson puts it, "Singer seems curious to learn how someone who is as good an atheist as he is could disagree with his entirely reasonable views."[1]

Johnson acknowledges that Singer is motivated by good intentions, that "he is trying to create a system of ethics derived from fact and rea-

1. Johnson, "Unspeakable Conversations."

son, that largely throws off the perspectives of religion, place, family, tribe, community and maybe even species." It is what Johnson calls a "grand heroic undertaking." But Johnson is also acutely aware that Singer "has his flaw." "As she explains, because of his "unexamined assumption" about people with disabilities and the way in which he takes this "all-too-common prejudice" to its logical conclusion, "catastrophe looms." One significant point that Johnson makes is that because Singer simply thinks that "the humans he is talking about aren't people, aren't persons," then he can impassively advocate the killing of disabled babies or individuals at any age "with cognitive impairments so severe that he doesn't consider them 'persons.'" In "the terrible purity of Singer's vision," he cannot see that this may be problematic.

Singer and Friends on the Person

In *Rethinking Life and Death*, Singer calls for a "Copernican revolution," which entails a radical change in perspective away from seeing human beings "as the centre of the ethical universe," a viewpoint that he says is part of the "crumbling" old ethics of Judaism and Christianity. Anticipating "fierce resistance" for being a "blow to our human pride" and acknowledging "for many the (new) ideas will be too shocking to take seriously," Singer contends that the new view will offer "a fresh and more promising approach."[2] Singer offers a practical approach to ethics where thinking about issues philosophically "should enable us to reach better-justified conclusions."[3] Part of his project is to articulate helpful definitions, in particular a definition of the person that no longer holds human beings to be uniquely special. As Singer explains, by focusing on "ethically relevant characteristics," decisions about anencephalics, the severely mentally disabled, patients in persistent vegetative state, cease to be problematic. How we define death also loses its importance.[4]

Singer's practical ethics focuses on what is wrong with killing. Although Singer remains unconvinced about the meaningfulness of rights

2. Singer, *Rethinking Life and Death*, 189, 206.
3. Singer, *Practical Ethics*, 3rd ed., viii.
4. Singer, *Writings on an Ethical Life*, 213.

language, he does recognize that "the idea that we have a right to life is a popular one,"[5] so he says that "if we want to put this in the language of rights, then it is reasonable to say that only a person has a right to life."[6] When it comes to specifying who counts as a person, Singer places Locke's definition of the person "as a being with reason and reflection that can consider itself as itself, the same thinking thing, in different times and places" at the center of his own thinking.[7] Thus for Singer the "two crucial characteristics," rationality and self-consciousness, are the core of his definition of the person.[8] Again, following Locke, Singer thinks that the special value in the life of a rational and self-conscious being has to do with having desires for the future. Harm is caused when these desires are thwarted.

Singer can then logically argue that just as killing a snail does not thwart any desires of this kind, since snails are incapable of having such desires, the same applies to human fetuses and newborn infants.[9] He does, however, accept that killing an infant could be viewed as a "terrible thing" if it had a negative impact on the parents. Singer goes on to say that the situation is "different" in the case of an infant born with serious disability: the difference between killing disabled and "normal" infants lies in "other considerations" about killing, and notably Singer thinks that a disabled infant is a threat to the happiness of others.[10] Moreover, he thinks that, for the "more severe" conditions, aiming for the death of the baby is the only humane course of action.[11] While Johnson may be concerned at Singer's discriminatory attitude, there is serious concern to be had at any suggestion of killing a human being on the grounds that the human being does not fit in with a specific and reductive definition of person. Singer's urge that we put aside our feelings against infanticide since they are based on thinking that infants have special value "because infants are small and cute" or "helpless"[12] is an example of imperson-

5. Singer, *Practical Ethics*, 81.
6. Singer, *Rethinking Life and Death*, 198.
7. Singer, *Rethinking Life and Death*, 197.
8. Singer, *Practical Ethics*, 74.
9. Singer, *Practical Ethics*, 77.
10. Singer, *Practical Ethics*, 161.
11. Singer, *Practical Ethics*, 180.
12. Singer, *Practical Ethics*, 152.

al and pure logic. Singer sees these feelings as emotionally moving but strictly irrelevant aspects of killing a baby.

Singer uses the logic of his reasoning in other cases, and he applies it in his discussion of involuntary euthanasia for people with profound disability because these cases are, he thinks, most nearly akin to his discussion on the status of fetuses.[13] Taking up the situation of the patient in vegetative state, Singer states that these patients "do not differ importantly from disabled infants. They are not self-conscious, rational, or autonomous, and so considerations of a right to life or of respecting autonomy do not apply." Singer adds, "if they have no experience at all, can never have any again, their lives have no intrinsic value." In his final analysis, "their life's journey has come to an end. They are biologically alive, but not biographically." The only reason he can find against euthanasia for this group of human beings is that it may cause irrational fear of euthanasia in others.[14]

In her exchange with Singer, Johnson says that Singer "insists he doesn't want to kill me," and that he does not think that she should feel threatened by his views. Indeed, Singer does not see himself as having a discriminatory attitude toward people with disabilities. Following Singer's logic, human beings who do not fall within his definition of a person are subject to the same level of concern as any other nonperson: infants are much like snails, disability is irrelevant, and so there is no discrimination. Singer also explains that he is "not an advocate of killing the disabled"; rather, he is an advocate of "giving parents a greater say on whether their severely disabled child lives or dies."[15] The misery and suffering that he thinks are entailed by a life of disability are merely added into the equation that informs the choices of others.

As for people like Johnson, who "at this stage" of her life "is a person,"[16] Singer is adamant that his view is not discriminatory. After all, he says that in his ethic there is "equal consideration" for people with disabilities who are "now living their own lives in accordance with their

13. Singer, *Practical Ethics*, 159.

14. Singer, *Practical Ethics*, 2nd ed., 191–92. Singer has a more extended discussion of vegetative state in the second edition of his book.

15. Singer, "Reply to Stephen Drake," 223.

16. Johnson, *Unspeakable Conversations*.

own wishes."[17] But Singer does think that "by definition" people with disabilities "are lacking at least some ability that normal people have," and that "these disabilities will sometimes mean that they should be treated differently from others." He gives the example of not hiring a blind person to be a proofreader.[18]

Johnson is at least confident that Singer "doesn't propose killing anyone who prefers to live." Nevertheless, a deeper exploration of Singer's logic may remove this confidence. Singer is well known for advocating preference utilitarianism, though in the third edition of *Practical Ethics*, he is less confident that preference utilitarianism can provide the necessary answers,[19] and he returns to a more classical utilitarian position. Preference utilitarianism holds that "an action contrary to the preference of any being is wrong, unless this preference is outweighed by contrary preferences. Killing a person who prefers to continue living is therefore wrong, other things being equal." Preference utilitarianism may provide "a direct reason" for not killing a person. Singer accepts that preferences are not decisive, however, and a person's preferences can be outweighed by the strong preferences of others, even by important "indirect reasons."[20] In the utilitarian scheme of things, the expression of preferences and the exercise of autonomy may have weight, but they are not respected for their own sakes. Both utilitarians and preference utilitarians may conclude that a person is mistaken about the level of misery in their life, in which case, for Singer, "it would be right to kill a person who does not choose to die."[21]

It would be a mistake to think that Singer is a lone voice in the conversation between disability and the status of being a nonperson. Singer acknowledges the influence of the philosopher Jonathan Glover, whose classes he attended when he was a student in Oxford.[22] Singer says that Glover's book *Causing Death and Saving Lives*, published in 1977, "blazed a trail" that he followed into applied ethics. In that book, Glover explains

17. Singer, *Practical Ethics*, 3rd ed., 165.
18. Singer, *Practical Ethics*, 45.
19. Singer, *Practical Ethics*, preface, x.
20. Singer, *Practical Ethics*, 80–81.
21. Singer, *Practical Ethics*, 84.
22. Singer, "Intellectual Autobiography," 12.

that although he writes "as though human beings are automatically persons," "it may be said that what is important is not the status of 'human being,' but of 'person.' "[23]

John Harris, a fellow student with Singer, also attended Glover's classes. Like Singer, Harris accepts as a given that a definition of "person" makes "features which depend upon the capacity for self-consciousness and a minimal rationality central." Harris thinks that it is speciesism to believe that members of the human species are "morally significant *per se*" and "more morally important than any other creature."[24] Instead, Harris uses person as "a shorthand term for all the reasons we have for thinking particular individuals morally important."[25] He rules out as irrelevant either species membership or potential to acquire the desired capacities.[26] Unlike Singer, however, Harris places more emphasis on liberty by embedding value and autonomy into his own definition of the person. According to Harris, persons "properly so called" are "human individuals who have developed the capacity to value their own existence." He claims this is the view held by "Locke and many philosophers since," thus ruling out embryos, fetuses, and neonates.[27] What gives our lives "special value" is autonomy in terms of the ability to make choices and to modify our lives through our preferences.[28] Harris thinks that Locke's "elegant account" of the combination of rationality and self-awareness identifies features of the person that we value.[29] Harris adds, because killing a person frustrates every wish that person has and so wrongs that person, "creatures that cannot value their own existence cannot be wronged" because "their death deprives them of nothing."[30]

Harris also assures his readers that Locke would have been "at home

23. Glover, *Causing Death*, 43.

24. Harris, "Embryos and Hedgehogs," 69–70.

25. See Harris, "Embryos and Hedgehogs," 66–67, where Harris also includes Mary Warnock as a supporter of this view. Harris points out, however, that Warnock thinks that a preference for the human species is "far from being arbitrary" and is "a supremely important moral principle" (69).

26. Harris, *Enhancing Evolution*, 96–97.

27. Harris, *Enhancing Evolution*, 96–97.

28. Harris, "Euthanasia and the Value of Life," 8–9.

29. Harris, *Value of Life*, 15.

30. Harris, *Value of Life*, 19.

with" the idea of improving human beings to a superhuman level.[31] In his argument for creating superhumans and avoiding bringing people with disabilities into existence, Harris is keen to point out that his position "depends at no point and in no part on possession or absence of disability": no embryo can be a person "properly so-called."[32] As far as Harris is concerned, there is no discrimination in attempts to "eradicate" disability by identifying and discarding disabled embryos, and he thinks that "abortion and even infanticide for disability are extensions of the legitimate, perhaps imperative ethics of combating disability."[33] Harris claims there is no discrimination because only persons can be unjustly discriminated against, and the grounds for distinguishing between persons and nonpersons are the "presence or absence of the capacities that make for moral significance."[34] Notably, Harris seems to think that existence begins sometime *after* birth. At times, Harris shifts from asserting objective criteria, based on Locke, such as self-consciousness and a minimal rationality for personhood,[35] to offering the more subjective criterion of autonomy, and what value an individual person places on his or her own life.[36]

Harris recognizes that his ethical thinking has negative implications for people with profound intellectual disabilities. Earlier in his career, Harris had suggested that "most people" would not think that people with intellectual disabilities were "somehow less valuable than others." Still, he argued that, on a practical level, those who accepted that abortion was justified on the grounds of disability "must accept that such an individual is, or will become, less valuable than one without such handicap, less valuable because less worth saving or less entitled to life."[37] In contrast perhaps to this earlier position, Harris claims in *Enhancing Evolution* to distance his view in favor of "selecting against disability" from discrimination on the grounds of disability. As he explains, his

31. Harris, *Enhancing Evolution*, 3.
32. Harris, *Enhancing Evolution*, 97.
33. Harris, *Enhancing Evolution*, 100.
34. Harris, *Enhancing Evolution*, 100.
35. Harris, *Enhancing Evolution*, 97.
36. Harris, *Enhancing Evolution*, 96.
37. Harris, *Value of Life*, 7.

own Lockean understanding of person "distinguishes persons with such capacities from embryos, foetuses, and neonates not on the grounds of presence or absence of disability but on the grounds of presence or absence of the capacities that make for moral significance."[38] Yet on a practical level, presumably, a profoundly disabled human being who does not have the required minimal rationality does not, in Harris's scheme, have the same moral significance as other human beings with capacity. After all, according to Harris, "creatures that cannot value their own existence cannot be wronged," and "their death deprives them of nothing that they can value."[39] As Johnson discovers to her dismay, Singer—and we can add Harris—seems to be clear that his definition of the person is entirely reasonable and indeed a given. This appears to be the case even though inevitably such definitions seem to rule out certain human beings, notably people with severe cognitive disability, from the category of persons. Glover is more tentative than his students, perhaps because his work is one of the early attempts to develop an account of a practical approach to life-and-death decisions that builds upon the key distinction between biological life and biographical life as well as the rejection of the principle of the sanctity of life.

Biological Life, Biographical Life, and the Sanctity of Life

The notion that a complete separation can be made between biological life and biographical life is key to definitions of the person that exclude some human beings. Although the precise formulation of this separation can be attributed to the philosopher James Rachels and his colleague William Ruddick,[40] this distinction can be found in the Lockean definition of the person. According to James Rachels, "the difference between biological and biographical life is the difference between *being alive* and *having a life*."[41] In an echo of the Lockean person, Rachels and Ruddick explain

38. Harris, *Enhancing Evolution*, 97.
39. Harris, *Value of Life*, 18.
40. See Ruddick, "'Biographical Lives' Revisited and Extended," 502.
41. Rachels, *Can Ethics Provide Answers?*, 73–79.

that biographical life involves having "self-referring attitudes," and these attitudes "presuppose a sense of oneself as having existence spread over past and future time," having plans, hopes and regrets.[42] For Rachels, continuing life in, for instance, a dreamless coma, is "*as if* we had died": we would still be alive biologically, but we would have no biographical life. Since it is only biographical life that is critical, then it is the loss of biographical life, not biological life, that is "the morally objectionable loss and is the proper object of moral protection."[43]

The separation of biological and biographical life has led to various reinterpretations of the significance of life and when life demands protection. And presenting these two aspects of human life as polarized has led many of its adherents to mischaracterize the important ethic of the sanctity or inviolability of life. The traditional ethic, as exemplified in the thought of Pope John Paul II, does not make a separation between biological and biographical life, and it calls for the life of a human being to be promoted, respected, and defended, "especially when it is weak or threatened."[44] Since there is no separation, the body is not "reduced to pure materiality" or "simply a complex of organs": the living body is perceived as "a properly personal reality."[45] Consequently, life is both protected and cherished, yet the limits of the human condition in the face of death can also be accepted.[46] In a polarized view of the human being that separates biological life from biographical life, there is the tendency to interpret the inviolability or sanctity of life ethic in vitalist terms, meaning that biological life is to be prolonged no matter what.[47] Vitalistic arguments are used on both sides of the euthanasia debate: by those who claim that any withholding, withdrawing, or limit of treatment is passive euthanasia, and by those who claim that in practice, passive euthanasia already takes place through limiting or stopping treatment, and that this then justifies active euthanasia. Vitalism is unworkable, and real, thoughtful proponents of the sanctity of life recognize that there are

42. Rachels and Ruddick, "Lives and Liberty," 91.
43. Rachels and Ruddick, "Lives and Liberty," 90.
44. Pope John Paul II, *Evangelium Vitae*, 77, 39–41, 60–61.
45. Pope John Paul II, *Evangelium Vitae*, 23.
46. See Pope John Paul II, *Evangelium Vitae*, 65.
47. See, e.g., Singer, *Rethinking Life and Death*, 188.

limits to the perpetuation of burdensome treatments and extraordinary means of preserving life without the licensing of direct killing.

Although the significant yet also limited nature of human life can be appreciated without a theological outlook, the inviolability or sanctity of life ethic is dismissed as an "old" ethic and an outmoded remnant of Christianity that can now be set aside because people no longer adhere to a religious outlook.[48] The sanctity of life ethic was mischaracterized as purely theological by the highly influential professor of law Glanville Williams in his book *The Sanctity of Life and the Criminal Law*, first published in 1957. Despite the painstaking analysis undertaken by Professor John Keown and Dr. David Jones that uncovered some of the many difficulties in Williams's thesis and demonstrated the philosophical underpinnings of the inviolability of life ethic,[49] the misconception remains. The term "sanctity" does have theological overtones. But even Keown's attempts to show its philosophical provenance by redescribing sanctity as inviolability does not seem to have altered perceptions.[50]

The inviolability of life ethic has also been finessed so that it does not actually protect human life. Singer advises that, in issues concerning the beginning of life, "more flexible adherents of the sanctity of life doctrine" can simply deny that an individual human being comes into existence before birth.[51] Rachels advocates a "sanctity of lives" principle, where what is valued is the different interests that people have at different times throughout their life story.[52] But Rachels distances the notion of value from any subjectivity. A person's interests are not valuable merely because that person believes they have value. Instead, Rachels interprets the value of interests in terms of the harm of loss. This is, he thinks, the "proper non-theological starting point for an ethic of life and death."[53] Rachels argues that killing is wrong when death would be a harm, a loss, for an individual.[54] Death is a harm for a person because it frustrates the

48. See, e.g., Singer, *Rethinking Life and Death*, 187–96.
49. Keown and Jones, "Surveying the Foundations of Medical Law," 85–126.
50. See Keown, *Law and Ethics of Medicine*.
51. Singer, *Rethinking Life and Death*, 187–96, 188.
52. Rachels, *End of Life*, 24–27.
53. Rachels, *End of Life*, 38.
54. Rachels, *End of Life*, 39–40.

hopes, aspirations, and desires that that person has for his life.[55] Naturally, to be able to suffer such a harm, a human being must have enough cognitive capacity to be able to hold hopes, aspirations, and desires: the kind of Lockean person who is a thinking thing with the capacities of reason, reflection, and memory.

Rachels and Ruddick further explain that there is a "close connection" between having a life and being a person: "only persons have lives."[56] In formulating his "new understanding of the sanctity of life," Rachels lists a number of human beings who are alive but with no life, and so who would fall outside the scope of a law against killing based on the new sanctity of lives principle. He calls them "human vegetables," giving examples of people with profound disabilities: a child born with a brain injury that leaves him blind, deaf, mute, and deformed; "defective infants" with a poor prognosis of a meaningful life; and the terminally ill.[57] According to Rachels, the death of a profoundly disabled human being, particularly a "mentally defective" human being, is less tragic than the death of a "normal" person because the disabled human being does not suffer the same loss as the normal person. Moreover, in the case of a nonhuman animal that has a more complex mental life than a mentally defective human being, "there would be reason to prefer the life of the animal to that of the human."[58]

Although Rachels does not use the language of disablism, he is keen to point out that his view is not against people with disabilities. Rachels explains that it is "misleading" to think of a human being with profound disability, especially severe mental disability, as "a handicapped person." He calls it "perverse" to categorize the profoundly disabled with the handicapped. This, he says, is a "clever rhetorical ploy," since "we all agree that handicapped people should receive every possible benefit."

55. Rachels, *End of Life*, 49.

56. Rachels and Ruddick, "Lives and Liberty," 91.

57. Rachels, *End of Life*, 28–32. After the early death of Rachels from cancer in 2003, Ruddick looked again at the notion of biographical lives. According to Ruddick, Rachels had recognized that his designation of severely disabled infants as "abiographical" was "disturbing." Ruddick then suggests that such infants may have some biographical life derived from their mothers, so they may be entitled to some protection on this basis. "'Biographical Lives" Revisited and Extended," 504, 514.

58. Rachels, *End of Life*, 58–59.

Instead, Rachels claims that a handicap such as blindness, deafness, or "even mild retardation" still leaves the human being "capable of having a human life," though it is made more difficult by the handicap. In the case of profound disability, the human being may be alive, but she at most has a subnormal life, so her death cannot harm her.[59] Once again, as with Singer, Harris, and Glover, it seems that there is no discrimination because there is no one who is being discriminated against.

From the seemingly unshakeable confidence of Singer, it appears that the notion that there are some human beings who are nonpersons has triumphed. Relying only on her experience to frame the argument in her "unspeakable conversations," Johnson concludes that she is still seeking "acceptance" for her humanity. The conversation between Johnson and Singer is not unique, however. It seems to mirror the tension between two competing visions of the person in bioethics as set out by two of the discipline's founding fathers, Paul Ramsey and Joseph Fletcher.

Paul Ramsey and Joseph Fletcher: Persons and Humans

Paul Ramsey first expressed the significance of the concept of the person for medical ethics in the 1969 Lyman Beecher Lectures, part of a conference that inaugurated bioethics. From these lectures, Ramsey wrote what became a foundational book in bioethics, *The Patient as Person*. Its central message called for a move away from a purely medical view of the patient as a body to be acted upon to seeing the life of a human being as biographical, as a personal story. In part, Ramsey was addressing the implicit problem of a separation between biological and biographical life, where medical practice had entirely neglected the biographical aspect of life. According to Ramsey, the practice of medicine is a covenantal relationship of one human being to another, and ethical questions concern the meaning of faithfulness within this relationship.[60] Alongside asking the patient, the principle of consent is a "canon of loy-

59. Rachels, *End of Life*, 64–67.
60. Ramsey, *Patient as Person*, xlv.

alty" expressing this covenant.[61] For Ramsey, it follows that those who are unable through disability or immaturity to consent also enjoy this canon of loyalty, since to experiment on them without their consent and without direct benefit to them is to no longer consider them a patient:[62] "the issue here is the wrong of making a human being an "object."[63] For Ramsey, there is no separation of biological and biographical life because the person is "an embodied soul or an ensouled body,"[64] an inseparable unity of mind, body, and soul.

In affirming the inseparable aspects of the person, Ramsey was also responding to his colleague Joseph Fletcher, for whom the body was something other than the person. According to Fletcher, the person is concerned with choice and control; it has to do with rationality and self-consciousness.[65] Inspired by American pragmatism,[66] Fletcher decided that the "acute question" in bioethics is "what is a *person,*" since "rights (such as survival) attach only to persons." Fletcher set about formulating indicators of "humanhood" or aspects of human beings that indicate persons,[67] with the expectation that these indicators would help to provide practical and workable solutions to difficult bioethical problems. Among these indicators of humanhood Fletcher lists a minimum intelligence quotient of 20, the level for profound intellectual disability. Fletcher's set of humanhood criteria provoked vigorous discussion, and as a result he refined his criteria by identifying four traits as the "singular *esse* of humanness": neocortical function, self-consciousness, relational ability, and happiness, happiness being introduced as a "lighter note."[68] Singer notes that Fletcher's definition of "human" is close to "person," and he is confident that Fletcher would agree that rationality and self-consciousness are core to the concept of the person.[69] Fletcher

61. Ramsey, *Patient as Person*, 10.
62. Ramsey, *Patient as Person*, 14, 18.
63. Ramsey, *Patient as Person*, 36.
64. Ramsey, *Patient as Person*, xiii.
65. Fletcher, *Humanhood*.
66. Fletcher, *Situation Ethics*, 40.
67. Fletcher, "Four Indicators of Humanhood," 377. In *Humanhood*, Fletcher lists some twenty indicators of humanhood (7–19).
68. Fletcher, "Four Indicators of Humanhood," 377.
69. Singer, *Writings on an Ethical Life*, 128.

thinks that those who do not possess the characteristics he originally listed are "objects," sub-personal beings.[70] He argues that "humans without some minimum of intelligence or mental capacity" are not persons, and "idiots" are not human; they have no rights and are "outside the pale of human integrity."[71]

After offering his list of characteristics for humanhood, Fletcher invited others "to add or subtract,"[72] as if by refining the list "we" might come to some agreement. Many bioethicists seem to follow philosopher Daniel Dennett's line: "we" recognize that most but not all human beings are persons since "we" recognize that some conditions exempt human beings from personhood (Dennett says infants, the mentally defective, and the insane are denied personhood); "we" may not have yet discovered the formula for a definition of personhood (there may be none to discover), yet "we" would not abandon the concept of personhood since "the idea that we might cease to view others and *ourselves* as persons.... is arguably self-contradictory."[73]

Fletcher's vision seems be dominant among academic bioethicists, and the success of this vision may be due in part to the hugely influential textbook *Principles of Biomedical Ethics*, by Tom Beauchamp and James Childress. First published in 1979 and now in its seventh edition, this textbook defends a specific approach to biomedical ethics. The book is also interesting because it accepts that the competing views of the concept of the person have led to confusion. Moreover, an analysis of how the authors interpret and reinterpret respect for persons over its many editions charts the shifting visions in the definitions of persons and nonpersons.

Definitions and Principles

In *Principles of Biomedical Ethics*, Beauchamp and Childress set out a framework of four defined principles—autonomy, beneficence, non-maleficence, and justice—that they say can form the basis for most

70. Fletcher, *Humanhood*, 16.
71. Fletcher, *Humanhood*, 19–20.
72. Fletcher, "Four Indicators of Humanhood," 377.
73. Dennett, "Conditions of Personhood," 175–76; italics original.

medical decision making. At the same time as Beauchamp was working on the first edition of the book, he was also working with the US National Commission for the Protection of Human Subjects of Biomedical and Behavioral Research.[74] The commission had been set up following scandals in the United States involving ethically questionable research on people, notably people with disabilities, without their full consent. In 1979, the commission wrote up its findings in the *Belmont Report*, where it named "respect for persons" as a primary principle alongside beneficence and justice. The *Belmont Report* held to two ethical convictions: first, individuals should be treated as autonomous agents, and therefore informed consent follows as a requirement in research; second, "persons with diminished autonomy" are entitled to protection.[75]

Beauchamp recognized that he and Childress had "major substantive disagreements" with the commission. In particular, Beauchamp thought that the *Belmont Report* was "confused" in the way in which it analyzed the principle of respect for persons, because the report appeared to "blend" the principle of autonomy with the principle of beneficence.[76] The *Belmont Report* had taken up the principle of respect for persons in part because the report had been commissioned in response to scandalous research conducted on sick, illiterate, weak, and powerless human beings. But even though Beauchamp and Childress recognized that the report's primary principle, respect for persons, included nonautonomous persons, they used the principle of autonomy in their textbook. According to Beauchamp and Childress, "in evaluating the self-regarding actions of others we ought to respect them as persons with the same right to their judgments as we have to our own. This aspect of the principle of autonomy is often referred to as the principle of respect for persons."[77] By equating respect for persons with the exercise of autonomy, Beauchamp and Childress accept that they and the *Belmont Report* have "developed substantially different moral visions."[78]

As the *Principles of Biomedical Ethics* has moved through its various

74. Beauchamp, *Standing on Principles*, ix, 3–5.
75. Jonsen et al., "*Belmont Report*," 22–28, B, B, 1.
76. Beauchamp, *Standing on Principles*, 7.
77. Beauchamp and Childress, *Principles of Biomedical Ethics*, 59.
78. Beauchamp, *Standing on Principles*, 7.

editions, the moral vision of Beauchamp and Childress has crystallized. By the second edition, Beauchamp and Childress had already stated that the principle of autonomy "does not apply to persons who are not in a position to act in a sufficiently autonomous manner."[79] Autonomy appears to be understood in the libertarian sense of noninterference,[80] and the principles of beneficence and non-maleficence are left to govern decision making toward the nonautonomous person. Justice appears to be understood merely as distributive and concerned with resource allocation. In setting up a different vision than the *Belmont Report* and ditching the principle of respect for persons in favor of the principle of autonomy, Beauchamp and Childress believe that their other principles give some protection to otherwise unprotected human beings. For instance, they say that given that personhood in the case of fetuses is difficult to resolve since there are competing ideas, they are confident that fetuses can be protected by other principles such as non-maleficence.[81] By the sixth edition, they avoid the concept of person altogether, and adhere to "respect for autonomy," leaving "respect for non-cognitive properties" grounded in the principles of non-maleficence and beneficence.[82] The book continues into a seventh edition and adds a new discussion on degrees of moral status based on capacities such as sentience and cognitive ability or characteristics or moral agency or relationships, thus furthering the commitment of the authors to autonomy rather than persons. Beauchamp and Childress do think that individuals such as infants, the immature, and the incapacitated have some moral status and so may be deserving of respect. Nevertheless, protection of these individuals falls under the other principles.[83]

One of the difficulties of leaving the protection of the profoundly disabled to the notions of non-maleficence and beneficence is that it is the autonomous who decide. Those who follow utilitarianism have no problem in seeing the killing of the profoundly disabled as non-maleficence so long as it is done painlessly, since they think that there is no person there to be harmed in the first place. Others find it easy to justify kill-

79. Beauchamp and Childress, *Principles of Biomedical Ethics*, 2nd ed., 64.
80. Beauchamp and Childress, *Principles of Biomedical Ethics*, 62.
81. Beauchamp and Childress, *Principles of Biomedical Ethics*, 3rd ed., 162–63.
82. Beauchamp and Childress, *Principles of Biomedical Ethics*, 6th ed., 74.
83. Beauchamp and Childress, *Principles of Biomedical Ethics*, 7th ed., 108.

ing on the grounds of beneficence: that it is an act of compassion to kill those whose lives are not worth living.

The focus on autonomy rather than on the human being as a person that Beauchamp and Childress present in various editions of their textbook offers an insubstantial account of the person, where personhood is associated with self-consciousness or mental experiences. Following this account, some bioethicists argue that there are some human beings, notably the profoundly disabled, who are not and never will be persons, or that some human beings can lose the status of personhood once they have lost the relevant characteristics marking them as persons: the death of the person can occur before the death of the human being, and therefore in such cases the goals of medicine no longer apply.[84]

The four-principle approach of Beauchamp and Childress comes out of a set of philosophical assumptions. This approach is not without its critics; after all, there is no ethical guidance for when principles collide, and the application of the principles seems to be nothing more than a formal checklist. Notably, the attempt at oversimplifying issues by reducing everything to a balance of four principles seems to forget that there are other factors at stake in specific decision-making situations. Beauchamp himself thinks that the concept of the person is vague and inherently contestable, so much so that "we would be better off if we eliminated the language of 'person' from moral theory altogether and replaced it with more specific concepts."[85] Presumably, this is the reason why in the seventh edition of their book Beauchamp and Childress deliberately "shy away from" the language of respect for persons.[86]

Confused Persons

The competing accounts of what it is to be a person, lack of agreement on what may or may not be essential characteristics, and the conflicts over the possibility of completely separating biological life from biographical life have caused considerable confusion. The implications

84. See, e.g., Cranford and Smith, "Consciousness," 242.

85. Beauchamp, *Standing on Principles*, xxv; idem, "Failure of Theories of Personhood," 247–60.

86. Beauchamp and Childress, *Principles of Biomedical Ethics*, 7th ed., 68.

of this confusion in the United Kingdom play out notably in the *Report of the Committee of Inquiry into Human Fertilisation and Embryology*, produced by a commission chaired by Mary Warnock. The *Warnock Report* became foundational for the subsequent setting up of the Human Fertilisation and Embryology Authority, which licenses and monitors fertility clinics and all research involving human embryos in the United Kingdom and provides "clear and impartial and information" to the public.[87] Warnock admits that, with all its philosophical layers, the term "person "has become confused. She then refers to Locke's idea of person as a "forensic" term, and she claims that this is tantamount to saying that a person is something that must be decided on.[88] Through this approach of "definition by committee," a bare majority of the Warnock commission members thought that "we" did not "necessarily wish" for the embryo to have the same status as a child or adult, so this status was designed to fall far short of the moral respect owed to other human beings, thus opening up the possibility of research.[89] Some members of the committee concluded that experimentation on embryos was unethical on the grounds that it is "wrong to create something with the potential for becoming a human person and then deliberately to destroy it," and embryos should only be created with a view to implantation.[90]

Confusion over the characteristics for being a person has also led to a weakening of the significance of being a person. On the one hand, as the approaches of Fletcher, Warnock, and Harris demonstrate, being a person is significant when it comes to certain protections or treatments. But who qualifies as a person appears to be grounded in arbitrary characteristics. On the other hand, according to some theories and as exemplified by Singer and at times Harris, being a person is not what counts. Rather, what matters is whether the entity in question has certain interests or desires that would otherwise be frustrated if not protected, thus adding to the amount of pain over pleasure calculus in the world. It does not ap-

87. Website of the Human Fertilisation and Embryology Authority, accessed September 12, 2019, https://www.hfea.gov.uk/.

88. Warnock, "In Vitro Fertilisation," 239, and 241; idem, "Do Human Cells Have Rights?," 2.

89. Warnock, *Warnock Report*, 11, 17.

90. Warnock, *Warnock Report*, Expression of Dissent, B, 3, 9–10.

pear that the person is taken seriously, and if it is, it is only a reduced and flimsy notion of person connected to a disembodied self-consciousness. Persons count, but only in the sense of adding up interests. Disablism is finessed away in the contention that there is no discrimination because there is no person there to be treated unjustly. In simple terms, for some bioethicists, the nonperson is not "one of us."

Confusion with Theological Persons

In this confusion over competing accounts of the person, some bioethicists have turned to theology to find support for their own approaches. But it soon becomes apparent that unreflective or reductive or mistaken interpretations of theology simply add to the confusion. The subsequent chapters of this book address some of these misapprehensions, but for the moment it may be useful to introduce some of these mistakes and the bioethicists who rely on them for defining who counts as a person.

Confusion with the Human Being as Image of God

Theological reflection on human beings as images of God is particularly relevant for the troubling questions of both speciesism and disablism. The idea that all human beings, however weak or small, have "special value" appears to privilege humans over other animals. Singer says that according to Christianity, human beings have complete power over all the rest of creation to do with it as they please. He thinks that this teaching "conveys a clear impression that only humans really count," that only human beings have protection from being killed. Singer points out, however, that since "these doctrines are no longer generally accepted," it is "time to reassess our belief in the sanctity of the lives of members of our species."[91] Singer then appeals to the notion of person to argue that killing is directly wrong only in the case of persons, that is, entities both human and nonhuman with the mental wherewithal to see themselves as existing over time.[92]

The view that human beings no longer have special value merely for

91. Singer, *Writings on an Ethical Life*, 129–30; idem, *Rethinking Life and Death*, 160.
92. Singer, "Killing Humans and Killing Animals," 112–22.

being human is also at the heart of Jeff McMahan's thinking. In his book *The Ethics of Killing: Problems at the Margins of Life*, McMahan seeks "to defend the permissibility of certain killings of beings below the threshold" of equal worth and respect. This threshold is based on our "common intuitions" that we have respect for the worth of persons, and this entails that killing persons is, at least usually, wrong. McMahan deals with the moral status of various beings that he calls "marginal" who fall below this threshold. These beings include "animals, human foetuses and infants, anencephalic infants, severely retarded human beings, and human beings with acquired cognitive deficiencies of varying degrees of severity"—in short, beings that are "very different in seemingly important ways from morally innocent, cognitively normal adult human beings."[93] McMahan thinks that these individuals are different because they are not persons, and for McMahan, the idea of person goes back to Locke and "refers to any entity with a mental life of a certain order of complexity and sophistication," "roughly speaking," possessing the actual capacity for self-consciousness.[94] These beings are only on "the margins of life" because McMahan places them at the fringe of a specific definition of personhood, which gives them no protection from being killed. McMahan takes great pains to argue that various theological theories about souls are "empty" or "really another form of materialism" or "incompatible with what we know about the mind."[95] Ultimately for McMahan, accounts of moral worth based on notions such as the possession of a soul or being made in the image of God are "vulnerable to the possibility, or probability, that the favoured attribute is in fact illusory."[96]

While ethicists like Singer and McMahan seek to ditch the *imago Dei* as speciesist and out of date, some theologians appeal to the *imago Dei* to justify treating some profoundly disabled people as less than persons. In formulating his list of features essential for personhood, Fletcher appeals directly to an interpretation of the image of God that centers on the actual possession of rational capacities.[97] Similarly, Nigel Biggar says

93. McMahan, *Ethics of Killing*, 247, 251.
94. McMahan, *Ethics of Killing*, 6.
95. McMahan, *Ethics of Killing*, 8–24.
96. McMahan, *Ethics of Killing*, 256.
97. Fletcher, *Morals and Medicine*, 218.

patients in persistent vegetative state exist merely in biological life since they can no longer respond to their God-given vocation.[98] Engelhardt points out that in a post-Christian age, seriously deformed infants may be regarded as "monstrosities" and no longer "officially regarded as a gift of God"[99] and are therefore fitting subjects for infanticide. Going a step further, the evangelical theologian Robert Rakestraw suggests that certain profoundly disabled patients such as those in persistent vegetative state are theologically speaking dead even though the body is still alive, since the image of God in human beings requires a level of self-awareness, and without this the "earthly life of a person" ends.[100] These claims seem to mirror the notion that the image of God in human beings resides in the possession of intellect and free will; indeed, some bioethicists like Thomas Shannon make this explicit.[101]

As David Clough notes, the image of God is widely used in some theological anthropologies to highlight differences between human beings and animals in order to promote a "not-animal" view of humans, and he cites Augustine and Origen as early examples. In some cases, rationality has been identified as a defining attribute, which has marginalized human beings; in other cases, humanity has been separated, and any context among other creatures has been ignored.[102] Singer is correct in the sense that these challenging concerns do connect with theological reflection on Genesis. But Singer's rather reductive and superficial interpretation of the tradition presents a caricature that may have some resonance with Locke's reward and punishment strand of theological thinking but does not do justice to the rich Christian tradition.[103] Similarly, McMahan's dismissal of the sanctity of life doctrine and Fletcher and Rakestraw's separation of the human being from the person rest on incomplete understandings of the image of God in human beings.

Chapter 2's fuller exploration of the image of God in human beings

98. Biggar, *Aiming to Kill*, 47.

99. See Engelhardt, "Infanticide in a Post-Christian Age," 82–84.

100. Rakestraw, "Persistent Vegetative State," 126–27.

101. Shannon, "Grounding Human Dignity," 114. (Shannon's only named reference is to the medieval theologian Bonaventure.)

102. Clough, "Not a Not-Animal," 4–17.

103. See Camosy, *For Love of Animals*, 19.

demonstrates that the human being considered as a whole is made in the image of God, and with regard to some of the implications of this in a practical application to bioethics, chapter 6 recalls that this image always remains no matter the condition or situation of a living human being. Not only are human persons always unique gifts, but they are also all called to solidarity with others and with the rest of the created world.

Confusion with the Trinity

Behind the assertion that some human lives need not have protection because they are not persons lies the argument that we can separate biological life from biographical life and associate the person only with biographical life, a life of mental sophistication, desires, and interests. While provenance for this view is usually located in Lockean thinking, Singer and his colleague Paola Cavalieri claim that self-awareness and rationality, the central characteristics of personhood and biographical life, are grounded in Trinitarian theology.[104] Chapter 3 explores patristic thinking on the Trinity in depth to test this claim. Because the claim of Singer and Cavalieri is significant, however, it is worth following their argument.

Cavalieri and Singer explain that Descartes first made the fundamental separation between human beings and animals, and his thinking underlies the "absolute dismissal of animals from the sphere of moral concern." In this at least, Singer appears to have moved away from his timeworn position of charging Christianity with starting the disregard of nonhuman animals. The authors continue, to achieve a "more enlightened ethics" that considers the interests of all animals equally, bioethicists use the "long-established, well-respected" moral notion of the person in the "philosophical sense of possessing certain characteristics like self-awareness and rationality" since it has "import," especially regarding the "wrongness of killing." The authors see "person" as being problematic only when it is understood in its "second" sense, the "biological" sense of "human."

Cavalieri and Singer briefly note that classical Latin used *persona* and classical Greek used *prosopon*, meaning "mask," with connotations of role

104. Cavalieri and Singer, "The Great Ape Project," 132–36.

or "task to accomplish," so that they can claim that ancient usage sees the person "in terms of a subject of relations." Emphasis on relation is, they say, "fundamental" and an "aspect of autonomy" because relation speaks about roles and the place a being occupies rather than about a being's nature. They assert that this relation as an aspect of autonomy was "heightened" by Trinitarian theology: the Council of Nicaea presented the Trinity as "one substance and three persons,"[105] and then a counterprocess removed relation from the aspect of person by insistence on substantiality as individuality; "hence the famous definition of person" by Boethius.

For the authors, the connection of person to God "saved the life of the concept" by preventing it from being simply another term for human being. So, "person" can "overcome the species barrier": a human being need not be a person and a person need not be human, thus opening the way for even higher primates to be considered persons. According to Cavalieri and Singer, "person," an "emblematic term," refers to the idea of being "a locus of relations and playing a role in the ongoing drama"; therefore "to regard an entity as a person is to attribute a special kind of value to that entity." The authors conclude that while person has connection with "the capacity for reasoning" through Boethius (and Aquinas), rationality is attendant on the more basic aspect of relation, that is, relation with others and self-relation. Abstracting from the theological framework,[106] the authors take self-relation to refer more specifically to self-awareness and the Lockean definition of person.

Arguably, Cavalieri and Singer overstate the significance of relations in the development of the person in classical Greek and Roman thought. But their suggestion that Trinitarian theology simply "heightened" this significance and then ditched it in favor of substance completely misses the mark. The perhaps novel use of Trinitarian theology by the authors as a firm underpinning for their notion of the person is an interesting departure from Singer's usual dismissal of the Christian tradition. Nevertheless, the swift moves they make to establish Trinitarian theology as a basis for the person as self-aware and with desires for the future, therefore ruling

105. Strictly speaking in terms of language, the authors are mistaken here.

106. Following Henry Sidgwick's method, Cavalieri and Singer say that "modern rational ethics" emerges from abstraction from preconceived frameworks and moves toward an "anonymous social arena." "The Great Ape Project," 135.

out certain human beings while admitting higher primates, are untenable.

Chapter 3 makes plain that the arguments of Cavalieri and Singer are simply untenable. Moreover, in chapter 6, the practical implications that Trinitarian patristic thinking brings to bioethics and people with profound disabilities challenge notions of the person as autonomous and strong-willed individuals.

Confusions in Christology

Chapter 4 investigates human beings through the prism of Christology, since it is in this area that much patristic work is done on the relationship between the different human aspects that make up the whole being of a human being. US bioethicist Robert Veatch disagrees with the kind of insubstantial self, offered by those like McMahan, and he is surely right in challenging "Manichaean" bioethicists who claim that to be alive, we just need mental functions.[107] Veatch stresses that the human being is more than a body. Rather, he or she is an integration of mind (where, says Veatch, mind can also be equated with soul) and body.[108] According to Veatch, however, the relationship of body to soul or mind is a fragile one. Veatch claims that the classic Judeo-Christian idea that a human being is essentially an integration of mind and body entails that the existence of one without the other, of body without mind or mind without body, is not enough to constitute a living human being. Moreover, he believes that Christian thought and its "secular spin-offs" share the same outlook and hold in "universal agreement" that the human is more than a body: "a human is not a mere body; it is a body combined with something else." That "something else," once called soul or spirit, is, he argues, essentially the same as the modern conception of mind or consciousness.[109] He adds that even though elements of this thinking come from "arcane" theological questions, Christian tradition and secular philosophical thought hold that the integration of mental function is critical: "when, and only when, this capacity for mental function is present is the minimal set of qualities present to treat the human as a living member of the moral community."

107. Veatch, "Dead Donor Rule."
108. Veatch, "Death of Whole-Brain Death," 353–78.
109. Veatch, "Death of Whole-Brain Death."

Veatch asserts that this approach should have broad application because where the tenets of Western religion and philosophical thought are held by a great many, any definitions should be allowed to reflect those tenets.[110] Instead, then, of somaticism, that human beings are just bodies, or mentalism, that human beings are minds, Veatch offers the "new defensible middle ground" of integrated mind and body, an "embodied capacity for consciousness" that grounds full moral standing.[111]

While Veatch may reject some interpretations that make it possible for some living human beings to be nonpersons, his reasoning is not directed in favor of profoundly disabled human beings. In Veatch's controversial and problematic view, the word "living" is significant because Veatch thinks there are no living nonpersons; rather, those who some claim to be nonpersons are, according to Veatch, in fact dead.[112] Personhood, he believes, is not a scientific question but an issue for moral, philosophical, and religious consideration.[113] Yet for Veatch this integration of mind and body takes the form of the body plus the soul/spirit/mind/consciousness. There is a person only when the capacity for mental function is present: the existence of a body without a mind, or a mind without a body, does not constitute a living human being.[114]

While it is important to distinguish the material and spiritual aspects of human beings, the exploration of Christological thinking in chapter 4 reminds us that the connection is not simply a fragile one that can be easily broken, nor are human beings bodies plus something else. This is further reinforced in chapter 6 by the practical implications that Christological arguments bring to bioethics. Patristic thinking demonstrates that human beings are embodied souls, which leads to a deeper understanding of what it is to be a human being.

Confusions with Boethius and Augustine

Chapter 5 sorts out some of the difficulties that the influential thinking of Augustine and Boethius seem to present for people with disabili-

110. Veatch, "Death of Whole-Brain Death," 375n21.
111. Veatch, "Death of Whole-Brain Death."
112. Veatch, "Death of Whole-Brain Death."
113. Veatch, "Impending Collapse," 18–24.
114. Veatch, "Death of Whole-Brain Death."

ties in bioethics. Certainly, some theologians assert that Western theology as represented by Augustine and Boethius leads to modern notions of the person as an isolated individual characterized by rationality.[115] For those bioethicists who claim that not all human beings are persons and who support this claim by arguing that there is a clear connection between the person and the capacity for reasoning, the philosopher Boethius seems to be a natural ally. The Boethian definition of the person as "the individual substance of a rational nature" allows writers like Cavalieri and Singer to extrapolate "capacity for reasoning" from "rational nature," and by tracing its journey through Aquinas to Locke, they believe they have a solid grounding for their interpretation.[116] Having isolated reasoning as an essential feature, Cavalieri and Singer are not the only authors to elevate certain animals to the status of persons while recognizing that some human beings, especially the intellectually disabled, will now fail to reach the standard required for personhood.[117]

But in attempting to give their interpretation of the person historical and traditional provenance, the authors have made an unwarranted leap from the thinking of Boethius to John Locke. Singer and Cavalieri show that they do not take account of the context in which Boethius was writing, nor do they appreciate the nuances of the terms he uses. The legalistic, reward-and-punishment-based Christianity rejected by Singer, and its theological anthropology, Pelagianism, which shares substantial affinity with Lockean thinking, had been already identified in the early Christian tradition as a problematic innovation of the fourth century, and it was soundly refuted. On the one hand, seeing the person in terms of reason and free will seems to characterize contemporary notions of the concept of the person, but on the other hand, the understandings of Christianity that many contemporary bioethicists critique seem to bear more than a passing resemblance to Pelagian Christianity.

An exploration of the concept of the person from Trinitarian theol-

115. Gunton, *Promise of Trinitarian Theology*, 42–43; Grenz, *The Social God and the Relational Self*, 67.

116. Cavalieri and Singer, "The Great Ape Project," 286.

117. Singer, *Rethinking Life and Death*, 183. See also Fletcher, *Humanhood*, 7–19; Mori, "Is the Human Embryo a Person?," 151–63; Harris, "Euthanasia and the Value of Life," 8–9; Lockwood, "Moral Status of the Embryo," 18; McMahan, *Ethics of Killing*, 6.

ogy and from Christology demonstrates beyond doubt that the notion of the person gains its profundity through the struggles of theology. But taking Boethius as the starting point for the concept of the person to the neglect of the rich tradition that gives the concept of the person its depth inevitably obscures its meaning. So, it is even more concerning that some contemporary interpretations of the person have a reductive view of the person, believing that the concept refers merely to the rather insubstantial notion of self-consciousness, autonomy, or the actual ability to have desires for the future. At the same time, some of these interpretations make brief reference to the definition provided by Boethius, as if that supports these interpretations. Thus the definition from Boethius has become influential for some contemporary concepts of the person, even though, arguably, it has been wrongly applied or it has not been given in all its nuances.[118]

Rather than being obstacles to seeing people with disabilities as persons, Augustine and Boethius stand in the patristic theological tradition as supporters of the full status as persons for all human beings, as discussed in chapters 5 and 6. When attention is drawn to some contemporary bioethical views, it soon becomes clear that Kuhse and Singer are correct when they urge "a better understanding of the issues," where practitioners are prepared to ask "deep philosophical questions."[119] The fact that theology is deeply imbedded into the concept of the person, and appeal is made to theology by even the most ardent of secular thinkers, shows how necessary it is to have a reflective and careful grasp of the theology behind the concept of the person. This deep reflection will unfold in the subsequent theological chapters, where theology and philosophy often come together in patristic thinking. Yet mistakes made by influential bioethicists like Singer filter through to the thinking of other bioethicists who may not appreciate that often erroneous extrapolations have been made from theology. This is the reason why the final chapter looks at some of the practical implications of discerning persons.

118. See, e.g., Camosy, *Peter Singer and Christian Ethics*, 23, 128.
119. Kuhse and Singer, *Companion to Bioethics*, 4.

2. Discerning Persons • *Biblically Speaking about Human Beings as Images of God*

Introduction

According to the Eastern Orthodox theologian John Zizioulas, the concept of person is historically and existentially "indissolubly bound up with theology." This is not only because the term "person" was first used in any significant way in Trinitarian theology. The concept of the person acquires its depth and force precisely because "*the being of God Himself* was identified with the person."[1] Certainly, God creates human beings in his image, and God creates persons, since God is Three Persons. But the revelation of God as Three unfolds over time: the New Testament is hidden in the Old Testament, and the Old Testament is made manifest in the New.[2] The foundation for understanding human beings as persons then lies in the Old Testament teaching of the *imago Dei*, and the *imago Dei* has moral implications: if we love God and see that God is imaged in others, then we are also called to love others.

There are many interpretations of the image of God, and perhaps this should come as no surprise because the being of God is, after all, a mystery. This chapter reflects on some of these interpretations where they may seem to exclude or at least prove problematic for people with disabilities. The idea that the image of God in human beings gives humans special value has been the target for anti-speciesism, as it implies a discriminatory attitude toward other animals. This chapter explores this special value and considers it in terms of the dominion human beings are called to hold over creation and accountability toward each other.

1. Zizioulas, *Being as Communion*, 27, 40.

2. Second Vatican Council, *Dei Verbum* IV,16, quoting Augustine, "Questions on the Heptateuch" 2, 73.

If dominion or accountability is seen as essential to the image of God, then it seems that people who are unable to exercise dominion, perhaps through lack of capacity, may be excluded. Interpretations that focus on the image of God as located in the mind or grounded only in rationality seem to exclude people with intellectual disabilities, especially when the body is bracketed out of the discussion. Interpretations that emphasize spiritual growth may seem to cause problems for those with learning disabilities or other profound disabilities.

This chapter draws attention to the idea that human beings are a particular kind of animal within the animal kingdom, and that there is solidarity between human beings as members of one family. Solidarity and this bond apply to all human beings no matter their status, age, gender, or condition in life, since they are grounded in the shared image of God and in Christ, who is the true image of that image. Because relationship to God and to others rather than rationality is characteristic of the image of God, this chapter focuses on how, for the writers of Genesis and later for the patristics, human beings are understood as theological and not merely biological or biographical beings. And the vocation to grow more perfectly into the likeness of God is a call to excellence, not physical or mental improvement.

The Special Value of All Human Beings

The "special value" that human beings have is rooted in Genesis 1:26, where Yahweh says, "Let us make man in our own image, in the likeness of ourselves." This text brings into immediate focus how God came to initiate a special relationship with all human beings so that we have duties toward ourselves and are each accountable before God for other human beings and for the rest of creation.[3] But the claim that human beings have a unique place in God's creation does not mean that God does not have a relationship with his other creatures, nor does it imply that the rest of creation is of no account. As Pope Francis points out, other creatures have a value of their own in God's eyes. Moreover, if hu-

3. See Pontifical Council for Justice and Peace, *Compendium of the Social Doctrine of the Church*, 451–52.

man beings are considered simply as beings among other beings or the products of chance, then "our overall sense of responsibility wanes."[4] What becomes clear is that human beings belong to the world and yet are unique in the world, and this theme surfaces throughout early reflection on human beings as images of God.

Although the human being as image of God is an abiding idea for theological anthropology, there are few Old Testament references.[5] The best-known reference, in Genesis 1:26–27, sets the idea of human beings as image of God in the broad context of primordial history, salvation history, and the history of the patriarchs. Given this wide context, and the shortage of actual references, it seems difficult to pinpoint what exactly was meant by image of God. Yet investigation into the stories that recount the creation of human beings indicates some of its significance and perhaps is a reminder that the image of God cannot be reduced to one interpretation.

There are two creation stories in Genesis: chapters 1:1–2:3 are ascribed to the Priestly tradition,[6] and chapters 2:4–3:24 belong to the earlier Yahwistic oral source. In the Priestly tradition, God commands entities and beings to come into existence in an ascending order of dignity: light and darkness, land and sea, followed by plants and animals, with human beings, created in God's image, coming last.[7] For the Yahwistic tradition, the creation of man from the dust appears to be more distinct from the

4. Pope Francis, *Laudato Si*, 69, 118.

5. Gn 1:26–27, 9:6; Ps 8:5–6. Even though Psalm 8 does not use the term "image," it does echo the image and dominion theme found in Genesis as well as in Ben Sira / Eccl 17:3 and Wis 2:23, 7:26. Roger Ruston notes the claim of the "great Genesis commentator," Claus Westermann, that the rest of the Old Testament virtually ignores the *imago Dei* because the Genesis text is describing the action of God, not the nature of human beings. Ruston adds that this allows Westermann to support a Barthian interpretation where there are thus no implications for a philosophical anthropology. But Ruston also points out that the theologian and the biblical critic are in different positions: the theologian "cannot rule out anthropological reflections on such a startling statement, since his or her task is to develop its meaning for divine-human relations in a post-biblical political and social environment." *Human Rights and the Image of God*, 277–79. In contrast to Westermann, in their analysis of the Book of Genesis, Richard Clifford and Roland Murphy describe Genesis chapters 1–11 as "a single story, an unusually sustained 'philosophical' and 'theological' explanation of the human race... and of God and God's justice and abiding fidelity to the race." "Genesis," 9.

6. Possibly formulated during the Exile (597–586 BCE). For differing dating, see Middleton, *Liberating Image*, 140–45.

7. See Camosy, *Peter Singer and Christian Ethics*, 103.

creation of the world and takes place before the creation of animals. It is clear from the creation accounts that there is kinship between human beings and the world,[8] though this has been interpreted in different ways.

One such way is to see the human being as just one more example of a living being, like any other organism yet at a higher stage of perfection. Approached in this way, mere difference of species does not determine moral status. Rather, what counts are what capacities and abilities the individual has, and if cognitive capacity is seen as the defining characteristic, then some profoundly disabled human beings will have a lower status than some other animals. This is one reason why Singer urges that a belief in the equal value of human life should be replaced by a "graduated view" that applies to animals as well as humans.[9] But there do not appear to be enough grounds for applying a characteristic that is seen as predominantly human to other animals.

Rather than simply give a graduated view, the Anglican theologian Andrew Linzey in his discussion on this apparent hierarchy accepts that there is a distinction between human beings and animals, and between animals and vegetables. Nevertheless, he thinks that the distinction stresses commonality between animals and humans in relation to the whole of creation. Linzey thinks that there is a "special proximity of some (predominantly mammalian) animals to humankind" because land animals are created on the same day, the sixth day, together with human beings.[10] It is not clear from this why he picks out only certain land animals, however.

The Priestly and Yahwistic accounts of the creation of humans seemingly contradict each other. Even so, the final redactor allowed them to stand together, perhaps because, for its authors, Genesis was not so much a history or a presentation of a hierarchy. Rather, it was intended to be a prehistorical theological reflection on how God had been involved in the world from its very beginning, and instead of being contradictory, the two accounts of the creation of humans may share a common core.

Both Priestly and Yahwistic writers are clear that from the beginning

8. See Pontifical Council for Justice and Peace, *Compendium of the Social Doctrine of the Church*, 464.

9. Singer, "Speciesism and Moral Status," 567–81.

10. Linzey, *Animal Theology*, 33–35.

God entered into a special relationship with humankind. Although in the Priestly account humans are created on the same day as other land animals (Gn 1:24–27), in the case of God's previous creative activity, God simply commands and it happens. But before creating humans, God deliberates first (Gn 1:26).[11] This suggests that God is not simply continuing the process of creation but is instead undertaking something new. Moreover, humans are the only creatures made in the image and likeness of God (Gn 1:26). Thus humans both belong to and are set apart from other animals and the rest of creation. This setting apart is compounded by the task God gives them: to have dominion over the world.[12] In the text, the verb expressing dominion (*kabas*) translates as "subdue," and it implies a level of force to bring something under control.[13]

Notably, humans and other animals are only given plants for their food.[14] As Linzey points out, for the early Hebrews, in this state of paradise, violence between humans and other animals was not part of God's original plan for creation.[15] The connection between humans and nonhuman animals is further made in the Yahwistic account, which uses a play on words to indicate that the first man, Adam, is formed from the ground (*adamah*), and as such he is part of the material world.[16] He became a living being (*nephesh*), when God breathed into him the breath of life (*ruah*). The breath of life as gift of God is source of all being and life,[17] and it gives humans "a certain affinity" with other creatures.[18] The Yahwistic Adam is also given the task of cultivation, though in cooperation with God who sends the rain,[19] and man's dominion over creation is further expressed by his naming of the animals.[20]

11. It is by no means certain who are his dialogue partners: theological speculation ranges from the suggestion that God speaks to his celestial court to God conversing as Trinity or using an honorific royal "we." See Middleton, *Liberating Image*, 55–57. See also Justin Martyr, "Dialogue with Trypho," in *First Apology*, 62.

12. Gn 1:26, 1:28.

13. Clifford and Murphy, "Genesis," 11; for a discussion of the nuances of "to rule over" and "subdue," see Middleton, *Liberating Image*, 50–55.

14. Gn 1:29–30.

15. Linzey, *Animal Theology*, 126.

16. Westermann, *Genesis 1–11*, 206.

17. See Ps 104:29–30.

18. Pope John Paul II, *Sollicitudo Rei Socialis*, 29; *General Audience (Psalm 150)*, 4.

19. Gn 2:5, 2:15.

20. Gn 2:20.

Although there is an affinity between humans and other animals, there also appears to be a difference. According to Camosy, and referring to Genesis 2:18–19, animals are created "because 'it is not good that man should be alone.' Animals are brought to Adam *to be his companions*."[21] In trying to find points of contact with Singer's anti-speciesism, Camosy is perhaps pressing the issue too far. The biblical passage goes on to make it clear that nonhuman animals are not suitable companions for man: man needs an other like himself, "bone of my bones and flesh of my flesh,"[22] a being who is equally the same. Man is made complete only by the creation of woman: human beings exist in relationship with each other.[23] The understanding that each human being recognizes the other human being as an other has been expressed in some philosophies as an ethic of responsibility where responsibility does not demand reciprocity. For people with profound disabilities, this is not an issue of inequality. Rather, it is a question of the recognition and acknowledgment of the dignity of the human person as a member of the human family.[24]

In Genesis 2:15–17, God forbids Adam to eat from the tree of the knowledge of good and evil, indicating that there are limits to human freedom and dominion: humans are not morally independent to decide for themselves what is good and what is evil.[25] An important point for people with intellectual disabilities, this also perhaps indicates that autonomy is not the only significant aspect of humanity. But the limitation to dominion has been overlooked principally by bioethicists who do seem to set the highest store on human autonomy. For instance, Fletcher thinks that our situation is rightly "Promethean," that subjugation of nature by science and technology is almost quasi-salvific, that biological nature as raw material is there to be used as the person, detached from his or her biological constitution, sees fit, and the only limits to this dominion over the body are the ones set by human beings themselves. All

21. Camosy, *Peter Singer and Christian Ethics*, 46–47; emphasis original.

22. Gn 2:23. See Clifford and Murphy, "Genesis," 12.

23. See Pontifical Council for Justice and Peace, *Compendium of the Social Doctrine of the Church*, 36–37; Clifford and Murphy explain that this passage indicates that God made marriage part of creation. "Genesis," 12.

24. Matthews, "Human Dignity and the Profoundly Disabled," 10.

25. Pope John Paul II, *Fides et Ratio*, 22.

we need do is foresee the consequences of "stealing fire."[26] Fletcher sees human dignity in terms of autonomy and power over creation, and he urges the autonomous and strong to take control through technology. Following this call to take charge, bioethicists like Julian Savulescu and Guy Kane speak of the moral obligation to create children who are "the best" and so who are clearly not disabled.[27] Moreover, because Savulescu and his colleague Ingmar Persson think that some people are morally myopic in their moral judgments, today's "formidable technological powers" should be entrusted to beings who are "morally enlightened."[28] Power and dominion in the eyes of some bioethicists are only for the elite.

In contrast to the certainties of some bioethicists, Pope John Paul II draws attention to how the rapid advances of technology have created both demand and fear.[29] The pope notes that life is accepted "only under certain conditions" and rejected when it is disabled and inconvenient. In a philosophy of dominion as power, there is a "notion of freedom which exalts the isolated individual in an absolute way, and gives no place to solidarity, to openness to others and service of them." This ends up by becoming "the freedom of 'the strong' against the weak."[30] In this mindset, people appear to be set against each other, never mind against creation, and there are no bonds that unite us.

Arguably, there are difficulties in reasoning from Genesis that the bond that does unite us, the image of God, is found in all human beings, since the description is of God creating Adam and Eve as rational adults.[31] Whether this image is found in embryos or in the profoundly intellectually disabled is not addressed. It may seem that people without the requisite capacities of rationality cannot exercise dominion and therefore are excluded from the image of God. As the biblical scholar Claus Westermann notes, however, the Genesis texts refer not to individuals or to a person as an exemplar of all, but rather to the species

26. Fletcher, *Ethics of Genetic Control*, 5–6.
27. Savulescu and Kahane, "Moral Obligation," 274–90.
28. Persson and Savulescu, *Unfit for the Future*, 4, 9–10.
29. Pope John Paul II, *Redemptor Hominis*, 15.
30. Pope John Paul II, *Evangelium Vitae*, 14, 19.
31. See Peterson, *Genetic Turning Points*, 128.

humankind, and the creation account implies that the image of God in human beings constitutes us as human.[32] If dominion is seen not as speciesist privileging or wielding power over other animals but rather as holding responsibility and acting with solidarity and justice[33] with and alongside others as the human family, where all are responsible for creation, then this interpretation of the image of God need not exclude any human being. Furthermore, Genesis 5:1–3 suggests that this special relationship is passed on from Adam to all his descendants as Adam passes on his likeness to his children.[34] This leads into thinking about humans and nonhuman animals after creation.

Genesis, after Creation: Killing Human and Nonhuman Animals

Much bioethical talk focuses on justifications for killing some humans. But the account of the first murder, of Abel by his brother Cain, illustrates that each human being is in relationship with God and with others, and that every unjust killing violates this relationship.[35] In ancient Jewish Rabbinic writings, Cain's response "am I my brother's guardian?" to Yahweh's question "where is your brother Abel?" is seen as going against the Torah's ethic of responsibility for one's kin and one's neighbor.[36] Nevertheless, even if humans fail in relationships, Yahweh hears and responds to victims (Gn 4:10), and Yahweh also hears Cain. Yahweh places a mark of protection on him so that no one would kill him in turn.[37]

God's unique relationship with human beings continues through the flood story and its aftermath. Human wickedness has tainted the whole of creation (Gn 6:5–7:24). Yet Noah, who has won God's favor, is charged with preserving other species from the devastating flood. After

32. Westermann, *Genesis 1–11*, 202, 206.

33. Pope Francis, *Laudato Si*, 67–69.

34. Westermann, *Genesis 1–11*, 356; Pontifical Council for Justice and Peace, *Compendium of the Social Doctrine of the Church*, 428; van Kooten, *Paul's Anthropology in Context*, 2; Garr, *In His Own Image and Likeness*, 13.

35. See Pope John Paul II, *Evangelium Vitae*, 8.

36. Lv 19:16; Dt 21:1–9. See Berlin et al., *Jewish Study Bible*, 19.

37. Westermann, *Genesis 1–11*, 307. Notably, when Yahweh confers this mark, he does not address Cain as "you" but instead uses the third person (Gn 4:15), thus creating a unilateral covenant with him.

the flood subsides, God makes a covenant that involves the whole of creation (Gn 8:21–22), but he also establishes a new world order for the fallen world. In the Garden of Eden, humans and animals were given plants for food (Gn 1:29–30); now humans can kill and eat animals (Gn 9:3).

In his criticism of what he sees as the damaging legacy of Christianity, Singer explores both the first account of the creation of human beings and the dominance God gives them over nonhuman animals and the account after the flood where Yahweh says that human beings are now "the terror and the dread of all the animals." He deplores this second text as "the grant of dominion in more ominous language," and from this he says, "the implication is clear: to act in a way that causes fear and dread to everything that moves on the earth is not improper; it is, in fact, in accordance with a God-given decree."[38] What Singer fails to appreciate is that in the Christian tradition, the world has changed as a result of the Fall and the continued disobedience of human beings, so much so that creation itself has been harmed by the actions of those who were called to be its stewards. According to Camosy and Linzey, the permission to use nonhuman animals in this way is an accommodation by God to human sinfulness and violence.[39] Camosy explains that "the Bible is clear that our current relationship with animals is not the moral ideal and, indeed, is only a temporary state of affairs." After all, he says, the prophets predict a return to the nonviolence of Eden.[40]

Although human beings are now allowed to kill and eat nonhuman animals, the killing of human beings is prohibited in strong terms: "He who sheds the blood of man, by man shall his blood be shed, for in the image of God was man created" (Gn 9:6). The idea of the image of God has now been placed in the moral realm: killing another human is prohibited because humans are made in the image of God.[41] In contrast to the conclusion of Cain's story, in the new but fallen world order, a murderer is to be punished by death.[42]

38. Singer, *Practical Ethics*, 266.

39. Camosy, *Peter Singer and Christian Ethics*, 105; Linzey, *Animal Theology*, 127.

40. Camosy, "Other Animals as Persons?," 263.

41. See van Kooten, *Paul's Anthropology in Context*, 2.

42. Anthony Hoekema suggests that this is indicative of the development of governmental order. *Created in God's Image*, 16.

Some bioethicists point to the apparent incompatibility of appeals to the sanctity of life in cases of suicide and euthanasia and the permissibility of killing in self-defense, just war, or punishment, claiming that this incompatibility shows that the sanctity of life doctrine can be outweighed by other considerations such as justice, and therefore it could also be outweighed by autonomy or competing interests.[43] Cases of legitimate self-defense may bring about paradoxical situations where protecting one's own life and not harming another's becomes difficult to reconcile.[44] The death penalty is placed in a similar context, though arguably it is becoming acceptable only in "cases of absolute necessity," and "such cases are very rare, if not practically non-existent."[45] Pope John Paul II considers that the care taken to respect the lives of criminals and unjust aggressors heightens the care to be taken to protect the lives of innocent persons, particularly the weak and defenseless.[46]

Rationality, Being, and Bodies

To add to uncertainty about what the authors of Genesis meant by image of God, the words "image" (*selem*) and "likeness" (*demut*) seem to bear a range of meanings,[47] and while they are often considered synonymous,[48] they may have had theological significance for the writers of Genesis. Indeed, the patristic writers compared them.[49] *Selem* tends toward a concrete, perhaps bodily idea and was used to describe idols; *demut* tends toward a more abstract idea that includes the notion of comparison. Therefore the words themselves cannot be said to disclose a precise notion how humanity reflects the image and likeness of God. But in contrast to the insubstantiality of some contemporary notions of person, or a focus on pure rationality, the image of God in human beings appears to be a concrete reality. Notably, the image of God constitutes

43. See McMahan, *Ethics of Killing*, 466–67; Glover, *Causing Death and Saving Lives*.

44. See Pope John Paul II, *Evangelium Vitae*, 55.

45. Pope John Paul II, *Evangelium Vitae*, 56.

46. Pope John Paul II, *Evangelium Vitae*, 57.

47. See Vine, *Vine's Complete Expository Dictionary*, and Middleton, *Liberating Image*, chap. 2.

48. See van Kooten, *Paul's Anthropology in Context*, 2.

49. Grenz, *Social God and the Relational Self*, 187.

human beings as a particular kind of animal, animals of a rational nature. It does not rest on the actual possession of certain attributes.

Moreover, when it comes to thinking about disability, Genesis 1:31 says that God saw all that he had made, and "indeed it was very good." A strand of disability theology critiques the view that when something has "gone wrong... disability quickly becomes a sign of imperfection, a flaw in God's good order, something to be undone."[50] In this critique, the search for perfection through reimplantation diagnosis, prenatal testing, and screening is seen as buying into the "cult of normalcy" that measures people in terms of normal and abnormal, perfect and imperfect. Instead, in theology, perfection is seen as fullness of life[51] rather than physical or mental perfection. When perfection is understood as excellence, then matching up to a physical or mental norm is no longer relevant. As Pope John Paul II explains in relation to people with cognitive disabilities who are equally made in the image of God, "for disabled people as for any human being, it is not important that they do what others do but that they do what is truly good for them, increasingly making the most of their talents and responding faithfully to their own human and supernatural vocation."[52] There is solidarity in the very diverse human family.

Solidarity in Jesus Christ: Image of the Living God in Spirit, Mind, and Body

For the earliest Christian writers, the unity of all humankind seems to be a given. All humanity is included, and the image of God extends equally to the whole race.[53] These writers offer a strong and common thread of thought that links Adam, the first man and the one who expresses our initial relationship with God, to Christ, the last because it is through him that our final relationship with God is expressed. There is then a solidarity that binds the whole human family regardless of situation or condition. The two poles of the theology of all humans and their

50. Reynolds, *Vulnerable Communion*, 30.
51. Pope John Paul II, *Evangelium Vitae*, 36, 2.
52. Pope John Paul II, "Mentally Ill Are Also Made in God's Image," 4.
53. Gregory of Nyssa, "On the Making of Man," XVI, 16, 17.

dignity as persons are expressed by their image and likeness in Adam and hope in divinization in Christ. But while the spiritual and relational aspects of the image of God in human beings may be in no doubt, it is important to counter suggestions that biological life plays no part whatsoever in that image.

Even though all human beings are made in the image of God, experience constantly reminds the early Christians that human beings had tarnished the gift of image through sin, and they frequently fall short (Rom 3:23). Christ, the true "image of the unseen God" (Col 1:15; 2 Cor 4:4),[54] restores the image (Rom 8:29–30) through union of the believer in baptism with him and through the believer's graced daily life of dying to his sinful ways (Col 3:10–11). For St. Paul, salvation involves being united to Christ (1 Thes 5:10)[55] by putting away their former lives, being renewed and clothing themselves with Christ (Eph 4:22–24), and by becoming "mature in Christ" (Col 1:28).

Significantly, salvation includes the bodily and biological aspects of human beings as well as the spiritual and biographical aspects. Acknowledging that he is passing on the *kerygma*, Paul explicitly links the fate of Christ to the fate of humanity: hope in Christ gives firm foundation to faith so that what happened in Christ, his bodily Resurrection, will happen for us too (1 Cor 15).[56] Against some in Corinth who rejected resurrection of the dead, and some Greeks who rejected it as overly concerned with materiality, Paul explains that our resurrection as whole persons is guaranteed by Christ, raised from the dead as "the first-fruits of all who have fallen asleep" for "just as all die in Adam, so in Christ all will be brought to life" (1 Cor 15:12–22). That this is greater than can be anticipated is expressed in the eschatological tone of the hymn in Colossians 1:15–20 linking Christ with not only all humanity but also with the reconciliation of "all things," in heaven and on earth, the whole universe, in him.[57]

54. St. Paul appears to be quoting an older Christian hymn; see Horgan, "Letter to the Colossians," 879.

55. For an overview of Paul's understanding of God's plan of salvation history, see Fitzmyer, "Pauline Theology," 1390–93.

56. See O'Connor, "First Letter to the Corinthians," 812–13.

57. See Horgan, "Letter to the Colossians," 879–80.

With his affirmation of Christ as Lord, and with the superabundance of grace that Christ brings, Paul demonstrates that he does not see the earthly likeness of Adam as equal to the heavenly likeness of Christ. Nor does Paul take a negative view of bodily or biological life, however, as evidenced by his assertions regarding bodily resurrection, even though he contrasts life in the flesh and life in the spirit (Rom 8:1–13). Although the resurrection of Christians is dependent on Christ's Resurrection, Paul sees that preparation begins with Christian baptism into the death of Christ and by dying to sin (Rom 6:1–11). Paul draws a contrast between living fleshily, that is, according to the world, and living in the spirit, that is, being captured by Christ.[58] Thus Paul's division of life in the flesh and life in the spirit reflects not opposing parts of the human being, but this sense of growing in Christ.[59] For Paul, body (*soma*, σωμα) refers to the living body, and flesh (*sarx*, σαρξ) is often related to bodily existence that leads away from God.[60] But body, as *soma* and *sarx*, is the whole person rather than body as contrasted with soul. Life lived in the flesh is where the whole person, spiritual and bodily, lives in bondage to the self and in denial of his dependence on God. Paul keeps the human being whole.[61]

As an indication of how Paul naturally regards the human being as a whole, Paul expresses the unity of all in Christ by analogy to the unity of the human being: "for as with the human body which is a unity although it has many parts . . . so it is with Christ" (1 Cor 12:12; Rom 12:4–5). Christ brings all into the unity of his Body. The solidarity of humankind is confirmed by the vocation to stewardship gifted in Genesis. Within that solidarity, as Paul explains, everyone has "a part to play in the whole" (1 Cor 12:27),[62] for everyone makes a unique contribution. Continuing with his

58. For a description of Paul's anthropology, see Dunn, *Theology of Paul the Apostle*, 51–78.

59. As Joseph Fitzmyer, professor of biblical studies, points out, Paul does not describe human beings in themselves. Rather, Paul "hints at" the relationship of humanity to God. "Pauline Theology," 1406.

60. Vine, *Vine's Complete Expository Dictionary*.

61. See Fitzmyer, "Pauline Theology," 1406–7; Runia, *Philo in Early Christian Literature*, 72.

62. See 1 Cor 12:27. For a discussion of the Pauline notion of the Body of Christ as the Christian community, its parallels in ancient thinking, and how Paul's understanding goes beyond simply cooperation in the pursuit of a common goal, see Fitzmyer, "Pauline Theology," 1409–10.

analogy, "it is precisely the parts of the body that seem to be the weakest which are the indispensable ones" (1 Cor 12:22). The idea that in the human family those who appear to be weakest are in fact indispensable is an interesting point of reflection for those who deny much to radically dependent human beings.

Later Philosophical and Christian Anthropology: With Image in Mind

While Paul's distinction between fleshly and spiritual persons is not a separation of the human being,[63] a gradual move to a more intellectual understanding of the image of God may have been made in ancient Jewish and early Christian writings under the influence of Greek ideas of body and soul.[64]

Even though the Greeks had already established colonies in the Near East, the conversation between Hellenism and Judaism grew with the conquests of Alexander the Great (356–323 BCE).[65] Moreover, as Jews moved away from Jerusalem and settled in other areas, external circumstances inevitably influenced their later reflections. One area, the thriving new cosmopolitan center of Alexandria, became especially important for the development of biblical exegesis. Changes in the Alexandrian Jewish community meant that Jews began to depend on Greek rather than Hebrew, which led to the gradual coming together of Greek philos-

63. As a Greek-speaking Jew, Paul has been seen as spanning two cultures, and there is much debate on whether to read him in primarily a Greco-Roman culture or a Jewish one. Sanders, "Paul between Judaism and Hellenism," 74–90. In the case of Paul's use of the image of God, van Kooten claims that Paul's view on the believer becoming conformed to the divine image has "an analogy in the Platonic ideal of becoming as much like God as possible." "Image, Form and Transformation," 240. Van Kooten believes that the Jewish philosophers Philo and Paul share a similar "trichotomic" anthropology, as they regard human beings to be composed of spirit, soul, and body. *Paul's Anthropology in Context*, 219. Nevertheless, as Runia points out in his extensive review of the literature, Paul's "flesh" does not correspond to Philo's "body," nor does Paul's "spirit" match Philo's "soul." *Philo in Early Christian Literature*, 69–73.

64. Van Kooten argues for the presence of a Greek influence from the first century BCE (*Paul's Anthropology in Context*, 219). The influence of philosophy, particularly Platonism, is evident in the Alexandrian tradition from at least the first century. Engberg-Pedersen, "Setting the Scene," 3.

65. For the effects of the Hellenistic period, see Jagersma, *History of Israel*, Part II, chap. 2.

ophy and Hebrew ideas. This merger of ideas was furthered by the translation into Greek (the Septuagint) of the main texts of Hebrew scripture and the incorporation into the canon of some non-Hebrew texts, the Wisdom literature. In addition, the call to Christians to preach the Good News to the gentiles and so to engage with other cultures and mind-sets led inevitably to openness to other thought.[66]

Following first-century intellectual trends, Plato rather than Aristotle appealed to philosophically minded writers,[67] though Stoicism also figured.[68] For Christians, this appeal may have been because Aristotle's notion of God, the Unmoved Mover, seemed to be more like an Eternal Mind enclosed in contemplation of itself and indifferent to the universe rather than a personal Creator. Plus it was not entirely clear where Aristotle stood on the issue of the soul's immortality.[69] In contrast, for some Christians and for some Jews, the appeal of Platonism lay in the Platonic belief that the soul, the truly real aspect of the human being, needs to transcend the visible universe to find where it truly belongs in the real world of Forms.[70] At any rate, in order to demonstrate the rationality of Christianity, some early Christians adopted and Christianized some ideas from philosophy, notably the predominant philosophy of Platonism, while retaining a world view focused on Christ.

The spiritual movement of Gnosticism exemplifies the eclecticism of this Jewish, Hellenistic, and Greco-Roman culture. The Gnostics were influential in paganism and Christianity, perhaps developing some of their ideas from Platonism and especially from the Neoplatonist Philo.[71] It is difficult to identify Gnostic beliefs with precision because available sources tend to come from writers who are hostile to their thought. Apparently, for the Gnostics who held the material in contempt, the soul

66. See MacDonald, *History of the Concept of the Mind*, 89.

67. See Runia, *Philo of Alexandria and the Timaeus of Plato*, 263. For an account of the "dialogue" between Christianity and Platonism and Aristotelianism, see McGrath, *Christian Theology*, 73–76.

68. Troels Engberg-Pedersen notes the influence of Stoic philosophy alongside Platonism on early Christian writings until Platonism became culturally dominant. "Setting the Scene," 1–14.

69. Knight, *Aristotelian Philosophy*, 42–43.

70. For this shift to dualism under the influence of Greek thinking, see MacDonald, *History of the Concept of the Mind*, 89–92.

71. See Runia, *Philo of Alexandria and the Timaeus of Plato*, 558.

or divine element in humanity seeks release from its necessary housing in the material world and longs to return to its true home in the divine world of light. This true divine identity is recognized, though only by a few, by Gnosis, or revealed insight.[72] For the Gnostics, however, the soul is not simply trapped in a material body, as it is for Plato or Philo. They seem to believe that the body and soul are made in the image of God, but not with a divine element. Instead, this image is an inferior copy made by lower powers that are in opposition to God. The true divine element is present only in the chosen few and located in the spirit, the spark or seed, the "inner man."[73] For the Gnostics, salvation lies in attaining knowledge of the true self, this divine spark, and knowledge of the transcendent God.[74]

In this mix of ideas there seems to have been both a move toward a spiritual understanding of the image of God and a countermove against it. The more intellectual interpretation may have been a response to pagan ideas of gods as bodies, which encouraged bodily notions of the image of God in human beings.[75] But a more physical notion of the image of God is simultaneously found in Christian writing, and it counters a purely spiritual or intellectual interpretation.[76]

Professor of religion George van Kooten suggests that both Irenaeus and Tertullian challenge an exclusively spiritual understanding of the image of God by their insistence that human beings as wholes image God.[77] Rather than simply being a reaction to prevalent philosophies or a response to certain tendencies, notably Gnostic ones,[78] this focus on the whole human being is rooted in Christianity. All Christians, whether influenced by specific philosophies or claiming otherwise, arrived at and

72. Turner, *Sethian Gnosticism and the Platonic Tradition*, 2.

73. Logan, *Gnostic Truth and Christian Heresy*, 167–68.

74. Logan, *Gnostic Truth and Christian Heresy*, 211.

75. Van Kooten, *Paul's Anthropology in Context*, 9, 38, 62.

76. Van Kooten finds this in some Jewish writing but argues it is more predominant in Christian writing. He regards the *Life of Adam and Eve*, *2 Enoch*, *The Sibylline Oracles (Books I and VIII)*, the *Testament of Naphtali*, and the *Testament of Isaac* as Christian. *Paul's Anthropology in Context*, 38–43.

77. Van Kooten, *Paul's Anthropology in Context*, 43.

78. Van Kooten rightly notes that the Gnostic contempt of the body caused both Irenaeus and Tertullian to assert that the body is also in God's image. *Paul's Anthropology in Context*, 43.

tested their understandings in the light of the Gospel message of Jesus Christ. Because the Son of God assumed true humanity and rose bodily from the dead, most Christians attempted to keep body and soul in human beings together. Some early Christian writers express this unity in the understanding that human beings never lose the gift of God's image. Yet the demands of living a life in Christ mean that human beings can grow more into that image, or grow away from it, and the relationship of body and soul in this process at times sets up tensions in how early Christians saw the human person.

Two classical writers provide useful contrasts on how ancient philosophy is used in reflection on the image of God, and especially how it is interpreted in the Christian tradition as opposed to a more Platonic tradition that locates the image of God purely in the soul. Although some 150 years apart, the Jewish writer Philo (20 BCE to 50 CE) and the Christian writer Clement of Alexandria[79] (d. ca. 214 CE) both inhabited Alexandria, where it was reputed the Septuagint was written, and both were greatly influenced by Platonism, Middle Platonism, and Stoicism.[80] Both writers assert that human beings are especially dear to God because they are made in his image.[81] For both, the image of the divine image is the *Logos*; however, their thinking on the *Logos* is very different. Moreover, the goal for human beings—immortality and a return to that likeness—is achieved in different ways. So, according to Philo, writing

79. For both the influence of Philo on Clement and the gulf that separates them, see Osborn, *Clement of Alexandria*.

80. In this section, a contrast is made between the thinking of Philo and Clement because both writers operate in the Alexandrian milieu yet demonstrate their own Platonic philosophical or Christian specificity. The writings of St. Paul and Philo are historically closer. however, so a comparison may not be useful. In his book *Paul's Anthropology in Context*, van Kooten argues for a Greek and specifically Platonic context for Paul's thinking. While much of van Kooten's book looks at Philo, whose thinking was clearly rooted in Greek philosophy and the Platonic tradition, van Kooten seems to assume rather than argue for the same influence on Paul. Instead of philosophy, however, Paul seems to be motivated by pastoral concerns in the light of the good news of Jesus (see, e.g., Fitzmyer, "Introduction to the New Testament Epistles," 770; Elford, *Pastoral Nature of Theology*, 72–73. Moreover, MacDonald notes the "bewildering variety of assertions" that have been made about Paul's apparent Platonic dualism. *History of the Concept of the Mind*, 104–7. David Runia's extensive literature survey concludes that although there are parallels between Philo and Paul, they occur simply on the level of terminology, and the differences are profound and significant. *Philo in Early Christian Literature*, 66–73.

81. Philo, *On the Creation*, 14.77; Clement of Alexandria, *Christ the Educator*, I, III.

in the Jewish tradition, the goal is reached through observance of the Mosaic Law that mirrors the order of nature imprinted by the *Logos*; for Clement, writing in the Christian tradition, salvation is gained through Jesus Christ, who is the *Logos* made flesh.[82] Clement demonstrates what Christianity had always recognized: that a new initiative by God was required to return human beings to their original destiny. Thus, for Christians, the coming in flesh of the Son of God, the *Logos*, gave a deeper perspective to the image of God. Christ has universal significance as the "second Adam"[83] who raises and renews humanity and represents the solidarity of all human beings.

Philo of Alexandria

According to Philo, God first makes an incorporeal heaven and invisible earth,[84] then he makes the sense-perceptible cosmos, and to "crown" his creation of the visible cosmos, God makes human beings[85] who are formed after his image.[86] God's idea or image is in the *Logos*, an apparently functional and impersonal instrument by which God orders the world out of a mass of lifeless matter.[87] Thus the whole universe is an image of the *Logos*, which is itself an image of the divine image.[88]

For Philo, in the hierarchy of living beings, what differentiates living beings with and without souls is their level of sense perception.[89] So, he argues that "the most sluggish and least delineated type of soul" is allotted to fishes as a kind, and "the most developed and in every respect best type" of soul is assigned to humankind.[90] Following Platonism and its desire to escape matter, Philo says that fish share more in the substance of body than soul: "they both are and are not living beings. They move, yet do not really have soul." Birds are "more sensitive," and land animals more so again. Finally, human beings are endowed with intellect as a

82. See Vine, *Vine's Complete Expository Dictionary*.
83. See 1 Cor 15; Rom 5:12–21.
84. Philo, *On the Creation*, 6.29.
85. Philo, *On the Creation*, 11.65.
86. Philo, *On the Creation*, 4.25.
87. Philo, *On the Creation*, 4.22.
88. Philo, *On the Creation*, 4.25; van Kooten, *Paul's Anthropology in Context*, 48.
89. Philo, *On the Creation*, 11.62.
90. Philo, *On the Creation*, 11.65.

"special gift, a kind of soul of the soul."[91] Regarding the image of God in humankind, Philo is clear that there is not a bodily likeness since God does not have a human shape.[92] Instead, image is used, he says, "with regard to the director of the soul, the intellect" for, "in a sense it is a god of the person who carries it and bears it around as a divine image."[93]

Philo appears to regard the two creation accounts in Genesis as two races of humans: the first, the "idea," is the heavenly man of Genesis 1, created as incorporeal and imperishable. But because God is blameless in all evil, God's "helpers," heavenly beings, then made humans of mixed nature out of clay, male or female with external senses, and consisting of body and soul.[94] This earthly human of Genesis 2 is clay, but God breathes in his soul and infuses into him a mind that would have been earthly also if God had not breathed life into it. The mind, the dominant portion of the soul and presumably the higher faculties, is the only part of the soul worthy of this inbreathing, and it is mind that is created according to the image and idea of God.[95]

Platonic dualism of body and soul is central to Philo's thought.[96] According to Philo, the human being is a composite of mind (νους), spirit (πνευμα), soul (ψυχη), and then with the addition of a body (σωμα). In his understanding of the relationship between these human aspects, Philo seems to follow Plato's understanding in the *Phaedrus* where Reason, the Charioteer, drives with the help of one tractable horse, the higher emotions, and together they struggle to control his second unruly horse, carnal lusts, both horses being necessary to the chariot's team. Thus, while the body[97] is purely passive, the real conflict in humans takes place in the soul's rational and irrational parts.[98] If anything, the body holds

91. Philo, *On the Creation*, 11.66.

92. Philo, *On the Creation*, 12.69.

93. Philo, *On the Creation*, 12.69. See van Kooten, *Paul's Anthropology in Context*, 51.

94. Philo, *On the Creation*, 13.73, 13:75, 18.134; Philo, "Allegorical Interpretation 1, 2 and 3," XII, 31.

95. Philo, "Allegorical Interpretation," XIII, 39, 42.

96. Runia, *Philo of Alexandria and the Timaeus of Plato*, 260.

97. Runia notes that in the *Timaeus*, Plato locates the parts of the soul in separate areas of the body. Similarly, Philo declares that the soul is tripartite: reason is located in the head; the higher emotions, like courage, in the chest; and baser emotions in the abdomen. *Philo of Alexandria and the Timaeus of Plato*, 302–3.

98. Runia, *Philo of Alexandria and the Timaeus of Plato*, 262–63.

the soul back; it is an impediment preventing the soul from attaining the truth, so the philosopher's task is, as far as possible, to live a life untainted by association with the body.[99] For Philo, the mind needs to be freed from corporeal necessities[100] because it is not possible for one who dwells in the body and belongs to the race of mortals to be united with God. The person needs to be delivered from "that prison house of the body,"[101] and the pursuit of philosophy and wisdom enables him or possibly her to achieve immortality.[102] As Philo explains, the souls of the athlete and the philosopher differ because the athlete attributes greatest importance to the condition of the body while the philosopher seeks to educate the higher part of his soul. Although the body is necessary, it is in fact "an evil and a dead thing."[103]

Clement of Alexandria

Like Philo, Clement speaks of the *Logos* as the image of God, and man's mind as the image of the image.[104] Nevertheless, the *Logos* is not the impersonal idea of Philo:[105] he is the "divine and royal Word, the impassible man,"[106] Christ who became man, our teacher and moral guide.[107] As images of God, we are to imitate Christ and fulfill God's commands.[108]

Unlike Philo, Clement does not see the body as evil or dead precisely because God himself becomes flesh and he heals the body.[109] Clement's Christ appears to lack usual human needs, however; he is dispassionate and eats not for nourishment but to show his disciples he is not a ghost.[110] In this, Clement's Christ seems to exhibit elements from Gnosticism and perhaps a disregard for bodily life.

99. Plato, *Phaedo*, 66. For the development of Plato's thinking on the soul and body, see Torchia, *Exploring Personhood*, 39–69.

100. Philo, "Allegorical Interpretation 3," XIII, 41.

101. Philo, "Allegorical Interpretation 3," XIV, 42.

102. Philo, *On the Creation*, 14, 77.

103. Philo, "Allegorical Interpretation 3," XXII, 72.

104. Clement of Alexandria, "*Stromata*," V, XIV.

105. See Holmes, *Building the Christian Academy*, 20.

106. Clement of Alexandria, "*Stromata*," V, XIV.

107. Clement of Alexandria, "Exhortation to the Heathen," XI.

108. Clement of Alexandria, *Christ the Educator*, I, III. See also Osborn, *Clement of Alexandria*, 234.

109. Clement of Alexandria, "*Stromata*," III, XVII.

110. Clement of Alexandria, "*Stromata*," VI, IX.

It seems that while Clement did not remain immune from some Gnostic thinking, he did aim to avoid the excesses of the then current Gnostic trends. Although in the same passage Clement suggests that the goal for humans is to reach this kind of liberation from bodily necessities, he does recognize that humans have basic needs, and he encourages his flock in exercise of the virtues and an asceticism that maintains the body. This "training for life" and regulation of the body in moderation and temperance seem to be in response to a rather overindulgent luxurious Alexandrian lifestyle.[111] Moreover, Clement turns around the philosophical claim that the body is the tomb of the soul since the soul is buried in it for this life. Instead, Clement argues that the body can be either a tomb or a temple: the body is intimately connected to the soul's learning[112] and is "the soul's consort and ally"[113] and so can either aid or hinder it.

For Clement, both the idea of a Gnostic elite who gain salvation through rarefied knowledge[114] and the claims of Platonists and Stoics that the assent to God is through their own powers of philosophy[115] are profoundly mistaken. There are not, he says, some "illuminated" Gnostics and some "animal" human beings, for all are equal. This is a telling reminder that there are not some enlightened beings who can take control and wield the power of technology. It also perhaps provides an interesting reflection on today's situation, which divides human beings into biological and mere animal life and biographical more illuminated personal life. According to Clement, it is by baptism that we become children of God; its grace brings illumination and salvation.[116] Knowledge of God is a divine gift that wakes our free will and admits faith.[117]

To counter the false Gnostics, Clement makes a distinction readily available in the tradition between the image that human beings receive immediately at their creation and the likeness that they grow into yet

111. Clement of Alexandria, *Christ the Educator*, II, 1.
112. Clement of Alexandria, "*Stromata*," III, XVII, XIX.
113. Clement of Alexandria, *Christ the Educator*, I, XIII.
114. Clement of Alexandria, *Christ the Educator*, I, VI.
115. Clement of Alexandria, "*Stromata*," II, XII.
116. Clement of Alexandria, *Christ the Educator*, I, VI.
117. Clement of Alexandria, "*Stromata*," V, XIII.

only receive, it seems, at their perfection.[118] Clement can make much of this distinction because he used the Septuagint.[119] In the Greek, image (*eikon*), perhaps like *selem*, implies some sort of concrete resemblance, but likeness (*homoiosis*) seems to go further than *demut* in that it excludes the idea of equality.[120] For Clement, the "true Gnostic" who is in the image and likeness of God imitates Christ, lives righteously in self-restraint, in cultivation of the virtues, in faith and repentance.[121] God bestows his gifts on those who follow Christ, who repent as they begin to live in the light, and who take spiritual nourishment in the Eucharist.[122] In contrast to later theologies influenced by legalism, such as those of Locke and Fletcher, and repeated by some bioethicists as representative of the whole of Christian theology, true Gnostics do not avoid evil out of fear of punishment, nor do they do good for reward. Rather, in living a life in imitation of Christ, they act out of love.[123]

Clement draws attention to one important factor that has perhaps additional significance for people with profound disabilities. Clement says that all human beings are made in the image of God and all are called to grow into God's likeness as far as they are able, and with the strength given to them by grace. One common strand of thought sees people with profound disabilities as pure and sinless as the angels.[124] Yet this does disservice to the fact that people with disabilities are human beings. As with all human beings, they are made in the image of God and can never lose that image, but they are also called to grow in God's likeness as far as they are able with the aid of grace.

118. Clement of Alexandria, "*Stromata*," II, XXII.

119. Clement of Alexandria, "*Stromata*," I, XXII.

120. See Westermann, *Genesis 1–11*, 146. Westermann also offers an overview of theological interpretations of *selem*, *eikon*, *demut*, and *homoiosis* (148–55).

121. Clement of Alexandria, "*Stromata*," II, XII, XIX.

122. Clement of Alexandria, *Christ the Educator*, I, VI.

123. Clement of Alexandria, "*Stromata*," IV, XXII.

124. See Black, *Healing Homiletic*, 20.

The Christian Tradition: Keeping Mind, Body, and Soul Together

The contrast between Philo and Clement may seem obvious. However, tension in some early Christian thinking remains noticeable in writers who appear to locate image solely in the spiritual or reasonable part of human beings, the "inner man." Origen (ca. 186–255), one of the most influential Greek theologians who is often associated with Platonism,[125] seems to make such a move. Origen died a year after he was tortured for his faith. After his death, the orthodoxy of his teachings began to be questioned. Many of his writings were eventually burned, and only a few fragments of Origen's original Greek works remain. The available writings are colored by interpolation, censorship, and freedom in translation, so that some speculation is inevitably involved in piecing together his thought. The biblical scholar Jerome (ca. 347–420) and the monk Rufinus of Aquileia (ca. 345–410) both translated Origen's *De Principiis*. Jerome's translation was intended to point out Origen's heresies, and Jerome complained that Rufinus had purged his own translation of Origen's errors. Jerome's translation is no longer extant, and only the very free Latin translation by Rufinus remains.[126]

Origen writes against those who think that image refers to the body because they argue that God is corporeal.[127] Origen also seeks to refute the teaching of Celsus (writing ca. 178), who suggests that there are no differences in the souls of any species, be they human or ant. Origen argues that irrationality is the mark of nonhuman creatures. Reason, he says, is "the common possession of men, and of divine and heavenly beings, and perhaps of the Supreme God himself, on account of which man is said to have been created in the image of God, for the image of the Supreme God is his reason [*Logos*]."[128]

125. For the difficulties of labelling Origen as a Platonist, see Corrigan, *Evagrius and Gregory*, 29–33. However, David Runia examines the considerable influence of Philo on Origen. *Philo in Early Christian Literature*, 174–77.

126. Corrigan draws attention to the different factions, as typified by the dispute between Jerome and Rufinus, that have complicated the Origenist controversy. *Evagrius and Gregory*, 34–35.

127. Origen, *Homilies on Genesis and Exodus*, I, XII, XIII.

128. Origen, "Against Celsus," IV, LXXXV.

Arguably, Origen emphasizes image as reason to counter specific heresies, and it seems he refers to rational nature rather than the actual possession of rationality in the life history of a human being. But Origen also seems to think Platonically that souls fell into bodies,[129] or at least that the body was given after the Fall. Later theologians criticize Origen for this, and when Cyril of Alexandria (ca. 378–444) discusses the absurdity of preexistent souls falling into bodies, he explains that if they go into bodies because they have sinned, then it would increase disease, not healing, and we would not praise the Creator for increasing sickness.[130] Cyril adds that Christians declare the resurrection of the flesh so the body cannot be a punishment.[131] Similarly, Methodius (ca. 260 to ca. 312) says the body is not a fetter of the soul as Origen thought, since that means God, the great artificer, adds a further wrong to remedy an error. Methodius explains that man is neither a soul without a body nor a body without a soul; rather, he is "a being composed out of the union of soul and body into one form of the beautiful."[132] The body, the material, shares in beauty of creation in the image of God.

Early views of martyrdom also make this point. Fletcher believes that the sanctity of life principle is not particularly Christian, otherwise the martyrs would be wrong.[133] For the early Fathers, however, genuine martyrs do not court death. Early writers certainly show admiration and praise of martyrdom, yet they clearly do not approve of Christians voluntarily offering themselves up to death: "we do not commend those who surrender themselves, for not such is the teaching of the gospel."[134] The importance of the Christian idea of bodily resurrection is illustrated by the fact that pagan authorities refused to allow collection of the remains of martyrs and often burnt and dispersed the bodies in an effort to prevent their resurrection.[135]

129. At least this is what Jerome claims is from Origen; see Corrigan, *Evagrius and Gregory*, 34.

130. Cyril of Alexandria, *Commentary on John*, I, 9, 4.

131. Cyril of Alexandria, *Commentary on John*, I, 9, 5.

132. Methodius, "From the Discourse on the Resurrection," III, 1–1V.

133. Fletcher, *Morals and Medicine*, 194.

134. "Martyrdom of Saint Polycarp," 4; Chadwick, *Early Church*, 30–31.

135. Ehrman, "Letter of the Churches of Lyons and Vienne," in *After the New Testament*; Augustine, *City of God against the Pagans*, Books 1–10, I, 12.

Yet such was Platonism's appeal that Christian theologians, even those who did not set much store by philosophy, used the pagan concept of the soul, and so appeared to set up a body-soul dualism. For instance, Tertullian, an educated convert from Carthage who had once held pagan aversion to Christianity, later writes a treatise on the soul to refute pagan philosophy that obscures the truth by fanciful notions of the soul's origin, destiny, and possibility of transmigration.[136] Nevertheless, Christians take a critical approach to Platonism and its rejection of the body in favor of the emancipation of the soul. For Christians, belief in the Incarnation and Resurrection of Jesus Christ explicitly affirms bodily life. The coming-in-flesh aspect of Redemptive Incarnation allows the Fathers to see the human being as embodied spirit, who has been promised to see God "from his own flesh"[137] in the resurrection of the body. So, they speak also on the resurrection of the dead rather than simply the immortality of the soul.

In his treatise *The Resurrection,*[138] the early Christian apologist Justin Martyr stresses that "God calls even the body to resurrection and promises it everlasting life." As Justin explains in terms echoed later by Thomas Aquinas, "Is the soul by itself a man? No, it is but the soul of a man. Can the body be called a man? No, it can but be called the body of a man. If, then, neither of these is by itself a man, but that which is composed of the two together is called a man, and God has called man to life and resurrection, He has called not a part, but the whole, which is the soul and body."[139] Justin likewise thinks that as Jesus healed those who were deformed on earth, so there will be healing in heaven: at the Resurrection, therefore, the flesh of all shall rise perfect and entire.[140]

As Candida Moss points out, there are problems for some with the notion of a healed body in heaven, especially for those who see their disability as a part of their identity.[141] Moss claims that in the New Testa-

136. Tertullian, "On the Soul," III..

137. Job 19:26.

138. There are four fragments of this treatise preserved in the *Sacra parallela* of John Damascene. The text can be found in Justin Martyr, "Fragments on the Resurrection," VIII.

139. Justin Martyr, "Fragments on the Resurrection," VIII.

140. Justin Martyr, "Fragments on the Resurrection," IV.

141. Moss, "Heavenly Healing," 991–1017.

ment healing and salvation are synonymous;[142] "disability is associated with sin, and healing is equated with divine forgiveness or salvation."[143] Yet Moss seems to have overlooked one of the earliest healing stories, when Jesus cures the paralytic man. Jesus tells the man that his sins are forgiven. He only cures the man when it seems that proof of his authority is required to satisfy the inward thoughts of the scribes (Mk 2:1–12).

In his treatise *On the Soul*, Tertullian treats body and soul as separate when he discusses the different philosophical approaches to the nature of the soul. Against these approaches, however, Tertullian is also clear that soul and body are not simply two natures united in some way. Instead, he argues that they exist in profound unity forming a single nature: God breathed on man, and he became a living soul as the breath passed to his internal structure, spread, and congealed into his shape; soul and shape are formed together.[144] Death is the outcome of the Fall and an evil that violates nature.[145] Even the easiest death is violence to our nature, for the "close companionship of soul and body" that is by nature "inseparable" is by death divided.[146] Tertullian also considers the fate of damaged human beings or those who die prematurely, and arguing possibly against the Homeric view that souls linger on in some shadowy fashion after death for various reasons, he suggests that souls receive back at the Resurrection the self-same bodies in which they died, the same condition and age, and they remain seemingly unchanged until the "promised perfection," presumably at the end of time.[147]

Tertullian raises the distinction between image and likeness in his treatise *On Baptism*.[148] He explains that likeness to God can be lost through sin, even though he is also certain that the image of God in man can never be lost. This idea of the permanence of the image in human beings is also found in Irenaeus (ca. 135–200). Irenaeus, bishop of Lyons, was regarded as a particularly significant theologian because as a boy

142. Moss, "Heavenly Healing," 1007.

143. Moss, "Heavenly Healing," 1010–11.

144. Tertullian, "On the Soul," IX. See Eric Osborn, *Tertullian*, 214. For Tertullian, it seems that God and souls are particularly rarefied material substances.

145. Tertullian, "On the Soul," LII.

146. Tertullian, "On the Soul," LII.

147. Tertullian, "On the Soul," LVI.

148. Tertullian, "On Baptism," V.

he had seen and heard Bishop Polycarp,[149] one of the most renowned of early martyrs who had also known the Apostles, thus establishing a link between Irenaeus and Christ's first disciples.[150] Irenaeus wrote his *Against Heresies* to address thinkers like Marcion, who expressed hatred for the material world, and to counter those Gnostics who claimed that they had access to a more authentic understanding of Scripture. In his discussion of the profound unity of body and soul and the distinction between image and likeness, Irenaeus focuses on the work of Christ. For Irenaeus, salvation concerns the whole nature of human beings, body and soul, since the *Logos* took on soul, body, and spirit.[151] Like Paul, Irenaeus explains that Christ sums up afresh and restores mankind.[152] Irenaeus adopts a tripartite of body, soul, and spirit. Although this seems at first sight to follow the scheme offered by Philo,[153] Irenaeus has more in common with Paul. Moreover, both Paul and Irenaeus see any division as a distinction not a separation into parts. As Irenaeus says, the whole human being, soul, body, and spirit, and not merely part of a human being, is made in the likeness of the *Logos*: the soul and spirit are part of a human being, but they are not the human being, "for the perfect man consists in the commingling and the union of the soul receiving the spirit of the Father, and the admixture of that fleshly nature which was moulded after the image of God."[154] Irenaeus places the likeness to God in the spirit, the divine life given to humans, whereas the image lies more in the body and soul. Hence, although likeness is lost through the sin of Adam and restored through the redemptive incarnation of Christ, the image in the human being is indestructible.[155]

149. See Osborn, *Irenaeus of Lyons*, 3.

150. Irenaeus contended with two heretical views in particular: one was advanced by Marcion, who rejected the Old Testament and much of the New Testament, accepting only the Gospel of John. The other was taken up by the followers of Valentinus who put forward their own compositions as additional gospels. The claim of Irenaeus to be linked to the Apostles through Polycarp therefore gave him added authority in his promotion of the four-Gospel canon as handed down in the tradition. See Osborn, *Irenaeus of Lyons*, 175–80.

151. Irenaeus, "Against Heresies," V, VI, 1.

152. Irenaeus, *Demonstration of the Apostolic Preaching*, 32.

153. As to whether Irenaeus knew the work of Philo, see Runia, *Philo in Early Christian Literature*, 117.

154. Irenaeus, "Against Heresies," V, VI, 1.

155. The thinking of Irenaeus on image and likeness is not wholly consistent, however; see Osborn, *Irenaeus of Lyons*, 212–16.

Although the image of God appears to be reflected in the whole human being, the distinction between image and likeness, and the focus on spiritual growth into the likeness of Christ, may be a threat to the unity of body and soul by giving an opening into situating image in the soul only. Reform theologian Colin Gunton argues that this distinction of image and likeness contributed significantly to a strand of thought that sees solely reason or mind as the place where the image of God is found.[156] This kind of thinking inevitably has a negative impact on profoundly intellectually disabled people.

An incomplete understanding of the tradition that sees only a focus on reason or the mind has led to some overstatements, however. Richard Middleton, professor of biblical studies, claims that all Christian writers up to Aquinas understood image as likeness between the rational soul and the being of God, thus excluding explicitly or by omission the body from the image. Middleton argues that this entrenches dualism in human nature and limits the image either to a set of properties of the soul or to human-divine relation while devaluing the concrete life of the body.[157] Similarly, Frederick McLeod, professor of religion, points out that there was a division between Alexandrian and Antiochene schools of exegesis where the Alexandrians, in taking up Platonic ideas of the soul existing in the body, stressed the spiritual and minimized the role of the body in the economy of salvation. He counts among these Alexandrians Origen and some theologians influential in Christian anthropology such as the Cappadocian Fathers, specifically Gregory of Nyssa, Cyril of Alexandria, and Augustine.[158] These Fathers, according to McLeod, saw "image" as a spiritual reality residing in the body, albeit as a temple, in the highest part of the rational soul. McLeod allows for the fact that such writers held the body as good, but this does not appear to detract from his central view. Conversely, he claims, without providing any literary examples, that the Antiochenes identified "image" with the person of clay of Genesis 2:7; thus they emphasized the composite nature of man as body and soul.

156. Gunton, "Trinity, Ontology and Anthropology," 48.

157. Middleton, *Liberating Image*, 18–19; 24.

158. McLeod, *Image of God in the Antiochene Tradition*, 50–51, 50n25, 80–81.

A polarization of the two "schools" of Alexandria and Antioch seems to miss the complexity of the situation. In exegesis and therefore reflection on Genesis and the image of God, there appear to be traditions of exegesis rather than a systematic approach: what is often referred to as the Alexandrian school seems to develop in the third century, and the Antiochene school seems to grow in the fourth century as a challenge to the Alexandrian approach.[159] Not much is known about early tendencies in the Antiochene tradition,[160] if indeed there was such a tradition in the first three centuries.[161] Without denying that Alexandria and Antioch developed different theological approaches, it seems that McLeod offers too sharp a distinction and, along with Middleton, presents too generalized a picture. Moreover, they do not appreciate that there appears to be shifts in focus within reflection on the image of God in humans as the developing tradition faced different challenges. Since the focus of early Christian writers, such as the author of Hebrews, seems to rest on their conviction that God became man in the Incarnation, these early writers concentrate on Christ, the *Logos*, as true image of God.[162] Their anthropology sees humans as image of that image. Later writers, reflecting on the "how" of the Incarnation, and faced with threats to the equality of the Son with the Father, are less inclined to talk of Christ as image and humans as images of the image. This phrasing might suggest some inequality in the relationship of the Son to the Father. Instead, they focus on the consubstantiality of the Son with the Father and the goodness of creation that was deified by Christ when he became man.

The Image of the Image and Growing in Likeness

The significance of the coming of Christ in the fullness of time may have contributed to the distinction between image and likeness that some early writers found and reflected on in Genesis 1:26 when they de-

159. See Stiver, *Philosophy of Religious Language*, 31; Young, "Alexandrian and Antiochene Exegesis," 334.

160. See ter Haar Romney, "Eusebius of Emessa's Commentary," 127.

161. Pointing to the variety of thought in Antioch, Rowan Williams doubts that there was a single tradition. *Arius*, 158.

162. Heb 1:3.

liberated on the economy of salvation. Writers like Irenaeus and Tertullian used it principally to explain that by the Fall, mankind lost likeness to God, but by his Incarnation and Resurrection, Christ, the true image, restored this likeness.[163] Furthermore, perhaps following the philosophical tradition of the time whereby the novice philosopher in search of truth requires a wise teacher, others used the distinction to illustrate that imitation of the true image, Christ, aids in the recovery of this likeness. Thus Justin Martyr explains that although human beings were created in God's image after the image of the *Logos*, this was not immediately apparent because the *Logos* remained invisible. Moreover, owing to their weakness, human beings easily lost their likeness to God. The true image of God was finally made visible at the Incarnation and restored to human beings at Christ's passion.[164]

The notion of growing into "the image and likeness of the Lord" is clearly found in early writers such as Clement of Alexandria, who urges his flock to follow "the training of Christ" to attain this "moral loveliness."[165] In his exhortations on the God-given importance of daily life, Clement sees the Christian as a full member of society whose life, manners, and body are sanctified along with his spirit.[166] Irenaeus also explains that human beings, though made in God's image, have the task to mature and grow into his likeness. Human beings, he says, were not made perfect from the beginning since, like infants, they need the nourishment first of milk so that they can grow to appreciate the greatness of God's glory.[167] Although such gradual maturation of human beings was not universally held,[168] Origen takes this further in his exegesis of Genesis and points out that God's final intention for humanity involves both image and likeness; however, simply "image" is used in Genesis 1:27, thus indicating that perfection in likeness is only attainable in the last days.[169]

163. Zimmermann, *Incarnational Humanism*, 74–76.

164. Justin Martyr, "Fragments on the Resurrection," I, III.

165. Clement of Alexandria, "*Stromata*," IV, XXII, CXXXVII; *Christ the Educator*, I, XII. See Osborn, *Clement of Alexandria*, 245; Russell, *Doctrine of Deification*, 127–34.

166. See Osborn, *Clement of Alexandria*, 151.

167. Irenaeus, "Against Heresies," IV, XXXVIII. See Russell, *Doctrine of Deification*, 105–10.

168. See Clement of Alexandria, "*Stromata*," II, XXII.

169. Origen, "*De Principiis, First Principles*," III, 6, 1. According to Frances Young, Origen

Nevertheless, from the earliest Christian teaching, as evidenced by Paul, the idea of human beings as image of the true image, Christ, does not refer merely to imitation of Jesus or simple moral improvement.[170] For the Fathers, this idea of human beings as images of Christ reflects their deification. As Athanasius (296–373), bishop of Alexandria, Doctor of the Church, and staunch defender of the Nicene faith, explains, union with Christ leads human beings to their fulfillment, for we are perfected in Christ and restored but with "greater grace."[171]

Christ the True Image

It seems that later writers become more hesitant when using the distinction between image and likeness.[172] Whereas Cyril of Alexandria makes many references to Christ as image of God in his commentary *On John*, written before the Nestorian controversy, Cyril notes that the use of image and likeness has become problematic because his opponents were using these notions to deny Christ's divine nature.[173] Specifically, the term *homoiosos* (ομοιοςος), meaning "like" or "likeness, resembling," could suggest dissimilarity.[174] The distinction of image and likeness may have also implied that there was a defect in created humanity, or that the mind purely reflected the image and the mind needed freedom from the body to gain the likeness. These notions were hotly contested as the Fathers sought to emphasize the goodness of creation from the outset against those who despised the material through their Gnostic and Man-

---

and Basil associated the image with creation and the likeness with eschatology. She argues, however, that in the case of Irenaeus, both image and likeness are related to the creation of human beings, and the goal is that both will be confirmed in a progressive realisation of image and likeness. *God's Presence*, 160.

170. For an account of what Russell terms "participatory union with Christ" in early Christianity, see *Doctrine of Deification*, 79–114.

171. Athanasius, "Against the Arians," II, 67. For the account of Athanasius on Christian deification, particularly in response to the Arians, see Russell, *Doctrine of Deification*, 169–78.

172. See Thunberg, "Human Person as Image of God," 298. Stanley Grenz notes that the Protestant reformers "rejected as exegetically unwarranted and theologically injurious the distinction between image and likeness of God, which lay at the foundation of the medieval view." *Theology for the Community of God*, 170.

173. Cyril of Alexandria, *Commentary on John*, 1:26.

174. See Vine, *Vine's Complete Expository Dictionary*.

ichaean tendencies,[175] and the unity of body and soul against Neoplatonic notions of the soul seeking flight from the prison of the body.[176]

Patristic reflection on the distinction between image and likeness does suggest that significance is placed on the soul, on reason and will, since growth toward likeness to Christ and conforming to him involve dying to one's sinful ways. For the Fathers, however, and following Genesis, all human beings are created in the image of God and never lose that image, though they are also called to grow in likeness to Christ. Reason and freedom are common attributes of human beings, and they do not depend on capacity or abilities.[177] Significantly perhaps for those who are profoundly disabled, the Fathers note that the process of deification begins as God's work: by his assuming a human nature, Christ raises up humanity to a dignity beyond compare, and he heals what he has assumed so no human being is outside God's care. For those who can imitate Christ, the body is also intimately involved in this process, as aptly illustrated by the ascetic life.

Perfection of Body and Soul as Excellence: The Ascetic Life

As belief in the *parousia*, the imminent Second Coming of Christ, faded, those who expected change with the coming of the new Kingdom were still faced with the realities of sin and death. For some, Gnostic or apocalyptic movements held out the offer of hope of perfection. The encratic movement of extreme asceticism based on *enkrateia* (εγκρατεια), meaning mastery or self-control,[178] provides one example. Encratism has a variety of nuances that range from a simple ascetic life to disciplined self-control, as ultimately expressed in the rising popularity of monasticism in the fourth century, to complete renunciation of bodily values.[179] In its extreme form, encratism became an excessive practice rather than

175. Irenaeus, "Against Heresies," I, XXIV, I.XXV; Justin Martyr, *Apology*, I, XXVI.

176. Jens Zimmermann argues that this holistic approach to the image of God in human beings can be found across the patristic tradition. *Humanism and Religion*, 64–65.

177. See Zimmermann, *Humanism and Religion*, 62.

178. Liddell and Scott, *Greek-English Lexicon*.

179. See Burns, "Cappadocian Encratism and the Macarian Community," 27.

the continuation of a tradition.[180] The implications of extreme encratism and its apparent hatred of the body, as played out, notably by mistrust of sex, fed into the idea that the body is a hindrance to the soul.[181] As the classical historian Ugo Bianchi explains, however, the Christian church could not accept an encratism that either condemned marriage for its link to procreation or that was essentially dualist in the way in which it opposed spirit and matter.[182]

In response to the way in which early monasticism has been linked to extreme encratic practices, Peter Brown, a prominent scholar of late antiquity, returns both to their cultural context.[183] Brown says that some encratites were convinced that their present age was coming to an end, yet they believed it their Christian duty to hasten this by overcoming the tyranny evil powers still held over humanity and the universe. Apparently, some members of pagan society regarded sex and procreation as ways to overcome death, since children carried on the immortality of their parents. So, for the extreme encratites, sex became a symbol of human bondage to the circle of birth and death and a curb on the longed-for end of the age.

In his discussion of the desert Fathers, Brown challenges the view that monasticism represented Church institutionalization of hatred of the body.[184] Brown claims that the desert, the "zone of the non-human,"[185] presents the believer with his greatest temptation: to betray his humanity and become like the beasts. The ascetic comes to realize that he is an organism that is tuned to needing only enough nourishment to keep healthy. But fallen Man's twisted will persuades him to overfill his body with unnecessary food that leads to a surplus of energy, releasing itself in fleshly urges. Thus Brown argues that for these monks

180. Burns, "Cappadocian Encratism and the Macarian Community," 27n2.

181. See Quispel, *Gnostica, Judaica, Catholica*, 329–63. Quispel notes that encratism cannot necessarily be identified with Gnosticism: it is present in some Jewish and Christian writings (342), and not all Gnostics disparaged the world excessively (142).

182. Bianchi, "Religio-Historical Relevance," 35. For the extent to which Gregory of Nyssa, Gregory of Nazianzus, and Basil may have been influenced by encratic elements in their approaches to sexuality, see pp. 35–36 and Quispel, *Gnostica, Judaica, Catholica*, 345–46.

183. Brown, *Body and Society*, 83–99.

184. Brown, *Body and Society*, 216–39.

185. Brown, *Body and Society*, 218.

the first sin of Adam, when he ate the fruit of the forbidden tree, was not sex but greed. Restraints must be put on the body because it is ruled by a twisted will; hence the need to fast. Moreover, these restraints are necessary because at the Resurrection, the body was destined for future glory.

The body, then, is "deeply implicated" in the transformation of the soul; indeed, it bears the greater burden.[186] It cannot be regarded as distant from the self, an accidental addition, or bracketed out of the life of the person. Instead, as Horsiesios (d. ca. 380), the desert Father and disciple of Pachomius, the founder of cenobitic monasticism, explains, for the ascetic monk, the body is a God-given "field to cultivate."[187] The desert, Brown says, reveals the inextricable interdependence of body and soul.

Regarded as the first monk,[188] Antony of Egypt (ca. 251–356) bears out Brown's view. Antony seems to follow the Platonic tradition in his understanding of the body as "heavy" and tying man down.[189] But he explains that we stay in the "house of the robber,"[190] we have been taken over by evil, and we need to be transformed, body, soul, and spirit. This is carried out through the workings of the Spirit and repentance so that "the whole body may be changed and placed under the authority of the Spirit," purified and sanctified.[191]

Theologian and Doctor of the Church Gregory of Nazianzus (329–90) makes a similar comment on the death of his brother Caesarius, a medical doctor. In his funeral oration, Gregory says that death has shaken off the "fetters" that bound and held down the "wings of the mind" of his brother.[192] Gregory does seem to think that the soul is in God's image and is bound to an inferior nature.[193] He also explains, however, that in life it is the task of the physician who labors with souls to help the soul to raise to heaven its lower nature. Thus the soul can lead on "the matter which ministers to it" and unite it "as its fellow-servant to God."[194]

186. Brown, *Body and Society*, 235.

187. Horsiesios, "Instructions," 1.6.

188. The difficulty of applying the title of first monk or first hermit, or abbot, to Antony is noted in Burns, *Butler's Lives of the Saints*, 116.

189. Antony of Egypt, "Letters of St Antony," 6, 42.

190. Antony of Egypt, "Letters of St Antony," 5 and 6, 97.

191. Antony of Egypt, "Letters of St Antony," 1, 50–70.

192. Gregory of Nazianzus, "Orations," 7, 21.

193. Gregory of Nazianzus, "Orations," 2, 17, 22.

194. Gregory of Nazianzus, "Orations," 2, 17.

The tradition sees this unity not only in the ongoing life and final eschatological end of all humans at the resurrection but also in the origin of each human being, even if, as Professor David Jones, director of the Anscombe Bioethics Centre, explains, early thinking here is much more uncertain.[195] Notably, in his treatise *On the Making of Man*, Gregory of Nyssa, labeled "Platonic" by McLeod,[196] refers to Genesis 2:7 to explain that a human being is not a clay figure with a soul added and then the soul is made better. Rather, human beings are a unity.[197] The Creed of Constantinople (381) crystallized this understanding of the integral unity of body and soul. Discussion on the origins of the soul were not clear-cut: after much debate, the Origenist position on the soul's preexistence was condemned at the Fifth Ecumenical Council at Constantinople 553, and the traditional doctrine that soul and body come into existence at the same time was declared the orthodox position. Still, at the time of the Council of Vienna (1311–12), most theologians supported delayed ensoulment. It seems safe to say, however, that in the early tradition, although the soul signifies the spiritual principle in humans, the body also partakes of the image of God, for a human body is a human body precisely because it is animated by a soul, and this makes up the whole human person: body and soul together constitute the human being.[198] When apart, body and soul do not exist properly, so that their separation at death can only be temporary. As Justin Martyr says, just like two oxen at the yoke, "neither of them can plough alone," so too do body and soul act together in complete unity.[199]

Unique Persons

Christian reflection on the image of God in human beings indicates their embodiment, and it also points to the unity of all human beings in solidarity with Christ. Moreover, it expresses relationship. The relationship with God, others, and with creation, where each human being has

195. Jones, *Soul of the Embryo*, chap. 7.
196. McLeod, *Image of God in the Antiochene Tradition*, 50n25.
197. Gregory of Nyssa, "On the Making of Man," XXIX.
198. Gregory of Nazianzus, "Orations," 45.
199. Justin Martyr, "Fragments on the Resurrection," VIII.

both an individual and a relational role, is found in the often neglected yet profound patristic vision of the human being as a microcosm, a little world, or rather a "second world, a great world in a little one."[200] Gregory of Nazianzus uses this phrase in deliberate and firm contrast to pagan philosophy that saw man as a microcosm, merely a little world, of the universe.[201] The idea of the universe, expressed by Marcus Aurelius as "one living organism, with a single substance and a single soul,"[202] was the foundation for Stoic thought: everything has its part to play in this universe because a bond unites all things,[203] and everyone shares in the cosmic process.[204] Human beings are part of this whole and will eventually dissolve back into the whole;[205] in this life they are like limbs of the whole system.[206] Thus, in Stoic understanding, human beings reflected the world.

In early Christian understanding, as Gregory of Nyssa points out, the human being was brought forth by God as a second world. Yet human beings are not so much each a smaller world; rather, they are each "a vast one in this small visible one," for human greatness does not lie in our likeness to the created world but in the fact that we are each made in the image of the Creator.[207] True greatness is not in having the highest biological existence or greatest rationality. Rather, as illustrated by the solidarity of all humans, of conforming to Christ, growing in likeness, it is in being a "deified animal."[208] Each new world, each person, has their own unique and unrepeatable perspective such that when that person dies, in earthly terms that world is also lost. Here the individual, both as a being who transcends the self and as a link to the rest of the created world, is found. Patristic understanding of human beings as microcosm expresses

200. Gregory of Nazianzus, "Orations," 45.

201. For an overview of understandings of microcosm related to the character of a human being in antiquity, see Thunberg, "Human Person as Image of God," 295–96.

202. Marcus Aurelius, *Meditations*, IV, 40.

203. Marcus Aurelius, *Meditations*, VI, 38.

204. Marcus Aurelius, *Meditations*, VI, 42.

205. Marcus Aurelius, *Meditations*, X, 6, 7.

206. Marcus Aurelius, *Meditations*, VII, 13. Marcia Colish explains some of the difficulties and inconsistencies in Stoic thinking on the fate of the soul after death in *Stoic Tradition*, 29–31.

207. Gregory of Nyssa, "On the Making of Man," XVI.

208. Gregory of Nazianzus, "Orations," 45, 7.

the idea that it is logical that human beings were made last, and creatures were made for them because they link the order of the intelligible with the phenomenal order.[209] The Lutheran scholar Lars Thunberg argues that in the tradition, the task of dominion is grounded within the nature of human beings as contemplative beings, capable of reflecting on the existence of creation. Crucially, he points out that this contemplative capacity is not an individual capacity. Rather, it belongs to the whole of humankind.[210] Alongside this responsibility, and to fulfill their vocation as this bridge between the two orders, human beings need to see themselves as each a single, undivided whole—a psychosomatic unity.

The interrelationship of humankind to the nonhuman world is one thing. But a return to a view of image of God as dominance, taken as a principal focus of the concept of image, raises a clear but different problem for the Fathers. On a basic level, there is the issue of how to identify an entity as human, though this does not seem to present itself as a particularly pressing problem for the Fathers. Moreover, it seems that a dominant interpretation of the image of God involves, as John Hull puts it, "the image of the perfectly normal human, but raised to an even higher level of perfection."[211] According to Moss, there is a "sinister theme in early Christian constructions of heaven," and it is "the nature of the perfected heavenly body." As far as she is concerned, "the perfection of the disabled body at the eschaton in the writings of the early church can be understood as an extension of Christian constructions of disability in general." She additionally claims that evidence from the early Fathers points to the belief that "human identity, as a reproduction of the divine image, is only fully present in the non-disabled."[212]

On a theoretical level, the psychologist Brian Watermeyer partly answers the critique presented by Moss and the preferred construction of disability that it implies. Watermeyer explains that there is no easy agreement on how to consider disability, and "no single theoretical narrative is able to mirror disability adequately." He notes "disability's emo-

209. Gregory of Nyssa, "On the Making of Man," XVI; Nemesius of Emesa, "Treatise on the Nature of Man," 4.

210. Thunberg, "Human Person as Image of God," 304–6.

211. Hull, "Blindness and the Face of God," 215.

212. Moss, "Heavenly Healing," 993–1011.

tive and multi-layered nature" and that the social model is "helpful, but limiting." Ultimately, he says, we all struggle with disability.[213] Returning to the early Fathers and the charge leveled by Moss that disability is "gradually written out of the Kingdom of God," however, Augustine recounts tales of monstrous races of men, one-eyed men, men with no mouths, of small stature, androgynous,[214] and conjoined twins.[215] According to Brian Brock, Augustine challenges his contemporaries to revise their judgments about people with disabilities, which "parallels the modern critique of disability as a social construction."[216] As far as Augustine is concerned, "the observer" may be offended by deformity, but this is because he does not see the whole picture, the rationale of all things. In fact, says Augustine, it would be foolish to think that the Creator made a mistake in the slightest variation from the normal, say, the number of human fingers a person has. Augustine continues, "even in cases of greater variations, God knows what He is doing and no one may rightly blame His work."[217] From the fantastical tales he has heard about the many and varied human beings, Augustine says that if such peoples exist, and if they are human, "they are descended from Adam." For Augustine, apparent "monsters" born of human parents are human beings. And at the Resurrection, they will be restored to the state that naturally belongs to them.

The problem, then, about locating the image of God, is not with people with any kind of impairment, intellectual or otherwise. Rather, for the Fathers, the problem is with women, and this is the reason why some of the Fathers speak of the image of God as residing in the mind.

Women: Image of God?

The relocation of the problem of image of God to women rather than physical or mental impairment indicates that disability is a recent con-

213. Watermeyer, *Towards a Contextual Psychology of Disability*, 1–6.

214. Augustine, *City of God*, XVI, 8.

215. By his description, this appears to be what he means. Augustine, "The Enchiridion on Faith, Hope and Charity," 273–343.

216. Brock, "Augustine's Hierarchies," 65.

217. Augustine, *City of God*, XVI, 8.

cept. As Christian Laes points out, being a woman, left-handed, or a twin could be disadvantageous in the ancient world.[218] And as Gregory of Nyssa explains, the present conditions of a world of inequalities do not alter the fact of goodness at creation.[219] But this does not mean that inequalities are simply accepted as part of the order of things, and this can be shown by how the Fathers thought of women as sharing in the image of God.

Although the image of God gives equality to all human beings, it seems that in practice both the social climate and ancient scriptural exegesis[220] counted against applying image of God in terms of dominance to women. The patriarchal culture, institutional structures, and notions of the relationship of men and women in Greco-Roman societies had already established inequality and a lower status of usefulness or value for women.[221] Gregory of Nyssa seemingly refused to see the body as part of the image of God, not because of possible disabilities but because of the differentiation of human beings into male and female. This, he says, does not reflect God because God is not male or female.[222] Augustine finds himself defending Paul against those who used the Apostle's writings to claim that women do not share in the image of God.[223] In attempting to reconcile various scriptural texts,[224] Augustine concludes

218. Laes, "Introduction," in *Disability in Antiquity*, 4, 6.

219. Gregory of Nyssa, "The Great Catechism," V.

220. Generic terms are used in the Genesis accounts of the creation of human beings. In Scripture, the Hebrew word *adam* refers to an indefinite someone, and the Greek version of Gn 1:26 uses the word ανθρωπος (*anthropos*), which is singular and means "human being." But other texts clearly made it problematic for some writers to assert categorically that women are made in God's image, notably the creation of Adam in Genesis 2, and the subsequent creation of Eve from his ribs in Gn 2:22 after God has granted dominion to Adam and the account of the Fall and the punishment of submission given to Eve in Gn 3:16. Carol Meyers argues that the term "Adam" in Gn 2:7 "can be understood as denoting a genderless or androgynous being," and that both man and woman are created as gendered beings when God divides the first human. Baskin, "Adam," in *Cambridge Dictionary of Judaism and Jewish Culture*, 4. Other scriptural texts, particularly from Paul and especially 1 Cor 11:7–10, where man is "the image of God" and "woman is the reflection of man's glory," are equally problematic.

221. See Brown, *Body and Society*; Rist, *Human Value*, 14.

222. Gregory of Nyssa, "On the Making of Man," XVI.8; see Karras, "Science and the Cappadocians," 29–40.

223. Hill, "Response," 503–4.

224. Using a series of texts, Frederick McLeod argues that the reason why writers such

that the body is not on the same level as the soul in its likeness to God, and he asserts that woman is not an image of God physically, though she is equal with man in her likeness to God in mind.[225] Augustine adds that the body does not receive God's image because God is incorporeal and God cannot be limited by bodily members.[226] Rather, man (human being) is made in God's image according to his (her) rational mind, that is, not any part of the mind but where the knowledge of God can exist. Renewal of the mind, a return to likeness to God, takes place at baptism, and women are "fellow heirs" in this renewal.[227]

If this context, and the problem early theologians had with interpreting and reconciling texts on the apparent subordination of women, is ignored, then it may lead to the conclusion that the image of God is not reflected in the whole human being. Instead, Augustine takes pains to point out that it is not a question of seeing women in bodily terms and men in terms of the mind, for they share both aspects.[228] Rather, Augustine sees the image of God in that aspect of the person that seeks to understand and behold God.[229] The mind is an image of God only when it contemplates the truth. That image, he argues, may be obscured or defaced, but it always remains.[230] Resurrection of the body moreover gives future likeness with the Son.[231] The claim that this aspect of the image

as the bishop of Tarsus, Diodore (d. ca. 390); the theologian and bishop of Cyrus, Theodoret (ca. 393–460); and the bishop of Constantinople and Doctor of the Church, John Chrysostom (ca. 345–407) insisted that God fashioned only men in his image was because they took the real creation of Adam and Eve from Genesis 2. McLeod claims that these Fathers considered Genesis 1 to be a foreshadowing of the later account, and they used texts such as 1 Cor 11:7 and notions of sovereign power to reinforce this interpretation. McLeod adds that John Chrysostom thought that women were to be respected and treated as "equal in honour," yet for practical purposes—that is, for peace in the household—the man had to be preeminent, and this subordination was ordained by God. *Image of God in the Antiochene Tradition*, 191–231. Rosemary Radford Ruether argues that the Fathers justified the subordination of women by choosing certain texts, such as Genesis 2, to the neglect of others, such as Genesis 1. According to Ruether, most of the Fathers, including Augustine, believed that only men and not women were in the image of God. " Liberation of Christianity from Patriarchy," 325–26.

225. Augustine, *The Trinity*, XII:9–10.

226. Augustine, *The Trinity*, XII:7, 12.

227. Augustine, *The Trinity*, XII:7, 12.

228. Augustine, *The Trinity*, XII:13, 20.

229. Augustine, *The Trinity*, XIV:4, 6.

230. Augustine, *The Trinity*, XIV:4, 6; XIV:8, 11.

231. Augustine, *The Trinity*, XIV:18, 24.

of God always remains perhaps contrasts with some modern thinkers like Robert Rakestraw, the Anglican theologian Nigel Biggar, and, albeit implicitly, the Catholic theologians Father Kevin O'Rourke and Father Patrick Norris, who say that a human being who no longer has the capacity to respond to God no longer bears his image.[232]

That God does not have a body and therefore the body is not made in his image does not in fact entail that the body can have no share in the image and likeness of God, once it is remembered that in Christian thinking the body and soul are not two parts of a human being, even if that is often a common way of speaking. Augustine makes this point clear in his work *On Genesis*:[233] God makes the spirit and the body, and they are joined as one. The human being is a unity, an embodied soul. Nevertheless, there is tension in early theology. The Fathers distanced themselves from Platonic thought that saw the body as a prison, and from approaches that rendered God's good material creation evil. Belief in the resurrection of the body affirmed its significance. The nature of this resurrected body is less certain, however, and the spiritual nature of human beings has prominence.

Image of God: A Word on Dominance and Speciesism

To be sure, an understanding of dominion in terms of power or strength might play into dominion and subordination roles of men and women. Moreover, the terms "subdue" and "dominion" in Genesis 1:28 carry connotations of force and mastery. But reflection on the idea of dominion as an aspect of the image of God suggests that humankind exercises this rule in a similar manner to God, or to Christ, as God's representative. The hymn in Philippians 2 emphasizes that Christ exercises his lordship not from a position of power and control, but from a position of weakness and service. The Lord of all creation is also the Suffering Servant. So, the meaning of "to rule" appears to be more com-

232. Rakestraw, "Persistent Vegetative State," 127–28; Biggar, *Aiming to Kill*, 39; O'Rourke and Norris, "Care of the PVS Patient," 207–17; O'Rourke, "Reflections on the Papal Allocution," 93. See also Matthews, *Pope John Paul II*, chap. 9.

233. Augustine, *On Genesis*, II:9.

plex than the modern understanding of kingship that usually involves notions of power over, the kind of dominion that Peter Singer attributes to Christian thinking.[234] God's activity in the creation stories of Genesis is described as the work of a wise artisan who forms and fills a complex universe and orders it in a rational way.[235] That creation simply follows from God's word perhaps deliberately contrasts to the ancient Near Eastern myths of creation, where the world comes about as a result of a clash of cosmic forces and where, more often than not, the cosmos is formed from the destruction of the primordial enemy: a woman.[236] It would appear that the writers of the Priestly source of Genesis 1 were well aware of such myths and that even though they came from a largely patriarchal society, they saw that image and its aspect of rule belonged to all human beings, men as well as women, abled and disabled. Moreover, in ancient Near Eastern temples, the cult image was placed last and prominently in its sanctuary. The creation of the first human beings similarly takes place as the crowning point of creation when God declares it to be not only "good" but "very good,"[237] with the implication that simply by being human all people, whatever their capacities or abilities, have access to God.

For some early Fathers, this dominance is expressed physically and mentally. The Christian apologist Lactantius (ca. 250–325) claims that God determined to make human beings alone "heavenly."[238] Thus God made human beings stand upright so that they can contemplate heaven.[239] The mind, being in the head and the highest part of the body, is "nearly divine" because human beings are to rule not only over animals but also over their own bodies.[240] According to cultural historian Marjorie O'Rourke Boyle, from classical antiquity onward, the ability to stand upright was what distinguished human beings from other animals. O'Rourke Boyle adds that in Christianity, this ability, rather than

234. For an illustration of how complex the notion of dominion is, and the complexity of exegesis of the Genesis text, see Conradie, *Christianity and Earthkeeping*, 85–92.

235. Middleton, *Liberating Image*, 77.

236. See C. Keller in Middleton, *Liberating Image*, 257; Clifford and Murphy, "Genesis," 11.

237. Gn 1:31. See Middleton, *Liberating Image*, 207.

238. Lactantius, "On the Workmanship of God," VIII; see also Gregory of Nyssa, "On the Making of Man," VII, I.

239. Lactantius, "On the Workmanship of God," VIII.

240. Lactantius, "On the Workmanship of God," VIII.

the possession of a rational soul, indicated spiritual dignity.[241] Although O'Rourke Boyle intends to demonstrate the significance of the body, her argument may appear detrimental to those who have certain physical disabilities. Nevertheless, O'Rourke Boyle recalls Augustine's understanding that all human beings, whatever their bodily form or their faculties, are fully human and in solidarity with the first man, Adam,[242] and so the last, Jesus.

In terms of the relationship of human beings to other animals, Gregory of Nyssa stresses the role of virtue and justice. For Gregory, God, the "best artificer," made our nature fit to rule: as image of God, humankind was created to be regal from the start with its superior advantage of the soul that owes governance only to itself. But man is "clothed in virtue" instead of a purple robe; he has the "bliss of immortality" instead of a scepter; and he wears a "crown of righteousness" instead of a diadem.[243] Gregory notes that humankind lacks natural weapons and covering usually associated with dominion such as sharp claws: human beings are naturally vulnerable. His point is that if we had such things as speed or fur, then we would neglect a correct rule over other creatures, since we would have no need of their cooperation: horses provide us with speed, sheep give us wool for warmth.[244] If we do hold dominion, then it has implications for the use of nonhuman creatures in the medical field, in xenotransplantation, in experimentation, in the creation of hybrids and cybrids, and in the wider ecological field by manipulating and altering our genetic material or very bodies.

The notion of dominion has been the center of modern controversy, as some secular writers, accusing Christianity of speciesism, have attempted to take the category of person out of the sphere of the human and apply it to any creature with the requisite capabilities of consciousness, while denying it to those humans who fall short of these capabilities. Those who understand dominion as power over creation tend to link it with rational abilities and capacities to exercise that power, which appears to be an extension of the Christian tradition that holds that the

241. O'Rourke Boyle, *Senses of Touch*, 31–39.
242. O'Rourke Boyle, *Senses of Touch*, 53.
243. Gregory of Nyssa, "On the Making of Man," IV, 1.
244. Gregory of Nyssa, "On the Making of Man," VII.

image of God resides in the possession of intellect and free will. But the tradition speaks of the rational nature of all human beings, not of individual capacities, and it seems that setting human beings over and above other animals does not reflect the fullness of the Christian tradition.

Christian responses to the exploitation of animals have led to a refreshed vision of dominion as stewardship that is arguably a return to the original Genesis and patristic views. In contrast to some interpretations of the absolute rule of kings, ruling as God rules with royal concern for creation does not allow for exploitation. The Christian bishop and philosopher Nemesius of Emesa (fl. late third century) underscores this regal idea of human dominance: humans can make temperate use of whatever is under their authority, but they cannot treat creation with tyranny; ill use of irrational beasts is sin.[245]

Following Singer's lead, writers now commonly criticize Augustine for asserting that the life and death of all nonhuman animals are subordinated to the use of human beings, since nonhuman animals "have no rational association with us."[246] Singer takes Augustine and the whole of the Christian tradition, bar a few "gentler spirits" like Francis of Assisi, as demonstrating that in the tradition God does not care how human beings treat creation, "nature itself is of no intrinsic value."[247] The tradition is certainly complex, there is not simply one strand, and early theologians do accept that human beings can use nonhuman animals for their own needs. Nevertheless, theologians like Augustine make a clear distinction between exploitation and good use. In his comment on the subordination of nonhuman animals, Augustine is talking in the context of suicide as self-killing and the injunction against killing human beings in Genesis 9:6. Yet he goes on to explain the difference between the attitudes of Cain and Abel to creation when they came to bring their gifts before God. Augustine says that God did not approve of Cain's gift because Cain offered it in a spirit of "lust of dominion" over the earth, whereas Abel's attitude was one of making good use of the world for God.[248]

245. Nemesius of Emesa, "Treatise on the Nature of Man," 8. For further discussion of the Fathers and virtuous use of creation, see Blowers, *Drama of the Divine Economy*, 361–66.

246. Augustine, *City of God*, I:20.

247. Singer, *Practical Ethics*, 265–68.

248. Augustine, *City of God*, XV:7.

Given that, for the Fathers, God designed and sustains the world, in patristic writing, appreciation for the beauty and wonder of creation, as well as its ordered harmony, is always related to praise and worship of God.[249] The individual beauty and harmonious functioning of all creatures are understood as contributing essentially to the beauty and order of the whole universe: as Basil, bishop of Caesarea and Doctor of the Church, exclaims, all constitute "an unbroken bond of attraction into one fellowship and harmony."[250] Augustine sees both that humans are the most wonderful of God's creatures yet each type of creature has a place in the splendor and order of creation,[251] and all "fit together to make a scheme of ordered beauty."[252] Augustine stresses the participation of humans in the created order to the extent that we cannot fully comprehend the universe because we are mortal and so embedded in creation: only God can transcend it and thus grasp it in its entirety.[253]

Patristic writers also hold that creation expresses something of God's presence to us.[254] As Athanasius explains, God wished to be known through his wondrous world, and many natural events, from rain to harvest, are witness to God and his providence.[255] Although patristic thinkers saw humans as the high point of creation, they were also open to the beauty, mystery, and sacramentality of the universe. This sacramental perspective on creation allows for a reverential approach to the universe, where reverence and awe are offered to God, who mediates his presence through his world. Notably, many people with intellectual disabilities and those who live radically in the present seem to be more open to the beauty of the world around them.[256]

Many contemporary philosophers reject the Christian view that humans are the crown of creation as speciesist. The tendency to order the

249. Basil, "On the Hexaemeron," 5, 9; 2, 6–7; Augustine, *Confessions*, 13, 19; idem, *City of God*, XXII:24. For the patristic appreciation of the beauty of creation, see Schaefer, *Theological Foundations for Environmental Ethics*, 44–50.

250. Basil, "On the Hexaemeron," 2, 2.

251. Augustine, *City of God*, XXII:24.

252. Augustine, *City of God*, XII:4.

253. Augustine, *City of God*, XII:4.

254. Basil, "On the Hexaemeron," 5, 9; 2, 6–7; Augustine, *City of God*, XII:4; idem, *Confessions*, 7, 17, 23.

255. Athanasius, "Against the Heathens," 35–37.

256. Matthews, *Pope John Paul II*, 53.

universe in some form of hierarchy does have its dangers. As Augustine recognizes, some may use utility as the criterion of value, are ignorant of the true placing of an entity, or subordinate an entity to their own convenience.[257] Yet in the process of criticizing the Christian ordering, some bioethicists may have fallen into the danger identified by Augustine when they blur the line between human beings and other animals while redrawing it on the grounds of a narrow view of personhood. Instead of value being attached to rational capacities and a counting of interests for everything, the Fathers see creation as witnessing to the wonders of God, and they see human beings in terms that are not measurable. An appreciation of the wonder of the world also lies at the heart of philosophy. Philosophy has long marveled at the fact that there is something rather than nothing. As the avowedly atheist philosopher Raymond Tallis explains, his very existence as a particular entity gives cause for his own sense of daily wonder.[258]

Summary

Christianity may have been influenced by Greek philosophy. But Christians were more firmly anchored in the Gospel tradition, the resurrection of the body, and the clear belief in the goodness of creation against those who saw only evil in the material world. Many early theologians highlighted the significance and priority of the soul. Nevertheless, their thinking on the resurrection of the body recognized that the body and soul are complementary and so form a unity. This belief in the eventual transformation of the body is also expressed in the conviction that here and now the body has a part to play in transforming the soul. Patristic reflection on human beings made in the image of God is not so much about the characteristics that set humans apart from the rest of creation or about biology or even about descriptive anthropology. Instead, it says something about the God who creates human beings and the relationship he establishes with them. The solidarity of humankind in sharing in the image of God is also a sharing in the fallen nature of

257. Augustine, *City of God*, XI:16.
258. Tallis, *In Defence of Wonder*, 1–2.

humanity through Adam, however. To renovate this disfigurement, the Gospel *kerygma* proclaims that the true image of God, Christ, enters into solidarity with us by assuming our humanity, restoring it, and raising it up beyond its original glory to share more completely in God's eternal life. The teaching of the image of God in humans, then, is principally a theological message of creation, relationship, and salvation.

Some of the early Fathers do offer a descriptive account of the person as they consider different aspects of human beings or discuss the soul's relationship to the body. Yet their anthropological insights do not seem to include an actual division. Even if they are influenced by philosophies that separate the soul from the body, for Christians, the very fact of the Incarnation and bodily Resurrection of Christ entails that human persons are embodied wholes. Early Christian thinkers then try to hold together the understanding that the soul, the spiritual aspect, is better and the body inferior, yet also that the soul is not good by nature and the body bad.[259] They are not so much opposites as complementary,[260] so that the whole person is the image of God. To be sure, the traditional position recognizes the importance of intellect, will, and freedom as an "outstanding manifestation of the divine image,"[261] but this is a seemingly significant aspect of human nature rather than a required criterion of each and every human being, who is said to be created in God's image. In this descriptive anthropology, the Fathers attempt to be faithful to the Genesis stories that speak of a human being as an animal of a rational nature who has the capacity to transcend the self, and that these two aspects are united in the one person.

Christian anthropology is necessarily personal, since it is a personal God who creates and enters into a particular relationship with every human being, each with their unique perspective, a new world. Yet, according to Christian theology, every human being is made in the image and likeness of God and that God is a tri-unity. From the Trinitarian aspect, the tradition of seeing the divine image in humans as an internal attribute such as reason, whereby human beings are said to be related

259. Clement of Alexandria, "*Stromata*," II.
260. Clement, "*Stromata*," XXVI.
261. Second Vatican Council, *Gaudium et Spes*, 17.

to God in their individuality, seems to offer a static reflection of human beings and, by implication, of God. As the *Report on the Trinity of the British Council of Churches* points out, "by concentrating on reason or freedom or our moral sense as the basis of our distinctive humanity, the tradition has been frequently tempted into an individualistic or merely secular anthropology: the image of God is that which human beings individually possess."[262]

Instead, Genesis 1:27 reminds us that human beings are not solitary individuals; rather, they belong to a community of persons, for God creates man and woman in a partnership. The insight that human beings are social beings and are each made in the image of God puts us into a personal relationship with God and each other, so it also places the concept of the person in the moral realm. Each human person counts before God and, as the Genesis stories of Cain and of the flood remind us, we are all responsible for all and ultimately accountable to God for each other. This accountability extends also to the environment and animal kingdom, as human beings are called to be stewards of God's creation.

Most of the early Fathers insist that even though the image of God in human beings may be defaced or obscured, it is indestructible. Although the Fathers were generally thinking of humans who had caused this disfigurement through their own evil choices, this may also give pause for thought for those who find it difficult to discern the image of God in certain human beings, particularly at the margins of life, who do not meet some expectations of what it is to be a person. Moreover, for Gregory of Nyssa, the nature of human beings is not completely open to contemplation because God is incomprehensible, and so his image in human beings is also incomprehensible.[263] This perhaps provides a focus for seeing the person not so much as a concept to be defined and understood but as a mystery to be discerned. As Tallis says, our relationship to our bodies is "the crowning mystery of biology."[264] Consideration of where the concept of the person took root, in Trinitarian theology, belongs, then, in the framework of approaching a mystery rather than defining

262. British Council of Churches, *Forgotten Trinity*, 23.
263. Gregory of Nyssa, "On the Making of Man," II.
264. Tallis, *In Defence of Wonder*, 3.

and solving a problem. It is about discerning persons. To ensure that this enterprise is not ahistoric, it seems necessary to add a note on the etymology and use of the term "person" before it was taken up in Trinitarian theology.

Being a "Person" in Greece and Rome

The etymology of "person" comes from the Latin *persona*.[265] Generally, *persona* is used infrequently in everyday Latin because, where in English we normally write "person," the Latin denotes it by using the word *homines*, or by putting the adjective in the masculine gender. Thus "many persons think" would be rendered *multi id sentiunt*. Similarly, the Greek *anthropos* is translated as "person," even though *homines* and *anthropos* do not carry any of the weight of modern concepts of person, such as the suggestion of an imperative to treat the subject as a person rather than an object. Thus a slave was considered *anthropos* or *homines*, but he or she did not have the kind of rights, in modern terms, normally associated with being a person, such as protection from being harmed or killed. Moreover, whereas the concept of person encompasses not only human beings but also spiritual beings such as angels, and is used in discussion of God, *homines* and *anthropos* do not.

The word *persona* seems to have originated from the action of wearing masks in role-play and from the Etruscan word for mask, *phersu*:[266] a mask is that through (*per*) which resounds (*sonare*) the voice of the actor.[267] The Greek προσοπον (*prosopon*) corresponds to *persona*, *pros ops*, meaning about or toward the eyes, and *prosopon* referred to face, front façade, mask, or dramatic character.[268] Mask wearing took place not only

265. See Barnhart, *Chambers Dictionary of Etymology*.

266. Mauss, "Category of the Human Mind," 15–16. According to Giuliano Bonfante and Larissa Bonfante, Phersu appears to have been a mythological masked figure involved in funeral games, singing and dancing. *Etruscan Language*, 203. For the use of masks in classical Greek theatre, see Rehm, *Greek Tragic Theatre*, 39–40, though Rehm is more cautious than Giuliano and Larissa Bonafante about ritual use of masks. In contrast, through research on depictions of scenes on ancient Greek vases, Claude Calame finds a clear link between actors and mask wearing, mythology and ritual. *Craft of Poetic Speech in Ancient Greece*, 132–35.

267. See Simpson, *Cassell's Latin Dictionary*.

268. Liddell and Scott, *Greek English Lexicon*.

in the theatre but also in religious rituals where only certain individuals had the right to wear a mask that possibly represented an ancestor. In Greek and Roman ritualistic action in the cults of gods of nature and vegetation, it may have had the added functions of protecting the wearer and his tribe from hostile powers as well as denoting a transfer of power from the god it represented to the wearer.[269] Perhaps as an offshoot of ritualistic action, plays began to appear, and a purely human mask began to replace the animal one.[270] In Greek theatre, masks tended simply to aid in the construction of a fictional identity.[271] Nevertheless, in both ritual and theatre, this early concept of the person was connected to role-play and representation, and so the person carried a somewhat artificial sense.[272]

The role-play aspect of "person" is also evident in the Roman art of declamation, where speeches "in character," *prosopopoeiae*, had to be delivered *in propria persona*, in character.[273] Still, the older idea that masks expressed the right to represent an ancestor continued in the self-understanding of the Roman Senate as a set group of *patres*, fathers, who represented the *personnes*, images of their dead ancestors, the *imago* being the wax death mask of the ancestor that was kept in the family shrine.[274] Perhaps building on the ancestral cult of the *patres*, whose role it was to represent the family clan, the Romans developed the notion of person beyond the right to assume a role or mask[275] when they adopted *persona* as a basic fact of law in the overriding legal authority of the *paterfamilias*.

Greek and Roman Disabled "Persons"

Neither Greek nor Latin appears to have a specific term for a disabled human being.[276] This may be because what was of concern was simply

269. See Albin Lesky, *Greek Tragedy*, 28.

270. Lesky, *Greek Tragedy*, 49–50.

271. Calame, *Craft of Poetic Speech in Ancient Greece*, 107–8.

272. Donald Pollock notes the confusion surrounding terms such as "person," "identity," and "self" when speaking of mask wearing. In his analysis of masking, he sees the mask as "iconic," that is, as a means to resemble and represent its object. "Masks and the Semiotics of Identity," 582.

273. Winterbottom, *Roman Declamation*, 52, 99.

274. Mauss, "Category of the Human Mind," 16–17.

275. See Mauss, "Category of the Human Mind," 14.

276. In *Eye of the Beholder*, Robert Garland offers an excellent account of disability in

whether people could fulfill their allotted roles, whether or not they had infirmities.[277] Moreover, it was not until nineteenth-century advances in medicine that the body was regarded as something that could be fixed, and therefore some bodies fell below a perceived norm. Nevertheless, in Greek and Latin, there were words for certain disabilities:[278] Hephaestus, the Greek god of blacksmiths, was called ἀμφιγύεις (*amphigúeis*), the lame one, or κυλλοποδίων (*kullopodion*), the halting one. Robert Garland points out that some Roman *cognomina*, family names, referred to an impairment had by the original bearer of the name, for instance, Strabo (Squinter) and Crassipes (splay foot). He notes that these appellations did not seem to have caused embarrassment either to the original bearer or to subsequent generations; after all, as the title of his book demonstrates, in antiquity, disability did not have the force that it has now. Instead, impairment was simply "in the eye of the beholder."[279] Individual human beings were described in general terms, also according to their physical and mental peculiarities. However, the term "person" was neither applied nor denied to human beings.

The Roman Law *ad Personas* and *Persona* in Declamations

In about 161 CE, the jurist and teacher Gaius began to write what appears to have been an influential textbook called *Institutes*. Gaius incorporated into his *Institutes* various existing sources of Roman law, from custom to the old written law of the *Twelve Tables*, and he used what may

---

ancient Greek and Rome and includes some of the terms used for people with disabilities. See also Edwards, "Constructions of Physical Disability in the Ancient Greek World," 35–50.

277. Laes, *Disability in Antiquity*, 4.

278. See Liddell and Scott, *Greek English Lexicon*; Simpson, *Cassell's Latin Dictionary*. Chris Goodley and M. Lynn Rose warn of the problems associated with any discussion of disability in ancient times. The authors draw attention to the impossibility of diagnosing people of the past with today's recognized medical conditions; they note cultural assumptions surrounding intellectual disability and presuppositions that arise from the framework within which modern authors work. In a survey of modern literature, the authors point to reductive interpretations of ancient thought and the problem of associating the Greek emphasis on wisdom and beauty with the apparent eradication of the disabled. "Mental States, Bodily Dispositions and Table Manners," 17–43.

279. Garland, *Eye of the Beholder*, 78–79.

have been an older classification to divide the law into three: the law of persons, *ad personas*; of things, *ad res;* and of actions, *ad actiones.*[280]

According to Andrew Borkowski, "status lay at the heart of the law of persons."[281] In Roman law, *persona* was used to distinguish entities that were considered persons, and so capable of legal actions, from entities that were considered objects. Freedom, citizenship, and the individual's position in the household were significant in the law of persons.[282] Children, slaves, the insane, the mentally impaired and lunatics, *furiosi*, possibly the deaf and dumb, and to a lesser extent women were not legal persons, and they required supervision or guardianship.[283] Legal persons might also be nonhuman entities such as *collegia* (private associations), the state, or charities.[284] Moreover, *persona* did not always adhere to the individual himself: under inheritance laws, property could be transferred from the deceased to his beneficiaries. In Roman times, however, one of the main reasons for appointing an heir was to ensure that the religious duties of the family, the *sacra*, and other legal duties would be carried out. To this end, the heir was regarded as continuing the *persona* of the deceased.[285]

On the human condition in general, Gaius writes that all men were either free or slaves;[286] those who were free were citizens, Latins, or *dediticii*. *Dediticii*, former enemies, could never become citizens or live

280. Jolowicz and Nicholas, *Historical Introduction to the Study of Roman Law*, 386–90; Nicholas, *Introduction to Roman Law*, 36. Gaius, *Institutes*, I, 2.8. A. M. Pritchard suggests this was not an innovation (*Leage's Roman Private Law*, 59), and Jolowicz and Nicholas also believe that Gaius borrowed the classification of law into persons, things, and actions (*Historical Introduction to the Study of Roman Law*, 389).

281. Borkowski, *Textbook on Roman Law*, 84. The problem of what precisely Gaius intended by his division of the law of persons, things, and actions is considered in some depth by Buckland, *Textbook of Roman Law*, 56–59. Borkowski appears to follow Buckland in associating the law of persons with status rather than, say, rights or privileges.

282. Frier and McGinn, *Casebook on Roman Family Law*, 12.

283. See Frier and McGinn, *Casebook on Roman Family Law*, chap. V.

284. See Borkowski, *Textbook on Roman Law*, 84–86. Borkowski says that for Roman jurists, "persons" essentially meant human beings; however, he is not equating "persons" with all human beings. Rather, he is showing that other nonhuman entities were recognized in the law of persons.

285. See Pritchard, *Leage's Roman Private Law*, 201, 256; Buckland, *Textbook of Roman Law*, 126–27, 808.

286. Gaius, *Institutes*, I, 3, 9.

within the city of Rome.[287] Slaves lacked privileges and legally were not persons.[288] According to Gaius, the law *ad personas* made a division between those who were their own masters, *sui iuris*—that is, legally independent—and those subject to the authority of others, *alieni iuris*, in the *potestas*, power of a *paterfamilias*.[289] So, an entity could belong to the category of the law *ad personas* yet not be an autonomous, self-governing subject in the legal sense. Typically, a person with full legal status was a Roman male citizen. He had some basic privileges, such as the right to appeal against a death sentence, to vote in assemblies, and to stand for public office. As the case of the Apostle Paul demonstrated, the status of citizen gave a person certain other privileges. Paul's appeal to his Roman citizenship spared him flogging without trial,[290] and tradition gives him the death of a citizen: beheading.

It seems, then, that the word *persona* was rarely used outside a legal framework. The Roman lawyer and statesman Cicero (ca. 106 to 43 BCE) is one of the few ancient writers to use the term *persona* when referring to individuals, though usually he used the term in reference to litigants, presumably in the context of legal declamation. Cicero is also noted for his "four *personae* theory," usually translated as a "character" theory, part of which seems at first sight to have some resonance with modern thought.[291] Using Stoic ideas in his advice on how to attain moral loveliness, Cicero reminds his son Marcus, and his reader, that there were four *personae* to bear in mind in order to help the reader achieve what was *decorum*, fitting: the first was the *persona* of rationality that was common to all human beings and delineated the rational human species from the irrational animal kingdom; the second *persona* was of the particular individual with his own capacities and skills; the third *persona* arose from chance or circumstance such as status at birth; the fourth *persona* concerned the individual's choice of role or way in life.[292] Initially, it would

287. Gaius, *Institutes*, I, 3, 26, 27. Borkowski, *Textbook on Roman Law*, 90.

288. Borkowski, *Textbook on Roman Law*, 93.

289. Gaius, *Institutes*, I, 48–49.

290. Acts 22:22–29.

291. Christopher Gill discusses Cicero's theory in relation to personhood and personality from its "markedly social perspective." "Personhood and Personality," 171.

292. Cicero, *De Officiis*, I.

seem that the second *persona* implied that there were certain capacities or abilities that might have defined personhood. But these *personae* were all concerned with social roles, and even the differences that Cicero describes for the second *persona* involved features that enabled men to succeed in their role in life rather than differences that indicated unique individuality. Cicero's theory, then, does not appear to have been designed to offer an analysis of the concept of person. Rather, it was to show that the wise man remembers that he is a human being with a rational nature yet with his own distinctive talents and social standing, and he thus mindfully chooses his way of life. Prior to theological reflection on the Trinity, the concept of the person was essentially contentless, which perhaps accounts for why it was taken up.

3. Discerning Persons • *Theologically Speaking about Divine Persons and Human Persons*

Introduction

Contemporary bioethical thinking on the person, particularly in the context of speciesism, is keen to point out that in early theology the word "person" was not reduced to human beings. This scope enables some bioethicists to expand the concept of person to include some non-human animals while contracting the concept so that it excludes some human beings, especially those with profound disabilities. In order to shore up a definition of the person as an individual possessing rationality and self-consciousness, writers like Cavalieri and Singer focus on self-consciousness as the essence of the Persons of the Trinity. While this bioethical thinking finds theology useful on certain points, a more considered reflection demonstrates the poverty of these oversimplifications.

Through an extensive analysis of how the term "person" was incorporated into Trinitarian theology, this chapter demonstrates that a person cannot be simply defined as a holder of interests or desires for the future, nor can the separation of biological life from biographical life find provenance in this theology. It also applies the insights from patristic theology to disability theologies that challenge some aspects of Trinitarian theology, such as God's impassibility. Much of this chapter aims to dispel some mistakes that have led to unwarranted claims about theology. Although some of the connections between disability and Trinitarian theology are more fully explored in chapter 6, this chapter highlights the significance of relationship and being as well as uniqueness and equality, themes that are vital for a theology of disability.

Struggles with Person Language

In the name of the Father and of the Son and of the Holy Spirit.

—Matthew 28:19

The term "person" comes into its own when it is taken up in early theology to express this profound mystery of God. For Christians, there is only one God. Yet early Christian *kerygma* and early liturgical practice also proclaim that Jesus is the Savior God and that the Holy Spirit is God: Christian baptism is not in the *names* of the Father, Son, and Spirit, as if there were three gods, it is in the name of the one God, who is Father, Son, and Spirit.[1] As the theologian Thomas Weinandy rightly points out, it is "this radical and unprecedented presence of God himself as a man" that challenged the early Fathers and forced the issue of how to account for the three-in-one.[2]

The early Christian community reiterates the commitment to monotheism, belief in one God, and unity in the godhead, not only in respect to the reality of the Son but also against other division in the godhead, notably that made by Marcion (ca. 144). Marcion, an early schismatic theologian influenced by Gnosticism and concerned with textual interpretations of Scripture, suggests that the "evil" God of the Old Testament is not the same as the "good" God of the New.[3] Dionysius, the bishop of Rome (259–68), suggests that Marcion makes a further attack on the unity of God when he divides the "good" God into three distinct godheads.[4]

1. "Didache," in *Apostolic Fathers*, 7; Justin Martyr, "Apology 1," in *First Apology*, 61, 65, 67; Tertullian, "On Baptism," 13, 3; Hilary, *The Trinity*, 2, 1; Gregory of Nazianzus, "Against the Arians," 33, 17.

2. Weinandy, *Does God Change?*, xxi.

3. Irenaeus, "Against Heresies," I, XXV, I. Sebastian Moll draws out an interesting distinction between the thinking of Adolf von Harnack on Marcion and the God of the Old Testament and Marcion's own view: according to Moll, Harnack wished to remove the Old Testament from the canon on the grounds that the uncomfortable traits of the God of the Old Testament meant that this God could not be reconciled with the God of the New. Harnack believed that he found in Marcion a "soul-mate." Moll correctly points out, however, that for Marcion, the god of the Old Testament was real but a very different god to the God of the New Testament. *Arch-Heretic Marcion*, 1–4.

4. Dionysius, "Letter against the Sabellians," 252–53. Although Marcion may have had links with Gnosticism, he probably did not accept emanation of aeons. Davis, *First Seven Ecumenical Councils*, 38.

Moreover, as demonstrated by the Apostle Paul in his speech to the Athenians at the Areopagus,[5] the early Fathers affirm that the "unknown God" of pagan philosophy was the God of Abraham and Moses, and the Father of Jesus. Engagement with the Greek philosophical culture of the time is reflected in theological language.[6] As patristic translator Norman Russell notes, in Greek philosophical thinking, the notion of "being" was not merely an issue of existence. Rather, "for the Greeks 'being' was contextual. Things did not just exist; they existed in a particular way."[7] Thus the conversation about God the Father and his Son Jesus also includes discussion on the attributes of God, such as immutability and impassibility. Immutability (ἀμετάθετος, *ametathetos*) means "unchangeable," and Lampe links it to "steadfast"; impassible (απαθως, *apatheos*) means "without passion," and Lampe notes that it also refers to the generation of the Son.[8]

It appears that the problem of a change in God or a suffering God threads through Trinitarian and Christological debates, especially when it comes to reflection on how there is a union of impassible divine and passible humanity in Christ.[9] For the Fathers, God's immutability and impassibility were taken as a given.[10] The patristic understanding of the immutability of God is related to the understanding, as revealed in Scripture, that God's goodness and his love cannot diminish or develop because God is Good and God is Love.[11] The understanding that God is impassible refers to the belief that there are no human passions in God, particularly negative ones that would diminish him as God. What pre-

5. Acts 17:23–34.

6. As Paul Gavrilyuk notes in *Suffering of the Impassible God*, the fact that the Fathers engaged with philosophy does not mean that the Fathers corrupted the biblical message with philosophical notions like divine impassibility.

7. Russell, *Doctrine of Deification*, 35.

8. Lampe, *Patristic Lexicon*.

9. O'Keefe, "Impassible Suffering?," 39–60. See Weinandy, *Does God Change?*, xxi. For a discussion of divine impassibility in classical and modern theology, see Keating and White, *Divine Impassibility*.

10. See Keating and White, "Introduction," in *Divine Impassibility*, 1–7. Keating and White suggest that classical thinking sought to safeguard divine transcendence. They argue that, in contrast, modern thinking is more concerned with theodicy and the problem of the nature of God in relation to human suffering, and hence there is a shift toward seeing God as suffering alongside the creation he loves.

11. For an account of Augustine's thought on divine immutability and its relation to God's goodness and wisdom, see Teske, *To Know God and the Soul*, 131–52.

cisely impassibility means was under consideration, however: as far as Tertullian is concerned, God is not impassive in the sense of the Stoic understanding of *apatheia* because God is immutable, but God is also loving and merciful to human beings.[12] Nevertheless, both immutability and impassibility reflect that God is infinitely perfect, "there is no change, nor shadow of alteration" in God.[13] Patristic debates then center on affirming unity in God and in reconciling understandings of the attributes of God with the reality of Christ.

Disability and the Impassible God

For disability writers like Nancy Eiesland, the idea of a God who is perfect and impassible has proved to be inaccessible and alienating. According to Eiesland, this idea of God is also part of a mind-set that requires people with disabilities to adjust to a norm. Instead, Eiesland presents the resurrected Jesus who bares his wounds as a "disabled God." For Eiesland, this image of God as a survivor is liberating because it has a connection with her own sense of embodiment and empowerment as a person with disabilities. In her theology, the disabled God shares in the human condition and is in solidarity with the disabled.[14] This reimaging of God is not without its problems. Eiesland's disabled God has physical wounds. It seems more challenging to envisage a God with mental impairment. As this chapter demonstrates, the issue of whether it is God who suffers and dies on the Cross is threaded throughout the patristic discussion on the Trinity and the relationship of the Father to his Divine Son. The mercy and compassion of God are not emotional states like those of human beings; rather, God is love and has infinite compassion. As Weinandy explains, precisely because God is ontologically distinct from the created order and so is not subject to the suffering and evil in that order, God can act within that order and deal with evil and suffering.[15]

In the struggles over divine impassibility, Christian faithfulness to the *kerygma* rejects the view that the Divine Son only appeared to be hu-

12. Tertullian, "Against Marcion," I.26, 2.27.
13. Jas 1:17.
14. Eiesland, *Disabled God*.
15. Weinandy, *Does God Suffer?*, 167.

man, a proposition advanced by the Docetists to preserve God's immutability and impassibility. The Docetists seemed to be influenced by Gnosticism and were already active and causing consternation for the early martyr Ignatius of Antioch (35–107) and possibly for John the Evangelist.[16] This faithfulness rules out subordinationism, an Ebionite strategy denying Christ's full divinity by calling him an inspired prophet whose adoptive sonship began at his baptism.[17] The Ebionites appeared to have links with the early remaining Jewish Christians.[18] These two extremes, the denial of Christ's humanity and the denial of his divinity, continue to reappear in subsequent controversies. Some of the difficulties with a disabled God, the resurrected Jesus, are that it seems to jeopardize the distinction between Father and Son, and that it may lay either Christ's humanity or divinity open to question.

Still, in early Christianity, there remained two issues: how to speak of Son and Spirit as divine yet not contradict belief in one God, and how to understand the relationship of Father and Son and Spirit. Early Christians operating out of a Judaic mentality could draw upon images from the Old Testament and apocalyptic literature to describe Christ. Justin Martyr uses such images in his dialogue with the Jew Trypho. It is not certain whether Trypho was a historical individual or an invention of Justin. If a real individual, he may have been a rabbi; however, it is more likely that he was a layman educated both in philosophy and Judaism.[19] Justin himself was first a pagan and then a follower of different philosophical schools until a chance and mysterious encounter with an elderly man on the seashore led to his conversion to Christianity. Justin explains to Trypho that the long-awaited expectations of the Jewish people have been fulfilled in God's new covenant and his sending of Jesus Christ as light to all, including the Gentiles.[20]

16. Ignatius of Antioch, "To the Smyrnaens" and "To the Trallians," in *Apostolic Fathers*, 1–8, 2, 10. See Brown, *Community of the Beloved Disciple*, 155–56. For an account of the docetists as opponents of John the Evangelist, see Strecker, *Theology of the New Testament*, 437–40. Michael Goulder suggests that there was a "docetic" threat, but he argues that the opponents of Ignatius were in fact Ebionites. "Ignatius' 'Docetists,'" 16–30.

17. Irenaeus, "Against Heresies," I, XXI–XXII. See Goulder, "Ignatius' 'Docetists.'"

18. See Bauckham, "Origin of the Ebionites," 162–81.

19. For more on this question, see Tellbe, *Christ-Believers in Ephesus*, 119.

20. Justin Martyr, "Dialogue with Trypho," in *First Apology*, 11. According to Tellbe,

To demonstrate this fulfillment of the Old Testament promise, Justin describes Christ as the Glory of the Lord or Law or Wisdom or Angel.[21] In the Old Testament, and notably in apocalyptic texts, angels accompany God, they are intermediaries with human beings, and the angelic hosts sing his glory. *Mal"ak* or αγγελος is also a supernatural messenger of the Lord sent with a specific message.[22] In some Jewish circles, the archangel Michael was the principal leader of the angelic host. To express the transcendence of Christ, Justin, along with some other early Christians, uses angel Christology: he calls Jesus *Christos angelos*.[23] Certainly, angel Christology is problematic if it is seen as denying either the humanity or divinity of Christ. A move in the disability discourse that calls some people with intellectual disabilities "angels" equally denies them their humanity. Nevertheless, Justin makes it clear that the Angel begotten of the Father is not the same as created angels.[24] Significantly, the many ways in which Justin describes Christ indicates that Christ is with God from the beginning. Christ does not have an angelic nature; rather, in Darrell Hannah's words, Christ is "God's messenger *par excellence*."[25] Similarly, Tertullian explains that although the term "angel" is used for Christ, he is not an actual angel like Gabriel or Michael.[26] Christ is not the same as Michael because, unlike the angel Michael, Christ is the divine *Logos*.[27]

The situation was further complicated as Christianity engaged with Hellenistic thought and Gnosticism, especially speculative theories of the emanation of aeons, divine entities that proceed from each other like human thoughts and desires proceed from the mind and will.[28] In Gnostic thought, the Demiurge, a god like Marcion's God of the Old Testament, creates the material world and breathes into earthly souls some

Justin was convinced that the Jews did not understand their own scriptures, and he set out to demonstrate their Christological interpretation. *Christ-Believers in Ephesus*, 121.

21. Justin Martyr, "Dialogue with Trypho," in *First Apology*, 61.

22. Vine, *Vine's Complete Expository Dictionary*.

23. For Jewish beliefs about angels and Christian angel Christologies, see Hannah, *Michael and Christ*.

24. Justin Martyr, "Dialogue with Trypho," in *First Apology*, 128.

25. Hannah, *Michael and Christ*, 214.

26. Tertullian, "On the Flesh of Christ." See Hannah, *Michael and Christ*, 170, 214–18.

27. See Hannah, *Michael and Christ*, 214–18.

28. See Davis, *First Seven Ecumenical Councils*, 37.

spark that is consubstantial with himself.[29] In this system of thought, there are material bodies (and souls) that are the result of fallen creation and the work of a lesser god. The spiritual element in the material longs to be freed from matter, and in the Gnostic system it is true knowledge, accessible only to the few, that leads to this freedom.[30] This system of thought is not unlike the modern view that sees the material body as raw datum to be manipulated, and the "person" who is self-conscious and can hold desires and interests as the true reality. Moreover, theories of disability that see the disabled as abnormal or falling below a supposed norm suggest that these humans are somehow less than other human beings. In an apparent hierarchy, people with intellectual impairment fall even farther.

Theologians like Irenaeus refute this Gnostic system and hierarchy by insisting on the one Creator God whose creation is good.[31] Nevertheless, there remains the question of the relationship of the Son to the Father and indeed, in Christology, the distinction some thinkers make between Jesus and Christ. In the lead-up to the Council of Nicaea in 325, the implications of some early Christian writings lean toward different degrees of subordinate divinity while also insisting on the simplicity and indivisibility of God. Some maintain that the divinity is unique and indivisible, but also that there are no mediating degrees between the Creator and creation.[32] The bishops at the Council of Nicaea affirmed the divinity of Christ, but as professor of historical theology Lewis Ayres points out, perhaps the real advance was made following the council by three theologians—Basil of Caesarea, his younger brother Gregory of Nyssa, and their friend Gregory of Nazianzus[33]—known since the mid-nineteenth century as the Cappadocian Fathers.[34] These three theo-

29. Moll points out that Marcion parallels Gnostic thinking, particularly when it comes to distrust of the material; however, he probably does not use the term *demiurge*, nor does he think of the demiurge as an assistant to the Supreme God. *Arch-Heretic Marcion*, 71–73.

30. Although Marcion himself did not appear to hold to a mythological system nor discuss the origins of the demiurge, this seems to be a feature of some Gnostic thinking; see Moll, *Arch-Heretic Marcion*, 18–19.

31. For Irenaeus and refutation of the Gnostics on creation, see Osborn, *Irenaeus of Lyons*, 54–61.

32. See Ayres, "Not Three People," 450.

33. Ayres, "Not Three People," 450.

34. Pope Benedict XVI, *Fathers of the Church*, 167.

logians made a significant contribution by helping to provide a way to express that the Father, Son, and Spirit are equal and real yet distinct. The term to express this is the Persons of the Trinity. At the very least, persons are real, not insubstantial. Persons are unique, distinct, and in relationship rather than isolated individuals, and equal in dignity. It is important to stress the depths of person language precisely in order to overcome the view that person is merely concerned with rationality. This is not simply for the sake of people with disabilities. It is rather a matter for all human beings and for a deeper understanding of the whole of theology.

That God is one-in-three is not a new or innovative idea worked out by early Christians. Rather, the One God who is Three Divine Persons is revealed in the Old Testament and made explicit in the New Testament with the coming of Jesus the God-man and the sending of the Spirit. A similar comment can be made about human beings and persons: the concept of the person cannot simply be defined, redefined, and made the subject of a list of characteristics or even determined by consensus in order to suit a specific agenda. Instead, the concept of the person is a matter of discernment.

To illustrate that the mystery of the person is not simply solved by definitions, long before the Council of Nicaea and the Cappadocians Fathers, early Trinitarian theology begins to grasp this mystery by finding ways to express it through misinterpretations and distortions that are tested against the *kerygma*.

Finding a Common Language

Monarchianism, referring to the unity of God as one sole ruler, is one early attempt before the Council of Nicaea, to reconcile biblical monotheism with the coming of Christ. Although Christianity holds to the unity of God, "Monarchianist" or "modalist" became the terms used to describe those who deny that in the one God there are three coequal Persons.[35] More accurately, those who denied the Trinity were known

35. J. N. D. Kelly distinguishes between "dynamic monarchianism," or Adoptionism, the theory that Christ was a mere man, and modalism, that blurred the distinctions between

as Theodotians, after the probable founder of the sect, Theodotus the Cobbler, who was working in Rome in about 190.[36] The term "Monarchianism" is possibly first used by Tertullian as a nickname for the patripassianists, who taught that it was the Father who had suffered and was crucified.[37] One strand of Monarchianism regards the Father and the Son as distinct modes of operation of the one God. This strand is held by Noetus (ca. 200), Sabellius (early third century), and Tertullian's opponent Praxeas. The other strand holds the divinity as one and elevates Jesus, a mere man, into the divine. This strand is presented by Theodotus the Cobbler, Theodotus the Money-changer (both fl. ca. 190) as reported by Eusebius (ca. 260 to ca. 339) in his *Ecclesiastical History*,[38] and by Paul of Samosata (fl. ca. 260).

Early Monarchian Christians wishing to stress the oneness of God are tempted to describe the distinction between Father, Son, and Spirit revealed in Scripture as energies or modes of the one God, so the distinction ceases to be real. For those wishing to maintain the distinction, the problem is how to describe a relationship that is real yet does not make Son and Spirit derivative or secondary. So, the context of the search for a common language involved avoiding the notion that there is no real distinction between the three and asserting that the three are all equally God. After some struggles and refinements, the search settled around the term "person" (πρόσωπον).[39] Although this term was used in the West by some, in the general vocabulary of theology, it appeared much later than the Council at Nicaea.

In the West

The initial locus of this search for a term to express the *kerygma* in Western theology is found with Tertullian, the first theologian to write in Latin rather than Greek in the West, and with Hippolytus (ca.

Father, Son, and Spirit. He explains that both were united by a concern for the divine unity. *Early Christian Doctrines*, 115.

36. Kelly, *Early Christian Doctrines*, 116–17. See also Behr, *Formation of Christian Theology*, 142–43.

37. Tertullian, "Against Praxeas," X.

38. Eusebius Pamphili, *Ecclesiastical History*, 5, 28.

39. See Lampe, *Patristic Lexicon*.

170–236), one of the last to write in Greek in the West. Tertullian writes his treatise against Praxeas sometime after 213, and Hippolytus writes against Noetus in about 200–210. It is difficult to determine whether Praxeas is a historical or fictional figure. Apart from Tertullian, no early writer, not even Hippolytus, writes about him. The name Praxeas seems to mean "busybody," and Tertullian may use it as a pseudonym for Callistus, bishop of Rome and a follower of Noetus, though why Tertullian should wish to disguise the person he attacks is not clear.[40] Hippolytus says that Noetus lived "not very long ago,"[41] and it seems that Noetus came to Rome from Smyrna. Noetus was accused of holding patripassian views, and despite his denials, he was expelled from the Church. He then apparently went on to establish his own school of thought.[42]

From the accounts available, both Praxeas and Noetus claim that the Son and the Spirit are not distinct from the Father.[43] To refute these two monarchists, Tertullian and Hippolytus use as their clinching argument the logic that if the Father and Son are the same, then Monarchians are committed to patripassianism: the Father suffered, which creates a contradiction for those who hold that God is impassible.

Unfortunately, as with many of those judged unorthodox, there is little original material left. Reports of what Praxeas and Noetus said come from their critics, so it is difficult to piece together their actual thought, and it is uncertain whether they promoted patripassianism. Apparently, while Noetus attributes passibility to the divine nature by holding that the Father suffered on the Cross, Praxeas claims that God as Father is illimitable and impassible, and as Son he becomes limitable and passible.[44] In later discussions, Athanasius, the fourth-century bishop of Alexandria, implies that the claim of Praxeas applies also to Noetus.[45] This form of patripassianism has problematic implications that surface in later Christological debates: an insistence on the unity of God without distinction suggests that the union of God with man in the Incarnation

40. See Stevenson, *New Eusebius*, 169; Davis, *First Seven Ecumenical Councils*, 41.
41. Hippolytus, *Contra Noetum*, 1.
42. See Behr, *Formation of Christian Theology*, 146.
43. Osborn, *Tertullian*, 127; Behr, *Formation of Christian Theology*, 147–48.
44. Hippolytus, *Contra Noetum*, 1; Tertullian, "Against Praxeas," I.
45. Athanasius, "De Synodis," 2, 26, 6.

is simply an indwelling, as suggested by Paul of Samosata, or a moral union as presented by Nestorius. This may in turn lead to the view that salvation depends on the goodness of the individual's moral will to follow the example of Christ, as offered in Pelagianism.

To counter early Monarchianism, some form of common language seemed necessary, and Tertullian is the writer credited with introducing the concept of person, *persona*, into theological language. Tertullian may possibly have been a Roman lawyer,[46] and interestingly, perhaps only some fifty years before, in his *Institutes*, Gaius had introduced the notion of *persona* when he classified Roman law into the law of persons, of things, and of legal actions.

Tertullian's approach and his appeal to credal methods of analysis suggest that for Tertullian, as a rule of faith, Trinitarian theology was a given.[47] Against those who see no difference between the Father and the Son, Tertullian argues that the Father, Son, and Spirit are inseparable yet distinct,[48] and he introduces the notion of *persona* to account for this sort of reality.[49] The idea that the faith is handed on in the tradition of the Church is important for early theologians, not least because they refuted the Gnostics who claimed to have their own access to unadulterated truth.[50] Tertullian himself argues in favor of unwritten traditions found in liturgical practice, "for how can anything come into use, if it has not first been handed down?"[51] Tertullian may have had another motive for stressing his continuity with the rule of faith, however: he joined the Montanists who may have been concerned initially with matters of discipline rather than orthodoxy, but later became the schismatic "New Prophecy."[52] Tertullian blames Praxeas not only for introducing heresy but also for ruining a possible concord between Rome and the new prophets.[53]

46. See Barnes, *Tertullian*; Dunn, *Tertullian*, 2–5.
47. Tertullian, "Against Praxeas," II.
48. Tertullian, "Against Praxeas," IX.
49. Tertullian, "Against Praxeas," VII, XII.
50. Irenaeus, "Against Heresies," III.
51. Tertullian, "On the Soldier's Crown," 3, 4.
52. According to Andrew B. McGowan, "'Orthodox' Theology," 437–57. If the bishop of Rome was about to recognize the Montanists, however, then in its early stages, Montanism may not have challenged orthodox thinking.
53. Tertullian, "Against Praxeas," I.

Tertullian explains that the Father, Son, and Spirit are not one person but rather "three coherent persons who are distinct yet one essence."[54] Tertullian further says that this is a scriptural distinction, for when God says, "let us make man," the plural is used because the Father already has his Son as "second person" and the Spirit as the "third person."[55] Moreover, to be a father, there must be a son.[56] There is one substance or essence, yet the persons denote a distinction but not a division.[57] Tertullian also asserts that this distinctness makes "an objective thing and a person" *res et persona*, a truly substantive being.[58] Although Tertullian does not suggest that his language is innovative, it is difficult to ascertain previous use, if any, of person language. Praxeas appears not to speak of persons: although in some English translations Tertullian states the "new-fangled" Praxeas claimed pure truth in thinking that a human being cannot believe in only one God in any other way than by saying that the Father, Son, and Spirit are "the very self-same *person*," "person" does not seem to appear in the Latin texts available.[59] The loose use of this term perhaps just goes to show that person language has not received the attention it merits.

Hippolytus lived in Rome, though he probably came from the East and had Alexandrian connections. He was elected bishop of Rome by his small band of followers, even though Callistus was already the bishop and so was in schism until his exile and death by martyrdom. Hippolytus answers the followers of Noetus who had been claiming that Christ was the Father himself and the Father was born, suffered, and died.[60] Again, apparently there is no "person" language: Father and Son are simply the same. Correcting Noetus, Hippolytus says the Father is indeed one, but there are two persons (*prosopa*, πρόσωπα) since there is also the Son and then a third, the Spirit.[61] Refuting the Noetian idea that the Fa-

54. Tertullian, "Against Praxeas," XXV.

55. Tertullian, "Against Praxeas," XII.

56. Tertullian, "Against Praxeas," X. Lewis Ayres argues that Origen introduces this as a new argument since he makes the relationship intrinsic to the life of God. *Nicaea and Its Legacy*, 27.

57. Tertullian, "Against Praxeas," XII.

58. Tertullian, "Against Praxeas," VII.

59. Tertullian, "Against Praxeas," II.

60. Hippolytus, *Contra Noetum*, 1.

61. Hippolytus, *Contra Noetum*, 14.

ther becomes the Son at the appropriate time, Hippolytus explains that this plurality is at the level of the eternal relationships of the Trinity, not just in the economy or plan of salvation. An expert in Patristic Greek, G. L. Prestige translates the *prosopa* of Hippolytus as "presentations" rather than "persons," presumably indicating that *prosopa* was not being used in any more developed sense than the classical Greek usage.[62] Yet it is also clear in its context that Hippolytus does not mean "mask" by his use of *prosopon*, since he wishes to assert the distinctive individuality of the Son against Callistus, follower of Noetus.[63]

It remains a matter of dispute whether Tertullian borrows the idea of "person" from Hippolytus.[64] Still, when faced with different doctrinal problems, Tertullian seems to find *persona* a valuable term for describing both the closeness of Christ and his distinction from the Father. Arguing against docetic views of a Christ separate from the Father in *Against Marcion,* Tertullian refers to the *persona* of Christ who spoke through the prophets as God's representative[65] or who, as perfect image, was the *persona*, countenance, of God[66] and revealer of the true God, the Creator.[67] Arguing against the view that Father and Son were so close it was the Father himself who was born as Son, suffered, and died, Tertullian in *Against Praxeas* uses *persona* to affirm the distinctness of the persons of the Trinity united in one nature. The understanding of *persona* for distinctness becomes prominent in the tradition perhaps because, at least in the West, it appears to solve the problem of describing the three-in-one.[68]

Living in Rome at the same time as Hippolytus, Sabellius became the leader of the monarchists, and through his development of the ideas of Noetus, he became for the Fathers the archetypal heretic. Sabellius may use *prosopa* in connection with the Persons of the Trinity, but it is unclear

62. Prestige, *God in Patristic Thought*, 106–7.

63. Hippolytus, *Contra Noetum*, 9, 12, 18–19.

64. According to Caroline Bammel, the heresy attacked by Hippolytus seems less developed and therefore earlier than that of Praxeas. "The State of Play," 197.

65. Tertullian, "Against Marcion," III, 6.

66. Tertullian, "Against Marcion," V, 11.

67. Tertullian, "Against Marcion," I, 19.

68. Richard Muller thinks that words in nontheological and non-Christian usage were acceptable precisely because they could act as problem solvers, though they were redefined in their theological setting. "Role of Church History," 84.

whether he uses the word in the sense of masks or to indicate presentations, if indeed he uses it at all. Historian J. N. D. Kelly argues against claims that Sabellius speaks of three *prosopa* in the sense of masks, not least because it would then have the opposite meaning to that used by Hippolytus.[69] Some texts reporting the writings of Sabellius quote the term "names," and some speak of *prosopa*.[70] But since Basil believes that *prosopon* has Sabellian connotations,[71] Sabellius may indeed use the word for "person" in connection with the Godhead. This uncertain usage perhaps indicates that a struggle was taking place over what meaning to give to terms that were beginning to gain acceptance for different reasons.

Possibly borrowing from the Stoics, Sabellius argues that the Monad, the One, dilates to become a Triad for the time of the economy of salvation: God is called Father for the giving of the law, Son for the work of redemption, and Spirit for the inspiration of believers. This is reported by Athanasius in his treatise *Against the Arians*,[72] and it indicates the lack of original evidence as well as the strategies used by theologians like Athanasius to taint their own opponents, in this case the Arians, by linking them to the thinking of notorious heretics. Unlike Praxeas and Noetus, for whom the Father is the Son, Sabellius seems to recognize a form of Trinity perhaps to avoid a charge of patripassianism,[73] though for Athanasius, Sabellianism is merely its Greek equivalent.[74]

Whereas Hippolytus intends to signify distinctiveness in his use of

69. Kelly, *Early Christian Doctrines*, 122.

70. Some texts—e.g., Bettenson, *Later Christian Fathers*, 38—refer to *prosopa*. Others—e.g., Williams, *Panarion of Epiphanius of Salamis*, 123—refer to "three names in one entity." The Latin and Greek versions of Epiphanius in J. P. Migne, *Patrologiae cursus completus: Series graeca*, vol. 41 (Paris: 1863), 173–1199, and Oehler *Corpus Haereseologicum II–III* (Berlin: 1859–61) refer to *appellationes* and *ovomasias*, so it would seem that Williams reflects a more accurate usage. In Migne's and Oehler's texts, however, there is also mention of *prosopon/persona* in connection with Sabellius, so the possibility he did use it cannot be ruled out. Apollinarius (see McCarthy Spoerl, "Apollinarius on the Holy Spirit," 584n65) and Basil (Letters 236, 210) believe *prosopon* has Sabellian connotations. Bettenson may be using "person" because he seems to think this best conveys what Sabellius means (the text is not critical), so he claims that Cyril of Jerusalem says, "Sabellius confuses the persons," whereas in other texts, e.g., *Nicene and Post Nicene Fathers*, vol. 7 (Cyril's Catechetical Lecture 16.4), it reads the Sabellians "work confusion," and there is no mention of persons.

71. Basil, *Letters* 186–368.

72. Athanasius, "Against the Arians," IV, 13, 25.

73. See Kelly, *Early Christian Doctrines*, 122.

74. Athanasius, "De Synodis," 2, 26, 6.

prosopon as well as plurality, not merely in the economy, God's plan of salvation, but also for the Godhead, Sabellius focuses on sameness but through presentations that last purely for the economy. Prestige suggests that before about the 250s, *prosopon* is rarely used with reference to the Trinity and becomes common only during the Arian controversy.[75] Instead, theologians speak more simply of "three" and "one," and according to Hippolytus, the Sabellians teach a doctrine of a single *prosopon* meaning, says Prestige, one individual or concrete presentation in the Godhead.[76]

The evidence of Hippolytus seems to contradict that of Bishop of Salamis Epiphanius (ca. 315–403), who writes a compendium of early heresies. Epiphanius states that Sabellius employs an analogy to the sun to show how there is one substance and three *prosopa*: the orb, represented by the Father, is the actual substance, the light is analogous to the Son, and heat to the Spirit. The Son was once emitted like a ray of light, and when he accomplished his work, he was taken back into heaven just as a ray is withdrawn again into the sun.[77] In this analogy, there is a sense of expansion and contraction in the sense of Gnostic emanation rather than distinction. This conflict of evidence seems to reflect the perennial problem of ascertaining what words were in fact used when all that remains are reports. Epiphanius and Hippolytus can perhaps be reconciled, however, if Hippolytus is understood as saying that according to Sabellius there is one *prosopon* before the dilation of Father into Son and Spirit and again after the return of Son to Father.

Following the evidence of Epiphanius, Tertullian and Sabellius use a similar analogy. To express the one nature of the Father and the Son, Tertullian also calls the Son light lit from light, a ray from the sun.[78] Tertullian wishes to assert that although the sun is the source, the ray is not separated from it; yet it is distinct, like a shoot is to a root or a river from

75. Prestige, *God in Patristic Thought*, 161–62. Prestige also claims that although Origen states that the Sabellians use *prosopon*, it is not with the sense of mask or role, and therefore its rare use is not due to it having been discredited in theology (113).

76. Prestige, *God in Patristic Thought*, 160, quoting Hippolytus, *Refutatio*, 10, 27, 4; 9, 12, 18–19.

77. Epiphanius, *Panarion of Epiphanius*, II, III, 62, 1–9.

78. Tertullian, "Apology 1," 21, 10–14.

a fountain.[79] Through this imagery, Tertullian seeks to establish a point of contact between Son and Father that does not imply division or absolute identity.[80] Tertullian is replying to the Gnostic system of emanations whereby an aeon was so separated that it could not know its source. Tertullian also explains that this distinction but not separation went beyond the economy of salvation: unlike some philosophies that held that God was alone with his *logos*, Tertullian asserts that before creation, the Word was truly in the beginning with God[81] and a personal being[82] active in the Old Testament.[83] To eliminate any patripassianism, Tertullian refers again to his analogy of river and fountain: just as pollution or injury that affects the stream does not affect the fountain, so too did Christ suffer but the Father did not.[84] This analogy, implying that the Son is dependent on the Father, becomes problematic for later theologians.

The analogy of the Son begotten of the Father as light from light is also taken up by Athanasius,[85] who recognizes that Sabellius dissolves not just the existence of the Father, Son, and Spirit once they had fulfilled their function in salvation history. According to Athanasius, the idea that the name of Son and Spirit cease once they have supplied the need means that the grace of baptism too ceases.[86]

The understanding of the person, then, references something distinct and concrete, though not radically separated and isolated from its source. Nevertheless, Sabellius perhaps recognizes a problem for Tertullian and Hippolytus: for those who maintain both the unity of God and that Christ is God, any suggestion that the Son has his own functions apart from the Father is too close to pagan arguments explaining the emanations coming from the One, and it leads to the temptation of having the Son (and Spirit) as secondary. Even though Tertullian seems to distance himself from the Gnostic system of emanations, he does not altogether avoid the impression that the Son (and Spirit) is subordinate.

79. Tertullian, "Against Praxeas," VIII, V, VI .
80. See McCruden, "Monarchy and Economy in Tertullian's *Adversus Praxeam*," 332.
81. Tertullian, "Against Praxeas," V.
82. Tertullian, "Against Praxeas," VII.
83. Tertullian, "Against Praxeas," XVI.
84. Tertullian, "Against Praxeas," XXIX.
85. Athanasius, "Against the Arians," I, 3, 9; III, 23, 3.
86. Athanasius, "Against the Arians," IV, 25.

In the East

While Western theologians seem more likely to accept the language of *persona*, Eastern theologians appear more circumspect. This may be because the evolution of *persona* to mean something distinct may have taken place earlier in the Latin tradition. In the Greek tradition, *prosopon* held on to a sense of mere presentation, and it implies impersonation far more than the legal Latin term *persona*.[87] According to Zizioulas, "*precisely because the term 'person' lacked an ontological content* and led towards Sabellianism," it was rejected in the East.[88]

Even if the Sabellians do not use *prosopon* as mask or role, some Fathers think that *prosopon* could be so used. The evidence for this comes from theologians who write sometime after the Council of Nicaea. Nevertheless, they comment upon what presumably was the position before the council. So, for instance, in his attempt to preclude Sabellianism and Ebionism, Hilary bishop of Poitiers (ca. 315–67) argues that the nature of the Son, the Word, is not subordinate like that of a sound that is uttered.[89] Rather, he is "God from God,"[90] and the Son does not deceive us by "theatrical transformation of names and aspects," nor is God a "single person who hides his features under a mask that we may imagine that two are present."[91] And while Basil's friend Gregory of Nazianzus seems less reluctant to use *prosopa* so long as the meaning of Three in Unity is maintained and the errors of Sabellius and Arius are avoided,[92] Basil sees *prosopon* as less appropriate than *hypostasis* (ὑπόστᾰσις, "subsistence").[93] Basil writes that Sabellius did not object to the word *prosopon* if it was not used as synonymous with *hypostasis*.[94] In the eyes of Sabellius, linking the two terms would naturally have led to confessing three-in-one, what Sabellius would regard as tritheism, as opposed to the

87. See Quasten, *Patrology*, 229.
88. Zizioulas, *Being as Communion*, 37; emphasis original.
89. Hilary, *The Trinity*, VII, 3.
90. Hilary, *The Trinity*, VII, 11.
91. Hilary, *The Trinity*, VII, 39.
92. Gregory of Nazianzus, "Oration," 40, 41.
93. Basil, *Letter* 236. For a definition and an account of the use of *hypostasis*, see Lampe, *Patristic Lexicon*.
94. Basil, *Letter* 210.

metamorphosing of the Father into the Son or Spirit as needs demanded, that Sabellius advocated. It is precisely this link of *prosopon* to *hypostasis* that Basil sees as vital to maintain the traditional faith that the Father, Son, and Spirit act in reality and not merely by appearance, trickery, or disguise. Moreover, it is the identification of *prosopon* and *hypostasis* that leads Boethius to define person as an individual nature that is real and distinct rather than a separate individual. Understanding that Boethius makes this identification is vital for a proper interpretation of the concept of the person because it clearly counters the surface meaning of person offered by bioethicists influenced by Locke.

Unlike the Roman West, whose Latin was characterized by a certain terseness, the Greeks, as Basil demonstrates, had available the terms *ousia* (οὐσία) and *hypostasis*, which may be another reason why Eastern theologians were slower to take up the language of *prosopon*. *Ousia* denoted what made a thing essentially what it was in terms of its internal characteristics. *Hypostasis* seemed to refer to a thing's external character as an empirical reality, and it broadly referred to what underlies something else, subsistence. It was used, for instance, to describe sediment in a wine cask or what gives support. *Hypostasis* was somewhat ambiguous, however, since it could stand for both the raw material that forms the foundation of something, substance, and subsistence, the individuating principle. The ambiguity surrounding *hypostasis* can be seen in the differing understandings of Dionysius, bishop of Rome, and the Greek theologian Origen.[95] Dionysius of Rome condemns those, among them possibly Dionysius of Alexandra, who divide the monarchy into separated substances, *hypostases*, "foreign to each other" to make three godheads, which divide the divine essence.[96] Here *hypostasis* appears to be the individuating principle. In contrast, Origen, to counter Sabellian modalism, uses *prosopon* in the sense of individual presentation or character and *hypostases* as the concrete realities (subsistencies) of Father, Son, and Spirit.[97]

The context of Origen's understanding of the *hypostases* of the Trin-

95. See O'Collins, *Tripersonal God*, 117–18.

96. Dionysius of Rome, "Letter of Dionysius of Rome to Dionysius of Alexandria," 248–49.

97. Origen, *Commentary on the Gospel According to John*, 2, 75. See Prestige, *God in Patristic Thought*, 161.

ity requires exploration. Before Origen's anthropology and cosmology were eventually rejected, his views were held in some respect by theologians like Athanasius.[98] Origen was also influential on all sides of the Trinitarian debate, not least because the unorthodox Arius partly comes from an Origenist tradition.[99] Origen's main concern seems to be to maintain the incorporeal nature of God against Stoic influences that see God as a form of rarified Spirit, a view that Tertullian had possibly held. To correct this materialistic view, Origen uses Platonism.[100] Origen starts with the absolute transcendence of God, who is unknowable not merely because of the weakness of our intellect but also because he is entirely other than created reality.[101] Origen then considers how God mediates knowledge of himself. He begins with God the Father, who alone is strictly God since he is not generated or spirated: as giver of existence, he is superior. To mediate between himself and creation, he brings forth the Son, who is truly God but second in rank since he is generated. The Son is less than the Father but superior to rational creatures. The Holy Spirit brought forth through the Word in the Father, spirated, is third.[102]

For Origen, the Son has a real existence, in *hypostasis*, not an existence merely in thought: "one cannot be a father apart from having a son."[103] Father, Son, and Spirit, then, are three distinct *hypostases*,[104] though for Origen this does not indicate three substances, nor does it imply ontological equality.[105] Although the Son does have a real existence and is somehow intrinsic to the being of God, Origen does not accept that the Son comes from the *ousia*, substance or essence, of the Father. For Origen, this would imply some sort of material conception.[106] Rather, Origen states that the Son is of the Father's will, not of his essence.[107] Yet it seems that for Origen this emphasizes the Son's eternal existence,

98. See Williams, *Arius*, 149.

99. There is continuity of tradition even if the actual relation of Origen's thought to Arianism is in dispute. Williams, *Arius*, 143.

100. See Trigg, *Origen*.

101. Origen, "*De Principiis*," 1, 1, 8.

102. Origen, "*De Principiis*," 1, 3, 5.

103. Origen, "*De Principiis*," 1, 2, 2, 3.

104. Origen, *Commentary on the Gospel According to John* 2, 75.

105. Origen, *Commentary on the Gospel According to John* 2, 10.

106. See Ayres, *Nicaea and Its Legacy*, 24.

107. Origen, "*De Principiis*," 1, 2, 6; 1, 2, 9.

as Origen has a sense of the Father's eternal will.[108] God's will produced this first act of creation, the Son. But this creation is not like the creation of the material world, for the Son is created as *ktisma* (κτίσμα), apparently some form of primary creation presumably of original rational beings, as opposed to *kosmos* (*κόσμος*), or material creation of the world.[109]

To add to the complexity of *hypostasis*, it seems that in the West *hypostasis* was taken to correspond to the Latin *substantia*, so the term was readily misunderstood: when Eastern theologians expressed the three *hypostases* of God, Western theologians heard tritheism; when Western theologians spoke of one divine *substantia*, Eastern theologians sensed modalism. Moreover, although in early theological thought the primarily philosophical term *hypostasis* was not equivalent to *persona* or *prosopon*, it was linked to *ousia*. This proved problematic, as it seems that Sabellianism understood both *ousia* and *hypostasis* to refer to an individual substance. The Latin West may have distinguished substance, the one, from persons, the three in the Godhead; however, this distinction held materialistic connotations. Until the East accepted that *ousia* referred to the one and *hypostasis* was exclusively for the three, there remained plenty of scope for misunderstanding.[110]

One Eastern theologian who admits the same substance, *ousia* for the Father and Son but not distinct *hypostases*, is Paul of Samosata.[111] Paul became bishop of Antioch and considers the Son or *Logos* as one of the powers coming from God. He teaches that the *Logos* takes up its dwelling on earth in the ordinary man Jesus. Paul seems to have been the first to use the term *homoousios*, of the same being *ousia*, to describe the relationship of the *Logos* to the Father, though by this Paul appears to mean that the *Logos* is not a distinct entity, *hypostasis*.[112] Rather, as God's eternal wisdom, the *Logos* is an attribute of God. After Paul was condemned, his influence began to wane. But the term Paul uses, *homoousios*, resurfaces at the Council of Nicaea. And the thinker who

108. Ayres, *Nicaea and Its Legacy*, 27.

109. Origen, "*De Principiis*," 4, 4, 1. Blosser, *Become Like the Angels*, 202.

110. See Davis, *First Seven Ecumenical Councils*, 48.

111. For Paul's Monarchian theology, see Pollard, *Johannine Christology*, 113–15.

112. For an account of the early use of the term *homoousios* and the confusion surrounding the term, see Hanson, *Search for the Christian Doctrine of God*, 190–98.

brought Trinitarian theology to a crisis point in a form that outlived him is Arius, who specifically does not like the term *homoousios*. According to Arius, who appeals not to Greek terms but to Scripture, the Son is a creature.[113]

The Council of Nicaea, 325 CE

Constantine initially summoned the Council of Nicaea in an attempt to deal with the "intellectual exercise," fostered by "misused leisure," of the Arian controversy. For Constantine, the controversy was grave principally because dissension threatened the Church's unity.[114] By the end of the council, Constantine became more aware of what was at stake theologically and, having seen Arianism condemned, was satisfied that the issues had been rigorously examined so that unity could be restored.[115] It appears that the settling of precise theological terminology did not form a part of the council's intention.[116]

At Nicaea, *homoousios*, of one essence or coessential, was introduced to express the relationship of the Son to the Father, and Constantine seemed particularly keen on the term perhaps because it was sufficiently vague to cover all views present.[117] Previously, both Irenaeus[118] and Origen[119] had regarded the term with suspicion because it had been used in Gnostic systems to explain the emanations.[120] Moreover, the council that deposed Paul of Samosata condemned its use. This meant that some fourth-century Fathers were embarrassed into explaining why the term was now appropriate. So, for instance, Athanasius explains that it was

113. For a discussion of Arius and Scripture, see Williams, *Arius*, 110–14. According to Williams, Arius aims to develop a "biblically-based *and* rationally consistent catechesis" (111; emphasis original).

114. Constantine, "Letter to Alexander and Arius," in Stevenson, *New Eusebius*, 332–34. See also Davis, *First Seven Ecumenical Councils*, 54–55.

115. Constantine, "Letter to the Alexandrians," in Stevenson, *New Eusebius*, 350–51.

116. Ayres, *Nicaea and Its Legacy*, 86.

117. See Davis, *First Seven Ecumenical Councils*, 62. Pier Franco Beatrice claims that Constantine did not adopt the term simply for political or for expedient reasons. Rather, he argues, Constantine used pagan theology gained from his pre-Christian days, and instead of seeing *homoousios* as empty or ambiguous, he regarded it as a technical term that had nothing to do with either Sabellianism or Monarchianism. "The Word '*Homoousios*,'" 269–70.

118. Irenaeus, "Against Heresies," I, V, I.

119. See Pamphilus, "Apology for Origen," 94.

120. Davis, *First Seven Ecumenical Councils*, 37.

coessential in a *bodily* sense that was rejected at the trial of Paul of Samosata.[121] Arius regards the term as Manichaean, indicating a portion of the Father therefore to be avoided.[122] Ambrose (339–97) suggests that the term was included in the Creed of Nicaea precisely because the Arians disliked it.[123] Arius had already said that the Son is not *homoousios* with the Father,[124] so its inclusion in the Creed of Nicaea clearly made Arius into a heretic. The inclusion of the phrase "begotten not made," where like comes from like, stresses that the Son "was not a work."[125] Yet, although *homoousios* may have excluded notions that the Son was created or was of God's will but not his essence, it did not define what the Fathers of the Council wished to include.[126] The result inevitably was that delegates from the council came away with different views as to the meaning of the term. After all, *homoousios* could imply that two things had the same ontological status, they were the same, or, in a materialistic way, they came from the underlying substance, they shared the substance.[127]

To unravel the terminological problems of *homoousios*, Athanasius recognizes that although many accepted what was defined at Nicaea, there remained a dispute about the word coessential.[128] Conciliatory toward those who were not Arian yet did not use Nicene terminology, Athanasius calls them "brothers" because they "mean what we mean" and are "not far from accepting the phrase co-essential." Athanasius examines the use of "of the essence" and "like in essence." Using the word examples of tin being like silver or wolf like dog—yet tin is not from silver nor is wolf the offspring of dog—Athanasius concludes that when they say the Son is "of the essence" of the Father, they must in fact mean coessential.[129]

Unlike Origen, Athanasius sees that the Father, Son, and Spirit are

121. Athanasius, "De Synodis," 45. See Hanson, *Search for the Christian Doctrine of God*, 193–94.

122. Arius, "Letter to Alexander," 326–27.

123. Ambrose, "Exposition of the Christian Faith," III, 15. See Williams, *Arius*, 68–69.

124. Arius, "The Banquet," 277.

125. Eusebius of Caesarea (260–340), "Letter to His Church on the Creed of Nicaea," in Stevenson, *New Eusebius*, 344–47.

126. Lewis Ayres claims that there was no intention to define the term. *Nicaea and Its Legacy*, 90.

127. See Davis, *First Seven Ecumenical Councils*, 61.

128. Athanasius, "De Synodis," 41, 43–5.

129. For an account of the defense Athanasius puts forward in favor of the term *homoousios*, see Ayres, *Nicaea and Its Legacy*, 140–44.

"all creative," "indivisible," and their "activity is one": "the Father does all things through the Word in the Holy Spirit."[130] He is likewise clear that "it is a Triad not only in name and form of speech, but in truth and actuality." Timothy Ware, now the Eastern Orthodox Metropolitan Kallistos of Diokleia, argues that Athanasius sees God's unity primarily in terms of substance; hence the significance he places on the term *homoousios*.[131] Given that Athanasius is responding to thinkers who were questioning the unity of the three-in-one, however, it seems natural that he should focus on *homoousios* as unity of substance rather than on the distinction between the members of the triunity. Yet in his efforts to confirm the solidity of the Nicene position, according to Athanasius, "*hypostasis* is *ousia* and means nothing else but simply being."[132] Athanasius does not have a word to express the distinction of Father and Son. This persistent confusion of *ousia* and *hypostasis* meant that even after the Council of Nicaea, its favored term, *homoousios*, could bear a Sabellian meaning.

Linguistic Consensus

For Basil, confusion in *homoousios* leads to the usual two grave misunderstandings: failure to confess identity of essence, *ousia*, means falling into polytheism, and failure to acknowledge distinction of the *hypostases* results in "Judaism" or Sabellianism and the changing of God from Father to Son or to Spirit as the moment required.[133] To adhere to the faith tradition, especially as expressed in liturgy and worship, Basil regards it as crucial to maintain the distinctive qualities of Fatherhood, Sonship, and power to sanctify within the unity of God.[134]

Basil is aware of the problems caused by using *ousia* and *hypostasis* as virtually synonymous.[135] Basil explains that in the West the two

130. Athanasius, *Letters Concerning the Holy Spirit*, First Letter to Serapion.

131. Ware, "Human Person as an Icon of the Trinity."

132. Athanasius, "Ad Afros Epistola Synodica," 4.

133. Basil, *Letter* 210, 236.

134. Basil, *Letter* 214. For the significance that worship and liturgy have for Basil, see Hanson, *Search for the Christian Doctrine of God*, 778–79.

135. Stephen Hildebrand charts a development in the thinking of Basil from seeing *homousios* as synonymous with *ousia* to noting a distinction. *Trinitarian Theology of Basil of Caesarea*, 57–64.

terms are not treated as identical, and Western theologians use *ousia* because they recognize the inadequacies of Latin.[136] Basil says many people think there is no difference, and so, when referring to the Trinity, they claim either that there is one *hypostasis* and therefore one essence or three *hypostases* and so also three substances.[137] Instead, Basil and Gregory of Nyssa argue for a distinction between *ousia* and *hypostasis* where *ousia* signifies the essence of God and *hypostasis* God's manner of being as three persons. This distinction means that *hypostasis* is not merely substance, *ousia*; rather, it is a unique subsistence.[138] Each *hypostasis* shares in the concrete divine nature that remains one. Basil continues, explicitly connecting *hypostasis* and *prosopon*, everything that the Father is is seen in the Son, and everything that the Son is belongs to the Father.[139] Basil regards *hypostasis* as person, though he also appears to be concerned about the Sabellian connotations of *prosopon*.[140] By this link, *prosopon* is seen as a proper existence instead of mere appearance: as Basil explains, for the persons to exist without *hypostases* would be absurd; rather, persons exist in real *hypostases*.[141] The term "person" does not refer to some sort of insubstantial or merely accorded existence. This is perhaps a salutary comment for those bioethicists who regard person as being an insubstantial holder of interests and desires or for those who merely decide who to call a person. For Basil and Gregory of Nyssa, the "union consists in the communion of the Godhead," the community of Father, Son, and Spirit.[142]

Augustine also is aware of language problems, and he too examines the terminology used to express the mystery of the Trinity from both the Latin and Greek perspective.[143] Augustine mentions both Basil and

136. Basil, *Letter* 214.

137. Basil, *Letter* 38. There is some controversy as to whether this is a letter from Basil or from Gregory of Nyssa. Agnes Way argues that Basil is the author (*Letters*, 84n1); Anna Silvas accepts the evidence that Gregory of Nyssa is the author (*Gregory of Nyssa*, 247–48). It is generally agreed, however, that Basil and Gregory of Nyssa hold the same theological viewpoint.

138. See Hildebrand, *Trinitarian Theology of Basil of Caesarea*, 61–62.

139. Basil, *Letter* 38, 8.

140. See Hildebrand, *Trinitarian Theology of Basil of Caesarea*, 87–89.

141. Basil, *Letter* 214.

142. Basil, "On the Holy Spirit," XVIII, 45.

143. Augustine, *The Trinity*, I:8, V:9–10.

Gregory of Nazianzus in his own writings against Julian of Eclanum, a follower of Pelagius, and he lists these two Fathers as among other authoritative bishops from the East who support his teachings against Pelagius since they all teach the Catholic truth.[144] Augustine may have had some of the homilies of Gregory of Nazianzus in Latin from a translation by Rufinus, and he himself translates some sentences from Basil, though he does not mention Gregory of Nyssa. Indeed, Augustine mistakes Gregory of Nazianzus for Gregory of Nyssa as the brother of Basil.[145] Augustine nevertheless independently confirms the moves made by Basil and Gregory of Nazianzus: the Greeks, he says, use *hypostasis* and accept a difference between *hypostasis* and *ousia*, and so confess one *ousia* and three *hypostases*; Latins use one essence and three substances. Augustine explains the clear source of confusion:[146] Latins understand by essence substance, so we cannot say one essence and three substances. Rather, one essence or substance and three persons is preferable and is the most suitable way Latin writers "whose authority carries weight" (possibly he is thinking here of Tertullian) found to enunciate in words what they understood without words. Gregory of Nazianzus had claimed that Latins had to use *persona* (*prosopa*) because of their limited vocabulary.[147] Augustine does accept that "human speech labours under a great dearth of words," but he says that "we say three persons, not in order to say that precisely, but in order not to be reduced to silence."[148] Augustine explains that this use of persons allows us to reflect on the mystery of the Father who is not the Son, the Son who is not the Father, and the Spirit who is neither Father nor Son; they are three. As Augustine points out, Christ says, "I and the Father are one. He did not say 'is one,' which the Sabellians say, but 'are one.'"[149] So, rather than emphasizing individuali-

144. Joseph Leinhard offers a comprehensive account of the connections between Augustine and Basil and Gregory in "Augustine of Hippo, Basil of Caesarea and Gregory Nazianzen," in *Orthodox Readings of Augustine*, 81–99. Leinhard points out that Augustine refers to Basil and Gregory not because they are Greek theologians but because they are teachers of the Catholic truth (99).

145. Augustine, "Answer to Julian," 1.19.

146. Augustine, *The Trinity*, V:9–10.

147. Gregory of Nazianzus, "Orations," 21, 35.

148. Augustine, *The Trinity*, V:10.

149. Augustine, *The Trinity*, V:10.

ty, Augustine focuses on the shared essence of the Persons of the Trinity, for he says the Godhead is "unity of the Trinity."[150]

Cavalieri and Singer are mistaken in their interpretation of *persona* as individual, and their historical excursion into the use of the term "person" by attributing person language to the Council of Nicaea: the Bishops at Nicaea do not use the formula "one substance and three *persons*." Tertullian may be the first theologian to refer to God as "one substance, three persons,"[151] and to use persons to suggest a concrete reality, but this is at a time when terms are imprecise. It is only at the Council of Constantinople in 381, when the connection of the terms *hypostasis* and *prosopon* to *persona* is clearly made, that the Church adopts the formula. At his oration to the council, Gregory of Nazianzus asks the assembly to "bid farewell to all contentious shiftings." He explains that the council avoids the extremes of Sabellianism and Arianism and is walking the "royal road" by confessing "one in substance" and "three in *hypostases* or persons—which term some prefer."[152]

Moving beyond Linguistics

The desire to avoid Sabellianism that denies the distinctiveness of persons, coupled with the recognition that there is a confusion of terms, leads to what Zizioulas calls a "radical change" in the use of the terms *ousia* and *hypostasis* plus the "momentous step" of the identification of *hypostasis* with "person."[153] For Zizioulas, the Cappadocians,[154] Basil, Gregory of Nazianzus, and Gregory of Nyssa take this step,[155] and in so doing, they go beyond the insights of Athanasius,[156] who looks primarily to the shared substance of the persons of the Godhead to ground the unity in God. Zizioulas argues that Basil's view that substance never

150. Augustine, *The Trinity*, VIII:8.

151. Tertullian, "Against Praxeas," XXV.

152. Gregory of Nazianzus, "Orations," 42, 16.

153. Zizioulas, *Being as Communion*, 38–39.

154. Although it has become commonplace to refer to Basil of Caesarea, Gregory of Nazianzus, and Gregory of Nyssa as the Cappadocians, Leinhard points out that this collective title has only been in use since the nineteenth century. *Orthodox Readings of Augustine*, 81.

155. Zizioulas, *Being as Communion*, 17.

156. Zizioulas, *Being as Communion*, 87.

exists without *hypostasis* is crucial for the concept of the person, and unlike Western theologians who follow Augustine in identifying the being of God with his substance, the Cappadocians place the unity of God in the *hypostasis*, the person of the Father who is the cause both of the generation of the Son and of the procession of the Spirit: "the being of God is identified with the person."[157] This gives what Zizioulas terms "ontological content" to each person of the Trinity[158] and thus to the concept of person itself. So, the identification of *hypostasis* with person becomes a momentous step also for anthropology. According to Zizioulas, "as a concept and as a living reality," person is "purely the product of patristic thought."[159]

The concept of the person is rooted in patristic theology, and linking the person to the being of God gives the concept a depth not apparent in ancient classical thinking.[160] Early Christian naming of God as Father, Son, and Spirit expresses a relationship of what Basil, Gregory of Nazianzus, and Gregory of Nyssa clarify as persons, indicating not a divine impersonal substance but a creative and dynamic communion of persons. Yet while Weinandy commends the view of Zizioulas that the Cappadocians offer a relational concept of person, by prioritizing person over substance, there remains the danger of seeing Father as the principle, giving rise "in linear fashion" to the Son and Spirit. Weinandy adds that the Cappadocians do not fully grasp the insight of Athanasius that *homoousios* demands that God is not the Father but is the Father begetting the Son and spirating the Spirit.[161] In contrast to the misapprehension of Cavalieri and Singer, who place significance only on their understanding of the person, there is neither priority of persons nor of substances because "what the one God is is a trinity of persons."[162] Cappadocian, Athanasian, and Augustinian insights work together.

Still, Zizioulas is correct in recognizing as crucial for anthropology Basil's insight that substance never exists without *hypostasis* and

157. Zizioulas, *Being as Communion*, 40–41.
158. Zizioulas, *Being as Communion*, 37–38.
159. Zizioulas, *Being as Communion*, 27.
160. See Long, *From Epicurus to Epictetus*, chap. 16.
161. Weinandy, "Zizioulas," 411.
162. Weinandy, "Zizioulas," 410–11.

his identification of *hypostasis* with person. In contrast, then, to disembodied Lockean insubstantial persons, and Cavalieri's and Singer's self-awareness, persons are real and substantial.

Athanasius, the Cappadocians, and Augustine frequently repeat the belief that although God is known from his operations, "his essence remains inaccessible."[163] We can have some grasp of what God is, yet our knowledge can only be faulty since "he exists, not as we are but as God is."[164] Person language became invaluable in speaking of the Trinity and, in turn, the term "person" came to be associated with the reality of God. In reflecting on how the relationships between the Trinitarian Persons are to be understood, the Fathers turned to analogy. Analogies from nature seem commonplace in earliest Christian thinking: Justin Martyr explains that the Son comes from the Father like fire from fire;[165] Athanasius like stream from fountain.[166] The Fathers also use human and divine analogy, since our most familiar resource is the human being. Yet what emerges is not so much possible likeness of human to divine, but rather radical dissimilarity, a point that is missing in the account offered by Cavalieri and Singer. Nevertheless, discussion takes place through concurrently exploring divine and human persons.

Relationships and the Personal: Insights and Analogies

On Analogy

While for Augustine "faith seeks, understanding finds," and the Creator can be partially known by his works,[167] when it comes to human beings made in the image of God, Augustine says there are grave lim-

163. Athanasius, "Against the Heathens," I, 35; Basil, *Letter* 234; Gregory of Nazianzus, "Orations," 28.17; Gregory of Nyssa, "Answer to Eunomius," Book II; Augustine, *The Trinity*, V:11.

164. Athanasius, "Against the Arians," I, 23.

165. Justin, "Dialogue with Trypho," in *First Apology*, LXI, 2.

166. Athanasius, "Against the Arians," I, 3, 9; III, 23, 3.

167. Lewis Ayres and Andrew Radd-Gallwitz explain that it was accepted that analogies could not fully grasp the nature of the divinity. Moreover, while analogies were discussed in a technical philosophical and rhetorical context, the character of analogy was not part of the debate in theology until after Boethius. "Doctrine of God," 876. See also Augustine, *The Trinity*, XV:2–3.

itations to analogy because there is a great disparity between the Trinity and human beings.[168] Augustine explains that analogies show both great unlikeness and some likeness because God is seen by us (quoting St. Paul) "through a mirror."[169] Even when we see him in heaven "as he is," we shall be like him but never equal.[170] Indeed, Augustine says analogies are made not so that it might be seen "face to face," but so that it might be seen albeit "in an enigma."[171]

There is an initial problem, however. Many commentators divide human and Trinitarian analogies into two often conflicting categories:[172] the category of psychological analogies attributed to Western theologians, especially Augustine, and the category of social analogies linked to Eastern theologians, particularly the Cappadocians.[173] Typically explained, psychological analogy compares the Trinity with a single human person who has distinct dimensions of personality, so the West begins from the unity in God; social analogy compares the Trinity with human community, so the East begins from the threefold in God.[174]

Zizioulas argues against the "Western" interpretation that has "unfortunately entered into modern Orthodox dogmatics."[175] Claiming that the notion of person as an individual goes back to Augustine and Boethius, this Western strand has led, Zizioulas says, to the "equation of person with the thinking, self-conscious individual," the "autonomous self who intends, thinks, decides, acts and produces results," and a culture where that thinking individual has become the highest concept in anthropology.[176] This seems to be the same leap made by Cavalieri and Singer[177] and is clearly to the detriment of people with intellectual disability. As Singer says, Boethius is often regarded as the exemplar of the "solid historical basis" that uses person "to mean a being with certain characteris-

168. Augustine, *The Trinity*, XV:7, 12.

169. Augustine, *The Trinity*, XV:16, 26; 20, 39; 24, 44.

170. Augustine, *The Trinity*, XV:16, 26.

171. Augustine, *The Trinity*, XV:21, 40.

172. See Placher, *Narratives of a Vulnerable God*, 68.

173. See, e.g., Fackre, *Christian Story*, 50; Olson, *Mosaic of Christian Belief*, 147–49; Migliore, *Faith Seeking Understanding*, 78.

174. Olson, *Mosaic of Christian Belief*, 147–49; see also Rolnick, *Person, Grace and God*, 36.

175. Zizioulas, *Being as Communion*, 40.

176. John Zizioulas, quoted in Fox, *God as Communion*, 41–42.

177. Cavalieri and Singer, "Great Ape Project," 136.

tics such as rationality and self-awareness." Moreover, either explicitly or implicitly, modern thought has presumed it is the intention of Boethius to confirm that a person is "an individual substance of rational nature," meaning an individual who actually possesses rationality.[178] Zizioulas adds that the Cappadocian insight is entirely the opposite, where true personhood arises not from one's individualistic isolation from others, but from love and relationship.[179]

But belief that the being of a human being is not important, rather the human being becomes a person through friendship or relationship, seems to be a version of a social construction of disability. Under this construction, there are not people with disabilities. Instead, people are disabled by social attitudes and behavior, and this disablement can be removed by attitudes of friendship.[180] This belief seems to neglect the actual situation of people where impairment is a real aspect of their lived experience. Notably for people with profound intellectual disability, it is precisely their impairment that cannot be overcome.[181]

In disability studies, different models of disability are often placed in opposition. The medical model is criticized for its focus on impairment, restriction, and lack of ability, and placing the "problem" is the medical condition of the individual, while ignoring social attitudes that contribute to disablement. The social model is criticized for its focus on society's attitudes and behavior while ignoring the real issue of impairment. Although these models may be helpful in the way they point out certain aspects of disability, too polarized an approach does not seem to do justice to the complexity of disability.

Similarly, for some, this relatively modern division[182] of East and West and of analogies into psychological and social is useful for analysis. Nevertheless, it allows some writers to draw too sharp a conclusion, and

178. Singer, *Rethinking Life and Death*, 180; Cavalieri and Singer, "Great Ape Project," 136.

179. Zizioulas, quoted in Fox, *God as Communion*, 41–42.

180. See Reinders, *Receiving the Gift of Friendship*, 54–58.

181. Matthews, *Pope John Paul II*, 25.

182. According to Michel Barnes, "only theologians of the last one hundred years" have ever thought that it is true that "Greek theology begins with the reality of the distinct persons while Latin theology begins with the unity of the divine nature." "Augustine in Contemporary Theology," 237–38.

it stereotypes Eastern and Western approaches to the Trinity.[183] Moreover, through exaggerating the difference between Augustine and the Cappadocians, it does not appreciate their considerable overlap: in his introduction to theology, Daniel Migliore, professor of theology, accepts the West linked to psychological and East linked to social distinction, and he places the analogy of lover, beloved, and bond of love between them clearly in the East linked to social camp when it is one of Augustine's analogies, although it is a relational analogy.[184] It is also difficult to argue that the Cappadocians offer a social analogy based on human community[185] since their discussions based on categories of the general and the particular, and on analogy of human and divine activity, are intended to illustrate how different the divine is from the human. Furthermore, the East social and the West psychological divisions do not take account of the context in which analogies are made: the Cappadocians answer Sabellian assertions of persons as appearances, so they focus on the reality of the persons; Augustine confronts Arianism,[186] so stresses the unity. Yet this does not mean either approach excludes the other: this artificial distinction may suggest a choice between the Eastern *person* approach and the Western *substance* approach, but it does so by forgetting the subtlety of the sources. Rather than seeing the approaches as opposed, it seems more informative to see them as complementary and mutually corrective. After all, each analogy reminds us of the limitations of the other.

Arguing from the Many: Father-Son and Fathers-Sons

The significance of family relationship language in Trinitarian theology and in general human discourse is clear and points to more than simply like coming from like. It demonstrates that this is an other, one like me. Denying the family relationship, the Father and Son, to Trini-

183. O'Collins, *Tripersonal God*, 135.

184. Migliore, *Faith Seeking Understanding*, 78.

185. Migliore, *Faith Seeking Understanding*, 78.

186. See Barnes, "Anti-Arian Works," 31–34. For the polemical aspect of Augustine's Trinitarian work against those who argue that the Latin West was free of such controversy, see Barnes, "Augustine in Contemporary Theology," 247.

tarian persons implies that there is an inequality in their relationship. The same can be said for the denial of relationship among certain categories of human beings. Failure to see certain human beings—particularly the embryo created by in vitro fertilization and those embryos who are subject to preimplantation diagnosis or prenatal testing—as in relationship to us, as someone's son or daughter, risks viewing those embryos, particularly disabled ones, as objects or products. As the experience of L'Arche communities[187] demonstrates, seeing people with disabilities simply as service users or individuals who are cared for neglects the significance of relationships and the riches that these relationships provide both for people with disabilities and those who live alongside them. Moreover, the neglect of the significance of relationships fails to appreciate the profundity of our common humanity and is myopic about the contribution that every person, whatever their capacities, makes to the growth in humanity of the other person. Writers in disability studies such as Hans Reinders recognize the importance of family caregivers; however, they are also inclined to view family relationships involving a person with disabilities as simply "a matter of natural necessity" and often a "burden of responsibility." As Reinders says, these relationships are not chosen as friendship.[188] While there is some truth in saying that the family caretaker relationship is not chosen, this view seems to forget the value of other relationships, and it overlooks the real significance of family bonds in the lived experience of people with disabilities that often provide a connection deeper than friendships.

Following Gospel tradition, when the Fathers speak of the one God, they also speak of God in his essence as "Father," a designation they say implies the existence of God the Son.[189] Origen's understanding that "one cannot be a father apart from having a son" and Tertullian's similar

187. The first L'Arche community was set up by the Canadian philosopher Jean Vanier in 1964 in France. Vanier invited two men with learning disabilities to leave their institution and join him in shared living accommodation in a house in Trosly-Breuil. The idea behind L'Arche is that people with disabilities have a great deal to contribute to society and that shared living in community helps all the members of that community, whether disabled or not, to grow and flourish as persons. L'Arche now has communities worldwide.

188. Reinders, *Receiving the Gift of Friendship*, 5.

189. Cyril of Jerusalem, "Catechetical Lectures" 6, 1; 7, 1–5.

understanding[190] represent this relationship as intrinsic to God. Apart from Origen's apparent subordination of the Son to the Father, use of the language of personal family relationships seems to stress the one nature of the three persons.

The Arians resist using "Father" and prefer to use the term "unoriginate" for precisely this reason: they intend to contrast the "unoriginate" to the "originate" Son in order to express subordination. In response, Athanasius insists that "unoriginate" is not a fitting title for the Father on the grounds that it is not scriptural, plus it does not convey the significance of the title Father: "Father" implies Son.[191] Athanasius seems to recognize that the titles of Father and Son denote a specific kind of relationship, today called a personal relationship, and this is destroyed by using impersonal or supposedly neutral terms. Furthermore, Athanasius notes its personal meaning for Christians who are baptized not into the name of unoriginate and originate, nor in the name of Creator and creature, but rather in the name of the Father, Son, and Spirit so that they are made sons.[192] For Athanasius, this familial relationship of persons focuses both on the same nature of the members and on their distinctness: "they are two, because the Father is Father and is not also the Son, and the Son is Son and not also the Father; but the nature is one; (for the offspring is not unlike its parent, for it is his image), and all that is the Father's is the Son's,"[193] perhaps reminding that the debate was not merely about language but also concerned deeper problems. Similarly, whether humans are called persons seems to matter not simply on a linguistic level.

Athanasius is also aware of the problems of likening Father and Son to a human family relationship. The Arians had argued that the Son had a beginning, whereas God was without beginning.[194] Athanasius uses Arius's the *Banquet* to illustrate this Arian insistence that "God was not always a Father; but once God was alone, and not yet a Father, but af-

190. Origen, *De Principiis*, 1, 2, 2, 3; Tertullian, "Against Praxeas," X.
191. Athanasius, "Against the Arians," I, 9, 34. See Leithart, *Athanasius*, 37–38.
192. Athanasius, "Against the Arians," I, 9, 34. See Leithart, *Athanasius*, 35.
193. Athanasius, "Against the Arians," III, 23, 4.
194. Arius, "Letter to Eusebius of Nicomedia," 279.

terwards He became a Father. The Son was not always."[195] According to Athanasius, Arius relies too heavily on relations found in created human realities because Arius interprets generation of the Son in time like human generation, so he can then assert there was a time when the Son was not. Athanasius believes it is not suitable to measure divine generation by human, however.[196] Thus he argues that God's fatherhood is unique and the type of human fatherhood,[197] and therefore that men are not really fathers and sons but rather "shadows of the True":[198] a father, born of his father, has a son, and the son in turn becomes a father. Father and son do not stay in their respective characters, so they are not properly speaking father and son. But it is different in the Godhead: the Father is properly Father since he is not from a father, and the Son is properly the Son; the Father is ever Father and the Son ever Son.[199] Athanasius does not seem to have considered that in human terms a man can be both father and son simultaneously, as Gregory of Nazianzus indicates.[200] But the point Athanasius makes against Arian thinking is that there is no change in God, for Father and Son exist eternally.

The generation of the Son proved to be the source of further controversy. One response to the Nicene *homoousios* was heterousian theology: that the Son is unlike the Father in essence, although he may be in some ways divine.[201] Those, like the Arians, notably Eunomius, who assert the essential difference of the ungenerated Father and generated Son coin the word *anomoios*.[202] Eunomius (ca. 325–95), a Cappadocian rhetor and constant critic of Basil, Gregory of Nazianzus, and Gregory of Nyssa, argues that God can be distinguished from all others because he is unbegotten.[203] But because the Son is begotten, he does not share the same nature. Eunomius distinguishes generation from essence, whereby what

195. Athanasius, "Against the Arians," I, 2, 5; I, 3, 9.
196. Athanasius, "Against the Arians," I, 8, 26.
197. See Ayres, *Nicaea and Its Legacy*, 111–13.
198. Athanasius, "Against the Arians," I, 6, 16.
199. Athanasius, "Against the Arians," I, 6, 21.
200. Gregory of Nazianzus, *Oration* 29, V.
201. See Ayres, *Nicaea and Its Legacy*, 144–49.
202. For an account of the theology of Eunomius and his hierarchy of language, see Barnes, *Power of God*, 173–219.
203. Eunomius, *Extant Works*, Apology 1.

is generated shares in that essence, from generation by will, generation by will being the position, he says, of Origen.[204] Having said the Son's generation is by will of the Father, Eunomius can then claim a subordinate status for the Son. Eunomius differs from Arius since Eunomius believes that Christ was adopted as Son from the very beginning. Echoing accusations made against Arius, however, Gregory of Nyssa claims that Eunomius asserts that there was a time when the Son was not and that he is a creature.[205]

According to Gregory, Eunomius implies that there are three beings, and Eunomius is then forced to make a difference in rank between them to avoid Sabellianism.[206] Gregory is faced with the traditional Arian position that confronted Athanasius: Eunomius is not prepared to use the biblical names Father, Son, and Spirit because they imply that God the Father has a divine Son. Instead, Eunomius prefers "the supreme and absolute Being" for Father and "another Being existing by reason of the First, but after It though before all others" for the Son, the Spirit being "a third Being not ranking with either of these, but inferior."[207] Arguing from tradition, Scripture, and liturgy, Gregory believes that in suppressing the names of Father, Son, and Spirit, Eunomius destroys the proper and natural relationship in the Godhead that the names imply.[208] Furthermore, Eunomius intends to deny that the Spirit properly exists as a person.[209] Eunomius also offers a belief in mere appearances or fiction rather than a real belief in persons who do properly exist.[210] If, Gregory questions, we rely on such fictions, then why be baptized into and live in Christ?[211]

Gregory is also aware that simple analogies of created existence with God's existence do not work,[212] still careful use of them seems neces-

204. Eunomius, Apology 15.
205. Gregory of Nyssa, "Against Eunomius," I, 10.
206. Gregory of Nyssa, "Against Eunomius," I, 19.
207. Gregory of Nyssa, "Against Eunomius," I, 13.
208. Gregory of Nyssa, "Against Eunomius," I, 13, 14.
209. Gregory of Nyssa, "Against Eunomius," I, 14.
210. Gregory of Nyssa, "Against Eunomius," I, 14, 20.
211. Gregory of Nyssa, "Against Eunomius," I, 22.
212. Gregory of Nyssa, "Against Eunomius," I, 18. Michel Barnes explains how, for Gregory of Nyssa, there is a unique type of generation for the Son and any analogy is limited. Gregory of Nyssa, "Contra Eunomium III.6," 369–82.

sary. According to Gregory, everything created is dependent on time and space, whereas God, whose existence is all-sufficient and everlasting, is not in time and space. Rather, he is above all things in an unknowable way. Although we share in existence, there is a whole difference of essence.[213] Since we cannot know God's nature other than he is one, undivided, and simple, when we speak of God as Father or unbegotten, we are speaking with reference not to his (unknowable) substance but to his being a person. And we come to some knowledge of the Father through the person of the Son. The fault of Eunomius lies in his speaking of beings instead of persons: if Eunomius had said that it was not right to confuse the persons in the Godhead, then that would be acceptable. But Eunomius errs by making the actual substantial being of each person different from the others. This leads not only to a plurality of beings with distinctive differences but also to their alienation from each other by those differences: Eunomius breaks their communion of relationship.[214]

Like Athanasius, Gregory of Nyssa sees real significance in the relationship of the Father, Son, and Spirit that does not translate into the more anonymous terms of "supreme Beings." Today, that relationship might be characterized as personal in order to highlight its significance. Contemporary language speaking of humans, particularly embryos, in an impersonal biological way, speaking of the disabled in discriminatory and depersonalizing ways that emphasize the disability over the person, masks the fact that inevitably they exist in relationship to other humans. Gregory's criticism of Eunomius recalls that human beings share a common nature. They exist not merely side by side in community, κοινότης. Rather, they are called to communion, κοινωνία, to recognize each other as persons. This goes beyond simply seeing people with disabilities as friends, as Reinders urges, important as friendship is. As the personalistic philosophies of thinkers like Emmanuel Levinas demonstrate, seeing the other as "an other" can be understood philosophically as well

213. Gregory of Nyssa, "Against Eunomius," I, 26.

214. Gregory of Nyssa, "Against Eunomius," I, 19. According to Lucian Turcescu and through his analysis of Gregory's other writings, "Gregory makes communion among the three persons the important factor that transforms them from mere collections of properties into persons." Turescu emphasizes that this is not simply a community, κοινότης, but a communion, κοινωνία. *Gregory of Nyssa*, 58–60.

as theologically,[215] and this concerns the being of the other as well as relationship in community.

On Not Three Gods

Some of the Fathers were initially concerned that "person" in relation to the Trinity could bear a Sabellian understanding of presentation and so fail to convey the distinction in the Godhead. But "person" now causes some modern theologians concern because it is often understood as a subject of individual self-consciousness and so implies tritheism. Basil, Gregory of Nyssa, Augustine, and Boethius explain that *hypostasis* and *persona* do not indicate separate individuals. Instead, the terms point to what is distinct and unique in the Godhead. Although this conversation takes place by showing the dissimilarity between God and humans, it also illustrates that instead of notions of individualism and its associations with autonomy, control, and having personal desires, the concept of the person highlights the notion of uniqueness.

Basil and Gregory of Nyssa

Hoping to bring further precision to Trinitarian discussion, Basil and Gregory of Nyssa explain that the distinction between *ousia* and *hypostasis* is the same as that between the general and particular. This is understood probably through the influences of Stoicism or Aristotelianism.[216] Using the example of "animal" and "a particular human" to illustrate what is common and what is particular, Basil says that only such a distinction can give a sound account of the faith that in the Godhead there is one essence or substance and three *hypostases*.[217] For Basil, what is in common is the Godhead, and the particular is the distinction made in the characteristics attributed to each: Fatherhood, Sonship, or the power to sanctify, and these define the persons as unique.[218] Moreover, Basil suggests it is insufficient merely to list the differences.[219] To

215. Nigel Zimmermann gives an account of the interrelationship of philosophy and theology in the thinking of Levinas on being and the other in *Levinas and Theology*, chap. 2.

216. See Turescu, *Gregory of Nyssa*, 50–51.

217. Basil, *Letter* 236, 6.

218. Basil, *Letter* 236, 6; 214, 4.

219. Basil, *Letter* 210, 5.

have a clear understanding, he insists that it be acknowledged that each Person has a natural existence in a real *hypostasis*.

To stress that there is no difference in degree for those who are of the same essence, Basil speaks of "man," what is common, and "a certain man," what is particular.[220] An individual, Peter, is no more "man" than Andrew, John, or James: "man" signifies all those alike who are included under the same name. To understand "Peter" or "John" requires a further subdivision.[221] Basil may say that we will "not go wrong" if we use the same standard of difference recognized in *ousia* and *hypsotasis* in human affairs to teaching on the divine,[222] and his explanation accounts for how we can speak of one substance, *ousia*, and three persons, *hypostases*. Basil's analogy with human nature proves problematic, however. When we speak of one human nature and three human beings, we are also speaking of three men. Yet in the Trinity, there is only one God, not three. It remains to explain why humans cannot be one and many, whereas we can say this of God.

Gregory of Nyssa's treatise *On Not Three Gods* provides a partial answer. Gregory explains that when we speak of "many men" because they share in a common nature, it is a mistake of language. Many share the nature of being disciples or martyrs, but "the man in them all is one" since "man" is to do with what is in common. Luke may be a man, but it does not follow that if someone is a man, he must be Luke.[223] Gregory's argument is not without its problems, however.[224] His analogy suggests that each person of the Trinity has a common substance plus an individualizing property, and so he does not escape charges of tritheism. Basil may urge to "count if you must" but do not do damage to the faith, for "the unapproachable is above number" and "we do not let an ignorant arithmetic carry us away to the idea of a plurality of Gods."[225] Still, even

220. Basil, *Letter* 38, 2.

221. For further discussion on Basil and the common and particular, see Hildebrand, *Trinitarian Theology of Basil of Caesarea*, 64–66.

222. Basil, *Letter* 38, 3.

223. Gregory of Nyssa, "On Not Three Gods."

224. Turescu agrees with Christopher Stead that, at this stage of Gregory's argument, it "resembles an accomplished conjuring trick more nearly than a valid theological demonstration." *Gregory of Nyssa and the Concept of Divine Persons*, 66.

225. Basil, "On the Holy Spirit," 18, 44.

though Basil tries to explain that the counting in this case is not "by way of addition" but "according to the distinction of persons, both (Father and Son) are one and one, and according to the community of nature, one,"[226] it seems that either the analogy holds and there appear to be three gods, or there is no satisfactory analogy owing to the difference between divine and human nature.

Turcescu argues that Basil and Gregory have a Neoplatonic understanding of the individual as a collection of properties, whereby some differences are (in Aristotelian terms) substantial: "rational, mortal, and being capable of knowledge belong to man *per se*"; and some, like "hook-nosed or snub-nosed," are accidental.[227] Basil and Gregory also state that each divine *hypostasis* has unique properties: uncaused and being Father, only begotten and Son, proceeding from the Father and Spirit,[228] and that "each of these properties (substance, mode of existence, power) makes the person known to us in part, but no property can be called a person apart from the other properties."[229] But Turcescu points out that the Father, Son, and Spirit are not mere collections of properties or individuals. Rather, they are divine *persons* since, according to Gregory, there is "a certain continuous and uninterrupted communion" in them.[230] This strong connection between them, like a chain where one who lays hold on one end of the chain pulls the other end to him, is "the communion among these persons that makes them persons."[231] This is not to say that persons are not individuals: Zizioulas argues that person is relational and is not to be taken to mean individual, as individuality implies isolation and the seeing of the other as an enemy.[232] But Zizioulas appears to read into the notion of individual person a modern, psychological understanding of person as center of consciousness, one that does not seem present in the Cappadocian context. It is this psychological understanding that Cavalieri and Singer also apply to their view

226. Basil, "On the Holy Spirit," 18, 45.
227. Turcescu, *Gregory of Nyssa*, 38–40 quoting Porphyry.
228. Basil, *Letter* 38, 4; see also Gregory of Nazianzus, "Fifth Theological Oration," II.
229. Turcescu, *Gregory of Nyssa*, 104.
230. Turcescu, *Gregory of Nyssa*, 57–58; Basil, *Letter* 38, 4.
231. Turcescu, *Gregory of Nyssa*, 59; Basil, *Letter* 38, 4.
232. Zizioulas, *Being as Communion*, 105–7.

of the person as a rational self-conscious individual. But the discussion does indicate that Basil and Gregory make a distinction between substance and persons by reference to individuality.

Augustine and Boethius

According to Ambrose, Augustine's mentor, by their division of the Godhead, the Arians were saying that there were two or three gods, and it is for this reason that the Latin West confesses a unity of essence.[233] Unlike Augustine, Ambrose knew Greek and had studied the Eastern Fathers. Ambrose explains that if we can say husband and wife are one flesh, an analogy already seemingly made by Origen in the context of the divine and human in Christ,[234] or all mortal men are of one substance as regards their general nature, then how much more are the Father and Son one in divinity, even if they are in fact beyond comparison.[235]

Augustine picks up this analogy to general nature, yet he is also aware of the problem of possible confusion with human beings as individuals. Whereas the Cappadocians investigate the question, Why not three gods?, Augustine asks the next question: If not three gods, then three what? Augustine explains that Abraham, Isaac, and Jacob are not the same but three. The answer to "what three" is three men, and what they have in common is "man." Regarding God, the answer to "what three" is "three persons," even though man is also called a person and there is a great difference between man and God. "Father" is not what is in common; rather, it is person, used as a generic word, and so there are three persons but, keeping to Scripture, not three gods.[236] As to the suitability of the term "person," it came about out of necessity: we cannot say three essences because that could imply a difference in equality; nor can we say "three somethings" (*tria quaedam*), since that implies Sabellianism.[237] Instead, we use "persons" because that best expresses unity and diversity in relationship. Father, Son, and Spirit are like three friends, three relations, or three neighbors, "for these terms are not said of each

233. Ambrose, "Exposition of the Christian Faith," 1, 1, 10.
234. Origen, *De Principiis*, II, 6, 3.
235. Ambrose, "Exposition of the Christian Faith," 1, 2, 18.
236. Augustine, *The Trinity*, VII:7–8, 11.
237. Augustine, *The Trinity*, VII:9.

one in respect to himself, but in relation to the others": these words "signify a relationship."[238] But if the focus is removed from the "relative" aspect, then the problem with comparing the three divine persons with three friends is that it implies tritheism. Augustine continues, three men share the nature of "man," but it is different for God. Each human person embodies only part of human nature. With God, however, it is the same thing to be, *esse*, and to subsist, *subsistere* (if indeed we can use the term "subsistent" for God at all): the Father, Son, and Spirit together are not a greater essence than the Father alone or the Son alone.[239] Perhaps Augustine erroneously connects Tertullian's *substantia* with *subsistere* instead of *substare*.[240] But if Augustine aims to show that what God is is a triunity, then he may have been careful in his choice of words.

Boethius says he writes in the same tradition as Augustine, following authority of faith and worship.[241] He uses and amplifies Augustine and the Cappadocian understanding of relation in the Trinity to explain that the Trinity is one God, not three gods: God is "predicated thrice," but this does not result in a plural number.[242] We can speak of things being the same, and we can speak of things being diverse in genus (man and horse have the same genus, animal), or species (Cato and Cicero are the same species), or number (Tully and Cicero are one in number).[243] Numerical difference is, Boethius says, caused by accidents, in the technical Aristotelian sense, such as place. However, there are no accidents in God since, unlike human beings, God is his own essence, as he does not depend for his existence on anything, and he is pure form.[244] Boethius uses Aristotelian ideas of matter and form to explain that whereas the Divine Substance is form without matter, a human being is soul and body, not soul or body separately.[245] Although body and soul do not simply equate with biological and biographical life, just as Boethius sees

238. Augustine, *The Trinity*, VII:11.

239. Augustine, *The Trinity*, VII:11.

240. Lancel, *St Augustine*, 379.

241. Boethius, "De Trinitate," I. For the extent to which Boethius may have been influenced by Augustine, see Bowery, "Boethius," 77–79.

242. Boethius, "De Trinitate," III.

243. Boethius, "De Trinitate," I.

244. Boethius, "De Trinitate," II.

245. Boethius, "De Trinitate," II.

the one human being as a unity of body and soul, so too is there no separation between biological and biographical life in the one human being. Moreover, what man is he owes to other things that are not man, such as time and space, as well as higher things such as qualities of virtue, for instance, "just."[246] Thus man is one thing, and a just man is another. But "God is simply and entirely God" and God is justice.[247]

Discussing number in the Trinity, Boethius explains that by using synonymous terms like sword, brand, and blade for the one sword, the speaker does not denote three different things but instead speaks of the identical thing. When using the names Father, Son, and Spirit, however, we are not using synonymous terms, for the Father is not the Trinity, nor is the Son, nor the Spirit.[248] Father, Son, and Spirit are the same but are not identical, and therefore the terms do not result in several different things.[249] They are the same God and are a unity since there is no difference of substance and the diversity of the Trinity is by relation.[250] Relationship is "supersubstantial,"[251] and this "relation of identical" Boethius admits is not found in other things.[252]

Gunton claims that Augustine pulls back Cappadocian teaching because Augustine presents a "view of an unknown substance *supporting* the three persons rather than *being constituted* by their relatedness."[253] Yet it seems that this is not how Boethius interprets Augustine. Moreover, unlike Cavalieri and Singer, who separate person from the being itself, Augustine speaks against seeing the substance of the Trinity as somehow different from the Persons: he says that Father, Son, and Spirit are the Trinity but only one God; there are three Persons, but the divinity, which they have in common, is not "a fourth something, not like

246. Boethius, "De Trinitate," IV.

247. Boethius, "De Trinitate," IV. For differing accounts of the view of Boethius on universals and particulars, see Marenbon, *Boethius*, 79–94; Richard Cross, "Form and Universal in Boethius," 439–58.

248. Boethius, "De Trinitate." Father, Son, and Holy Spirit are substantially predicated of the divinity.

249. Boethius, "De Trinitate," III.

250. Boethius, "De Trinitate," VI.

251. Boethius, "De Trinitate," IV, V.

252. Boethius, "De Trinitate," VI. David Bradshaw also points to some gaps in the thinking of Boethius. "The *Opuscula Sacra*," 108–12.

253. Gunton, *Promise of Trinitarian Theology*, 43; emphasis original.

one of them." Because of this one divinity, "the same Trinity is said to be one God."[254] Augustine speaks of Father and Son as eternally and unchangeably Father and Son.[255] Augustine points out, although "unbegotten" and "begotten" differ in terms of relationship, this does not indicate a different substance because "what is stated relationship-wise does not designate substance."[256] Augustine explains that "every being that is called something by way of relationship is also something besides the relationship." This is an important point to make with regard to the idea that it is relationship or a social theory of being human that is the foundation for a positive understanding of people with disabilities who are radically dependent on others and that a shift away from a Christian anthropology focused on "self-conscious subjectivity as the center of being human, but now conditioned by sociability" is required if relationality is to make a difference.[257] Being and relationality are significant for Augustine, who is concerned that "if being is predicated by way of relationship, then being is not being," and he does want to uphold the view that "each, Father and Son, is substance, and each one is substance."[258] Nevertheless, for Augustine, this analysis of substance and relationship is to assert the real distinction of the persons.[259] Because Augustine is answering the Arians and those who question the consubstantiality of the persons of the Trinity, whereas the Cappadocians are confronting the Sabellians and those who believe that the notion of person is mere presentation, it thus may be that their positions are complementary rather than in opposition. It also appears that in engaging in the "on not three gods" debate, Augustine seeks to avoid the static language of object precisely because of the personal in God.

254. Augustine, *Letter* 120:7. See Ayres, *Nicaea and Its Legacy*, 375.
255. Augustine, *The Trinity*, V:6.
256. Augustine, *The Trinity*, V:8.
257. See Reinders, *Receiving the Gift of Friendship*, 248–52.
258. Augustine, *The Trinity*, VII:2.
259. See Rolnick, *Person, Grace and God*, 25–26.

Mode of Operation

Basil and Gregory of Nyssa

For the Cappadocians, each of the Divine Persons has a distinct mode of existence: the Father is ungenerated and generator, the Son is begotten, the Spirit proceeds from the Father.[260] In contrast to human activity, however, the mode of operation of the Three Divine Persons guarantees their oneness. Whereas when workmen are engaged on a project they remain separated in their own environment in pursuit of the same form of action, the Father, Son, and Spirit do not each have their own special operation apart from the others.[261] Rather, every operation "has its origin from the Father, and proceeds through the Son, and is perfected in the Holy Spirit." This unity of action spills over into creation so that "the Father, the Son and the Holy Spirit alike give sanctification, and life, and light and comfort, and all similar graces."[262]

Augustine

Augustine accepts that the idea of inseparable operations is an inherited part of the tradition; however, he realizes this may lead some to believe that the whole Trinity assumes human nature and thus perhaps to patripassianism.[263] This was one of the problems facing Tertullian, and Augustine seems to operate out of the Latin tradition and Tertullian's three persons one substance formula.[264] To offer a partial explanation against patripassianism, Augustine comments on Christ's baptism: the Trinity is distinguished by Father as voice, Son as man, and Spirit as dove. The Father does nothing without the Son nor the Son without the Father—indeed, the Birth, Passion, and Resurrection are the work of both—yet the distinction of the persons is expressed for the sake of our

260. See Gregory of Nazianzus, "Fifth Theological Oration (Oration 31)." For the Creed of Constantinople, 381, see Kelly, *Early Christian Creeds*, 297–98. See also Turcescu, *Gregory of Nyssa*, 103–6.

261. Gregory of Nyssa, "On Not Three Gods."

262. Gregory of Nyssa, "On the Holy Trinity"; Gregory of Nazianzus, "Second Theological Oration (Oration 28)." See Ayres, *Nicaea and Its Legacy*, 216–17.

263. Augustine, *Letter* 11; idem, *Sermon* 2, 6. See also Ayres, *Nicaea and Its Legacy*, 373–74.

264. See Ayres, *Augustine and the Trinity*, 78–81.

weakness. Of course, for Augustine, if we can understand this fully, then we cannot be speaking about the unknowable God.[265]

Arguing from Inside: The Word and Words

Given the creative act of the Word in Genesis, its personification in Wisdom, and the Word of God become flesh of St. John's Gospel, it seems natural for the early Fathers to use the analogy of word and the Word to reflect on the relationship of Father and Son in the Trinity. Justin Martyr compares what happens in human beings and the generation of the Son, for as when we speak "we beget a word," so too with God's Word the Father speaks and it comes to be.[266] Yet more considered opinion seems guarded: like Justin Martyr, Irenaeus accepts that the generation of Son from Father is often likened to human speech, yet he also seems to feel that further conjecture about the infinite being of God is futile.[267]

Although there is this early understanding of the Son as Word of the Father, there does not appear to be any connection made between this analogy to human speech and the *per sonare* of theatrical roles, and the mask through, *per*, which resounds, *sonare*, the voice of the actor. Apparent failure to pursue the analogy may have been due to unease at its implications of subordinating the Son. In Platonic thought, the internal word as intelligible rather than sensible was thought to be superior to the spoken word.[268] Similarly, the Stoics made a distinction between internal speech and uttered speech, and they thought that the possibility of making this distinction differentiated human beings from animals. For the Stoics, speech appears to have manifested rationality.[269] Athanasius seems to confirm that the analogy to human speech is problematic and may imply subordinationism when he suggests that the controversial bishop Marcellus of Ancyra incorrectly taught that the Son was the "mere Word of God and non-existent" until expressed later. To reassert the Son's dis-

265. Augustine, *Sermon* 2, 1–14.
266. Justin Martyr, "Dialogue with Trypho," in *First Apology*, 61.
267. Irenaeus, "Against Heresies," II, XXVIII, VI.
268. Toom, "Potential of a Condemned Analogy," 205–6.
269. Long, *From Epicurus to Epictetus*, 242.

tinctness and preexistence, Athanasius explains instead that orthodoxy holds the Son to be "Living God and Word, existing by himself. . . . being and abiding with his Father before all ages."[270]

A century before Marcellus and Athanasius, Tertullian uses the analogy when arguing for the reasonableness of holding that the Son was with the Father eternally. But he does so by stressing the difference between the Word and human words.[271] Tertullian compares the Father and Word with human thought and consciousness: just as our word or thought is like a second person within us, so too was God not alone. Instead, he was in dialogue with the *Logos*, his Reason. Tertullian, however, arguably influenced by Stoic materialism, also explains that unlike sounds that are air, made intelligible to the ear but otherwise void, the substantiality of the Word is from the Father, for nothing insubstantial can come from the Father.

For Gregory of Nazianzus, the Son is called Word "because he is to the Father what a word is to the mind; not only because of his passionless generation, but also because of his union and because of his conveying information."[272] Gregory of Nyssa stresses the difference between the human word that is limited and transient, and the divine *Logos* that has an independent life, activity, and will.[273] Augustine also discusses the Word and human words; however, he uses the analogy specifically for the Incarnation. He explains that although our words are greatly unlike the Word, as our word becomes an articulate sound but is not changed into one, so does the Word become flesh but is not changed into it.[274]

The Fathers, then, seem to be wary of using analogy of human words to the Word unless clear distinctions are made. Setting too much store on speech may also be problematic in bioethics. Like the Stoics, the seventeenth-century philosophers Descartes, Hobbes, and Locke also believe that speech marks the difference between human beings and animals, but on the grounds that speech indicates the presence of

270. Athanasius, "De Synodis," 26, 15–17.
271. Tertullian, "Against Praxeas," 5.
272. Gregory of Nazianzus, "Oration" 30, 32.
273. Gregory of Nyssa, "Great Catechism," I.
274. Augustine, *The Trinity*, XV:20.

thought.[275] This link between the spoken word and rationality can be found well into the late nineteenth century in understandings of disability where those who could not speak—notably the deaf, who it was believed could not learn communication—were regarded as inhuman and below the animals.[276] Moreover, this seems to filter through to some contemporary disablist views of some disabled people, where assumptions are made about lack of mental capacity based on lack of speech and where such patients are treated as "less valuable" than nondisabled people.[277]

Looking to the Self Within

A charge made against some Western patristic theology is that it has decisively influenced the modern view of the person as essentially a rational individual. This is at the expense of the more relational approach found in Eastern patristic theology.[278] Gunton claims that Augustine's turn toward the inner self in particular marks the start of intellectualism and leads to modern individualism.[279] Notably, however, Basil and Gregory of Nyssa in their Trinitarian theology also reflect on the inner person. This reflection on the inner person found in both Eastern and Western theology perhaps indicates not so much individualism as the significance of the "spirit of man."[280] This is not to denigrate the whole person as embodied soul. Rather, it illustrates that the soul takes priority.

Basil and Gregory of Nyssa

In advance of Augustine, and quoting 1 Corinthians 2:11, Basil makes the turn inward to self and explores the usefulness of mind as a point of reflection: "the greatest proof of the conjunction of the Spirit with the Father and the Son is that He is said to have the same relation to God

275. Descartes, "Discourse on Method," in *Descartes*, 46–82, Discourse Part 5; Hobbes, *Leviathan with Selected Variants*, III, 11; IV, 22; Locke, *Essay Concerning Human*, III, VI, 22.

276. Albrecht, *Encyclopedia of Disability*, 142.

277. Scope, "Memorandum from Scope," 79–80.

278. See Reinders, *Receiving the Gift of Friendship*, 227–75.

279. Gunton, *Promise of Trinitarian Theology*, 37, 39.

280. Basil, "On the Holy Spirit," 16, 40.

which the spirit in us has to each of us: 'for what man it is said, knows the things of a man, save the spirit of man which is in him? Even so the things of God knows no man but the Spirit of God.' "[281] Similarly, Gregory of Nyssa speaks of the human mind in terms of its ability to do many operations while remaining one, which allows us to reason that God's many operations do not destroy his unity. Nevertheless, Gregory of Nyssa also considers that the disunity in us highlights the distinction between our existence and that of God.[282]

Augustine

Augustine also reflects on the "inner man," specifically in the context of his search for something in creation that proves that three things can be exhibited separately yet whose operation is inseparable. It appears that Gunton does not appreciate this specific context. Instead, Gunton says Augustine is "well-known" for being suspicious of the material world and is "rather embarrassed by too close an involvement of God in matter," such that anything containing matter is least suitable as an image of the Trinity.[283] According to Gunton, owing to "spectacles so strongly tinted with neoplatonic assumptions," Augustine finds it difficult to believe the material world can "either be truly real or the object or vehicle of knowledge," so he either misunderstands or distorts his predecessors and then relies on intellectualism and individualism for his own approach.[284] But bearing in mind the context, and examining what Augustine has to say on creation and analogy, the situation may not be as clear as Gunton makes out. After all, Augustine explains that we could "roam over the creation" to find instances of three separate things showing inseparable operations, or we could try something more familiar and "search for it first in your own self."[285] Reinder's view that the relationships described by Augustine are "exclusively intrapersonal rather than interpersonal"[286] requires more nuance.

281. Basil, "On the Holy Spirit," 16, 40.
282. Gregory of Nyssa, "On the Making of Man," VI, 1–2.
283. Gunton, *Promise of Trinitarian Theology*, 33, 35, 44.
284. Gunton, *Promise of Trinitarian Theology*, 33, 37, 39.
285. Augustine, *Sermon* 2, 17.
286. Reinders, *Receiving the Gift of Friendship*, 264–65.

In his *Confessions*, Augustine charts his move away from Stoicism that saw everything, including the divine, in material terms. It may also be that Augustine is aware of Tertullian's material views concerning God, even though he argues that it was not for these that Tertullian was considered a heretic.[287] Yet Stoic influences perhaps modify Augustine's apparent Neoplatonism.[288] Augustine also distances himself from the Manichaean view he once held, that all matter is evil. Augustine insists on the difference between God and his creation while also exclaiming how creation points to God: the very presence of heaven and earth speaks, "it was you who made them, Lord: you are beautiful, so it must have been you, because they are beautiful; you who are good must have made them, because they are good; you who are, because they are. Yet not in the same way as you, their creator, are they beautiful and good, nor do they exist as you exist; compared with you they have neither goodness nor beauty nor being."[289] There is then a hint of the Trinity in the created world.[290]

Although he sees the created world as good and reflective of God's goodness, Augustine is asking, "from what likeness or comparison of things known to us we are able to believe, so that we may love the as yet unknown God?"[291] Augustine's chief concern is that we cannot love what we do not know.[292] In his search for some likeness, he moves from creation and its hints of the Trinity to human beings who, as image of God, bear traces of the Trinity, even if, as Augustine always adds, that image is different from the divine and "falls far short" of God.[293]

Augustine considers that love holds the key, because in loving one's neighbor, one loves God, because if one loves, one knows love, and God is love. In other words, you see the Trinity if you see love.[294] He then identifies as a trace of the Trinity three things in love: the one that loves,

287. Augustine, *De Haeresibus of St. Augustine*, 86.
288. See Colish, *Stoic Tradition*, 144–45.
289. Augustine, *Confessions*, XI:6.
290. Augustine, *City of God*, XI:24.
291. Augustine, *The Trinity*, VIII:8.
292. Augustine, *The Trinity*, IX:3.
293. Augustine, *City of God*, XI:26; *Sermon* 2, 17; *The Trinity*, IX:2.
294. Augustine, *The Trinity*, VIII:12.

the beloved and love.[295] The Holy Spirit is "gift" of both the Father and the Son and signifies the unity of love between them.[296] But Augustine moves away from the lover, beloved, and love analogy to one within the mind itself, since the lover and beloved can be separated totally.[297] His intention is to discover three separate things whose operation remains inseparable.

Augustine next identifies two traces of the Trinity in the mind: first, the mind, the knowledge whereby the mind knows itself, and the love whereby it loves both itself and its knowledge of itself, and, second, memory, understanding, and will.[298] He argues that, unlike a drink made up from water, wine, and honey that makes up one completely mixed drink yet its ingredients are not of one substance, mind, love, and knowledge exist as one and the same essence, yet they are not confounded by the comingling.[299]

Like the analogy of general and particular, the analogy of the mind is also problematic. Augustine himself is aware it is not perfect,[300] as perhaps his many attempts to find different analogies indicate. An analogy of mind may give the impression of a close unity, yet it is not at all clear that there is not one entity, the mind, with two of its activities, or that each remain permanently distinct. Thus the analogy casts doubt on the distinctness of the Persons by tending toward a form of Sabellianism;[301] the general and particular analogy tends toward tritheism. Moreover, Gunton points out that Augustine's designation of the Spirit as gift or bond between the lover and beloved does not appear to give enough weight to the Spirit[302] and may depersonalize the third Person. In his criticism of Augustine's theology in comparison to Eastern theology, however, Gunton does not seem to be aware that Gregory of Nyssa calls the Son the Father's glory and the Holy Spirit the glory of them both.[303]

295. Augustine, *The Trinity*, VIII:14.
296. Augustine, *The Trinity*, V:12; VI:7.
297. Augustine, *The Trinity*, IX:6.
298. Augustine, *The Trinity*, X:17–19.
299. Augustine, *The Trinity*, IX:7.
300. See Ayres, *Nicaea and Its Legacy*, 381.
301. See Brown, *Divine Trinity*, 273–74.
302. Gunton, *Promise of Trinitarian Theology*, 51.
303. Gregory of Nyssa, *Homily* 15.

Augustine likewise makes it clear that he is speaking of the Spirit as gift "relationship-wise." If, however, the relationship between Father and Son is concretized in the Spirit, then that may point not only to the persons but also the relationships that are personal.

Basil of Caesarea, Gregory of Nyssa, and Augustine: Comment on Their Analogies

Analogies looking at the relationship between human beings and between the Persons of the Trinity seem to focus on the significance of communion, of seeing in the other an other. What is also apparent is that the distinctions between the Divine Persons point to uniqueness or incommunicability, not to individuality. As Boethius explains, however, the "relation of identical" only applies mysteriously to the Godhead.[304] After all, God is a unity, and for thinkers who take the Aristotelian position that it is matter that is the individuating principle, this can only apply to material beings.[305] In the case of human beings, there is a separation and a measure of individualization, as Gregory of Nyssa realizes in his treatise *On Not Three Gods* and when he discusses the divine mode of operation. For some theologians, like Gunton and Zizioulas, this individuality in both the divine and human is disastrously overemphasized by (exclusively) Augustine's analogy to the "inner man." Certainly, analogies of the Trinity to the "inner man," made not only by Augustine but also by Basil and Gregory, indicate the significance of self-reflection, self-awareness, and understanding as well as willing and desiring. But instead of representing a turn toward intellectualism and individualism, as Gunton and Zizioulas charge against Augustine, for Basil, Gregory, and Augustine, this is merely another way of deepening reflection on what is, ultimately a mystery where words are inadequate. Perhaps Augustine's further exhortation on how human beings grow as persons by imitation of the self-giving communion of the Trinity can offset the charge of individualism by its focus on the relational aspect of human persons.

304. Boethius, "De Trinitate," VI.
305. See Hill's comment in in Augustine, *The Trinity*, 230n36.

Image of God: As Trinity

The Fathers took seriously the idea of the image of God in human beings, and part of their thinking included growing into that likeness through grace and a life of prayer and virtue. Carol Harrison, who has written extensively on Augustine, suggests that Augustine's *The Trinity* was "intended as a work on the Christian life as it should be lived in relation to man's creator, reformer and redeemer,"[306] rather than reflection on the Trinity itself. Augustine's analogies seem to encourage a conversion process, where the journey inward leads to the journey upward, and we are brought from love of self toward love of God and neighbor. Augustine takes the Holy Spirit, a bond of absolute love that unites the Father and the Son, and applies it to humans. He explains that just as the Spirit joins the Father and the Son, so "we are bidden to imitate this mutuality by grace, both with reference to God and to each other, in the two precepts on which the whole law and the prophets depend."[307]

Unlike Pelagius, for whom grace seems to be knowledge of the law, and pure obedience to the law through the person's unfettered free choice leads to salvation,[308] Augustine recognizes that human beings are not self-sufficient but are dependent throughout on grace and the fellowship of others. For a theology of disability, this dependence is central, since it connects all human beings no matter their situation or condition to each other and to God. Notably in theology, the problem for humanity is not impairment or disability but spiritual disfigurement. For Augustine, the start of every sin is pride, the exaltation of self, where the human being "as if he were the light turns himself away from that true Light which, had man loved it, would have made him a sharer in the light."[309] Pride's denial of dependence characterizes the "earthly city" whose inhabitants seek dominion over others; the people of the city of God show "a loving concern for others."[310] This aspect of the Persons of the Trinity, becoming a model for the way human persons are to relate

306. Harrison, *Augustine*, 38.
307. Augustine, *The Trinity*, VI:7.
308. See Augustine, "Deeds of Pelagius."
309. Augustine, *City of God*, XIV:13.
310. Augustine, *City of God*, XV: 7.

to each other, seems a valuable reflection for how we are to be concerned with all humans, particularly the small, weak, marginalized, and disabled.

Modern Divine Persons

If person is taken to refer to rational self-consciousness, as some bioethical thinking has it, then this has serious repercussions for Trinitarian theology. In a somewhat modalistic approach, the theism of the philosopher Richard Swinburne readily presents God as "in some sense *a person*," and by "person" Swinburne means "an individual with basic powers (to act intentionally), purposes and beliefs."[311] His theism supposes that God is like us in having basic powers, but only more so: they are infinite,[312] so God is a person "in a somewhat extended sense."[313] For Swinburne, a person is "essentially a soul, a subject of mental properties, someone with a capacity for feeling, thought or intentional action."[314] He then "loosens up" this meaning so that he has a "stretched sense of 'person'" for the divine[315] to account, for instance, for his "supreme form."[316] In contrast to the Fathers, Swinburne focuses on the similarity rather than the difference between human and divine persons. He also claims that this theism, a view he says is common to Christianity, Judaism, and Islam, presents the "existence of one divine being, a person on whom all else depends" that is compatible with belief in the Trinity "given that any other divine person depends on the first person for his existence and for the delimitation of the sphere within which it would be good for him to act."[317] Swinburne maintains that he offers "a moderate form of social Trinitarianism" in that the divine Persons "would be the same individual but for the relational properties which are distinct from the divine essence and which distinguish them."[318] Swinburne's person as "a subject

311. Swinburne, *Is There a God?*, 4; emphasis original.
312. Swinburne, *Is There a God?*, 5.
313. Swinburne, *Coherence of Theism*, 101n1.
314. Swinburne, *Christian God*, 31.
315. Swinburne, *Coherence of Theism*, 286–87.
316. Swinburne, *Coherence of Theism*, 157.
317. Swinburne, *Existence of God*, 344.
318. Swinburne, *Christian God*, 189.

of mental properties" seems to chime with some bioethical approaches to the person to the detriment of people with profound disabilities.

In response to Swinburne, the philosopher Brian Davies points out that if we see God as a person in terms of being an immaterial, conscious individual with mental changes and as one who acts, then God merely becomes an invisible inhabitant of the universe, an "extraordinary person,"[319] and in this sense Davies argues that God is not a person at all. But other writers have also indicated the problems of understanding Divine Persons as centers of consciousness.

According to the Swiss Reformed theologian Karl Barth, in contrast to the modern idea of person, the Trinity is not "three divine I's, but thrice of the one divine I."[320] The addition of self-consciousness to the notion of person means, for Barth, that the older concept, a concept that embraced incommunicability and relationality, has, outside "monastic and a few other studies," "become completely obsolete and is now unintelligible." According to Barth, among strategies used for thinking about the Trinity are some Protestant views that embrace modern ideas by seeing the Persons as three independently thinking and willing subjects, some neo-Protestants who take a Sabellian view that God takes on three roles, and Roman Catholics who speak of persons as though the modern concept of person and personality did not exist. Instead, Barth prefers to refer to the divine Persons as "mode (or way) of being," since he says this is a more literal translation of *modus entitatiuus*, what he sees as the traditional context for referring to *prosopon* or *subsistentia*, a concept that expresses the idea that God is One but in three ways of being: Father, Son, and Spirit.[321]

Similarly, the German Catholic theologian Karl Rahner writes of the danger of thinking of the Trinity in terms of three different consciousnesses. The modern person, he argues, developed independently of the doctrine of the Trinity and holds the existential meaning of the ego opposed to every other person in its independent, proper, and distinctive freedom. Yet, he says, it is then incorrectly applied to God.[322] The question arises whether the arguments for abandoning the term "person" re-

319. Davies, *Reality of God*, 61–62.
320. Barth, *Church Dogmatics*, 351.
321. Barth, *Church Dogmatics*, 357–58.
322. Rahner, *Theological Investigations*, 101.

garding the Trinity greatly outweigh the arguments in favor of retaining it. Still, Rahner claims, unlike Barth, not to suggest that the person is no longer apt and should be replaced, but he does wish to point out its present ambiguity. Rahner seems mistaken in thinking that Barth wants to replace person in Trinitarian theology, however, for Barth says that the present confusion does not support outlawing or abandoning the concept but only applying it "in a sense of a practical abbreviation."[323]

Both Barth and Rahner clearly point to the difficulty, in a modern context, of using person for the Persons of the Trinity, though the Fathers were also aware of the dangers of using human persons as models for the divine. Yet both Barth and Rahner seem reluctant to give up the word entirely, even though they may suggest alternative ways of speaking. This perhaps finds a parallel with some bioethical confusion about human persons. Apart from the few writers, like the philosopher Derek Parfit, who seek the disintegration of the concept of the person,[324] contemporary thought seems convinced that there is something to being a person, whether that is expressed in rights, protection, or privilege of preference and satisfaction of desires. Similarly, in theology, alternative terms like "mode of being" or "principle," "source" or "ground of being" simply do not do the work expected from the word person. As Rahner explains, the word "person" has been sanctioned by usage, and "there is no other word which would be really better, more generally understandable and less exposed to misconceptions."[325]

The language of "three Persons in one God" persists precisely because the concept of person bears the kind of resonance theology is in search of when reflecting on a God who is personally involved with his creation. Independently of its technical or philosophical use, person immediately conveys some sort of meaning to every human being.[326] Reducing the person to rational self-consciousness seems an unwarranted extrapolation of its theological development; abandoning or replacing the idea of person does not seem to do justice to the Christian insight that God is a personal God. For the Dominican theologian Herbert McCabe, it seems

323. Barth, *Church Dogmatics*, 359.
324. Parfit, *Reasons and Persons*, 215, 217, 445.
325. Rahner, *Theological Investigations*, 101.
326. Kasper, *God of Jesus Christ*, 288.

"absurd" to say God is impersonal, since in principle what is impersonal can always become subject to us and is therefore limited,[327] a point worth considering if the profoundly disabled are regarded as nonpersons.

Modern Human Persons

The evangelical theologian Stanley Grenz accepts that Boethius's understanding of the person is "tied to Greek philosophy and not identical to the modern idea." But he also argues that Augustine's focus on the mind in the person's inward journey to God and Boethius's connection of person with "being an individual" both give the "impetus" to the "modern elevation of individuality" and the modern "inner self."[328] Grenz then says that Descartes merely raises the "first person" standpoint inherited from Augustine "to a new level."[329] Gunton claims that Boethius lies at "the heart of the trouble"[330] and Augustine bequeathed this "baneful legacy"[331] of radical individualism and rationalism. These are serious charges, given the repercussions that holding to an overly rational account of the human person has for the profoundly disabled human being.

As the philosopher Charles Taylor points out, "radical reflexivity," the "turn to self," the way I experience my activity, thought, and feeling, may begin with Augustine.[332] After all, Augustine's *Confessions* seems to be an entirely new genre of writing, part autobiography, part praise offered by a Christian from his very being to God. So, Augustine perhaps is the "inventor of the argument we know as 'cogito.'"[333] Nevertheless, with Descartes, the argument appears to change. Augustine makes the first-person standpoint fundamental for the search for the truth. Yet, for Augustine, this inward turn leads to the recognition that we are called to image God as the self-giving Trinity, but, he adds, we cannot do this ourselves: we need grace.

327. McCabe, *God Matters*, 8–9.
328. Grenz, *Social God and the Relational Self*, 61, 67.
329. Grenz, *Social God and the Relational Self*, 70.
330. Gunton, *Promise of Trinitarian Theology*, 92.
331. Gunton, *Promise of Trinitarian Theology*, 43.
332. Taylor, *Sources of the Self*, 131.
333. Taylor, *Sources of the Self*, 133.

Summary

The Persons of the Trinity are not insubstantial or fictional or like something that masks another reality, like the desires and interests of contemporary bioethical persons. Rather, the Divine Persons are distinct, concrete realities, but not separate. They are in relation, but they are not like individual centers of consciousness: there are not three gods. Reflection on early Trinitarian theology demonstrates the significance of holding both to the one and to the three of the One God in three Divine Persons. For human anthropology, this points to the importance of seeing human beings both as relational beings and beings that are unique in their own right. People with disabilities, like all other people, belong to the human family, and they have their own irreplaceable uniqueness as persons.

The significance of the Fathers' debates rests not on linguistics but on the issues of salvation and divinization: as Athanasius says, the Son is God and so can save us. "He was made man that we might be made God."[334] Moreover, this divinization of human beings is not the result of our own efforts: since only God is holy by nature, only a divine agent can make us creatures holy.[335] As Norman Russell explains from the thinking of Cyril of Alexandria, humanity is raised through Christ and the exaltation of Christ's humanity to participation in the divine life.[336] Thus, in theology, being a human person is significant, and it also has direction: it involves the call to grow to the best of our abilities and with the aid of grace into the likeness of God, who is Trinity.

A constant theme in both East and West is that all analogies or explanations limp where reflection focuses on what is after all the mystery of God and, as made in his image, the mystery of the human person. Yet while Trinitarian reflection highlights dissimilarity of God and humanity, it is with Christ, God and Man, both in one genuine Person, that the dialogue of divine and human persons continues even more directly.

334. Athanasius, "On the Incarnation," 54, 3.

335. Athanasius, *Letters of Saint Athanasius*, 1, 24; Basil, "On Psalm 32," 4.

336. Russell, *Doctrine of Deification*, 164–205.

4. Discerning Persons ❧ *The Word*

Introduction

"In whatever way the clay was pressed out, He was thinking of Christ, the Man who was one day to be: because the Word, too, was to be both clay and flesh."[1] This quotation from Tertullian sets up reflection on how the person of Christ brings light to the concept of human persons. "In whatever way" may be a reminder that different thinkers have different ways of speaking about human beings. The Fathers, and those with whom they debate, use their anthropological beliefs to elucidate their thoughts on the God-made-man. But "in whatever way" is also a salutary reminder that this image of Christ applies to all human beings, no matter what their condition or situation. And the modern tendency of seeing the person purely as a center of consciousness has parallels in mistakes made in how the two natures of Christ were seen, mistakes corrected by some profound and carefully worked out patristic thinking.

This chapter draws attention to the way in which patristic discussion on the human and divine in Christ occurs alongside discussion of the reality of the human being. Since it is important for the clarity of later chapters, this chapter gives a lengthy and painstaking account of human anthropology. Although some aspects of the discussion seem to have specific relevance to people with disabilities, the focus in this chapter is deliberately on human beings. This is because people with disabilities are in fact not different from other people, and theological insights apply as much to the disabled as to all: there is no "them" and "us."

1. Tertullian, "On the Resurrection of the Flesh," 6. The quotation is from the *Corpus Christianorum* translation in Jurgens, *Faith of the Early Fathers*, 1:149 where the treatise is known as *The Resurrection of the Dead*; general reference is made to the more widely available *On the Resurrection of the Flesh*, in *Ante-Nicene Fathers*, vol. III. Although the meaning is the same, the turn of phrase in the *Corpus Christianorum* is less unwieldy.

Difficulties and Opportunities in Speaking about the Word

The God-made-man presents the Fathers with the problem of expressing how the divine immutable nature can be united to a human mutable nature.[2] Stress on a real unity risks blurring the distinction, emphasis on the distinction jeopardizes a real unity. For the Fathers, a natural point of reference is the union of what some of them take to be the two separate substances of body and soul in human beings. Although not the same, the separation made by some bioethicists between biological life and biographical life has parallels in this early theological conversation. As early thinkers struggle with Christology, often because of their anthropologies, they offer descriptive discussion on what the human person is like. Again, as a parallel with some modern thinking on people with disabilities, some consider whether the locus of the human person is exclusively in the human mind or soul, and almost all reflect on the relationship of body to soul. Early Christian anthropologies and Christologies draw attention to some blind spots, contrasts, distortions, and corrections. These provide fruitful ground for reflection on the human person, particularly since some of their concerns have resonance with some bioethical thought and with disability.

In their Pastoral Constitution *Gaudium et Spes, On the Church in the Modern World*, the Fathers of the Second Vatican Council clarify the focus that Christ places on the human person: "in reality it is only in the mystery of the Word made flesh that the mystery of man truly becomes clear."[3] In addition to descriptive anthropology, early Christology offers theological anthropology. Many of the insights reached through reflection on Christ speak also to human persons, and so the concept of the person can be deepened by relating that mystery to the mystery of Christ. But it is not so much about refining or redefining characteristics or attributes so that another instance of a person can be identified more accurately. The mystery of the Word made flesh speaks of the paradox of

2. Apparently, for early thinkers, although the species of humanity was fixed, individual humans were mutable; see Shults, *Christology and Science*, 26.

3. Second Vatican Council, *Gaudium et Spes*, nn. 903–1001.

strength in weakness, of total self-giving, as the Word empties himself and takes on human littleness in order to raise humanity up to God.

In early Christological thinking, there is a clear shift in focus from attention to certain particularly significant aspects of the human being, such as soul or mind, to being attentive to the actual person of Christ. The anthropology and Christology of Irenaeus and Tertullian develop in relation to salvation and resurrection. Their thinking reflects the preoccupation of the earliest Christians about how to understand salvation in the light of the Incarnation, Passion, Death, and Resurrection of Christ rather than reflection on the human person. Nevertheless, following St. Paul, Christ is the "last Adam" and our pattern,[4] and just as Jesus rose again, so too will those who have died in Christ be risen:[5] "as we have borne the likeness of the earthly man, so we shall bear the likeness of the heavenly one."[6] So, two issues intertwine: belief in Christ's Incarnation and Resurrection confirms that the whole person and not merely some higher human aspect is the subject of salvation; moreover, who Christ is, and not simply what he does, matters for salvation. Inextricably linked to salvation, the Christologies of Irenaeus and Tertullian reflect on the two natures of Christ, his divinity and his humanity, as these writers establish the reality of both in Jesus. While engaged in this enterprise, these two champions of early Christianity make parallels with the reality of the human person.

There is a change in gear with Origen's perspective on resurrection, and his focus on the human rational soul. However, the event that sets the scene appears to be the debate between Paul of Samosata and Malchion, where reflection on Christ, true God, and true man turns into a more detailed investigation, and Christian thinkers look more toward the familiar analogy of the relationship between body and soul to help them clarify the relationship between divine and human in Jesus. For many, this analogy seems most appropriate because it appears to explain how two disparate elements are united in one. So, some assert this unity of two natures in Jesus on a seemingly unquestioned parallel with the unity of body and soul in human beings.

4. 1 Cor 15:45–49.
5. 1 Thes 4:13–18.
6. 1 Cor 15:47–49.

The debate between Paul and Malchion as well as reactions to Origen lead into the traditionally named *logos-sarx*, or Alexandrian, and *logos-anthropos*, or Antiochene, Christologies. Some early thinkers from both Christologies ask "What is a real human being like?" as a preparation for considering the God-made-man. Since the philosophical climate of the time was broadly based on responses to Platonism or to Aristotelianism, an oversimplified view is to see the *logos-sarx* Alexandrian approach as influenced by Platonic anthropology and the *logos-anthropos* Antiochene approach as approximating Aristotelian anthropology. The Platonic approach regards the human person as not having anything truly to do with the body or the animal soul that causes the body to function.[7] Rather, the person is mind, *nous*. The Aristotelian approach sees the human person in terms of a whole though composite nature. But the latter tends toward seeing a fragile union of soul and flesh or sometimes of soul, flesh, and spirit.[8]

Although the two approaches illustrate the kind of thinking behind early Christology and anthropology, it seems easy to overstate philosophical influences, and there are difficulties in making too neat a distinction between the two approaches or characterizing one as Platonic and one as Aristotelian: the Alexandrian approach is influenced by Platonism, yet it also seems to have an Aristotelian understanding of human persons, with its strong emphasis on the unity of the body and soul; although more Aristotelian, the Antiochene approach has Platonic elements since body and soul are seen as separate substances in relation.[9] Moreover, although Platonism was highly influential, Christian theologians from the very beginning checked and countered philosophy

7. See Annas, *Platonic Ethics Old and New*, 63.

8. See McGuckin, *St Cyril of Alexandria*, 224–25.

9. Shults argues that the Alexandrian approach has an Aristotelian understanding of human persons, with its strong emphasis on the unity of the body and soul, whereas the Antiochene approach is Platonic since body and soul are seen as separate substances in relation (*Christology and Science*, 32). McGuckin suggests the Alexandrian approach is influenced by Platonism (*St Cyril of Alexandria*, 224–25). But McGuckin's analysis keeps with the exegetical tendencies of the two centers of thought and so seems preferable. McGuckin's characterization of Antiochene Christology as "semitic" may be problematic in that Hebrew thinking seems to have a holistic view of the human being that does not always reduce to a tripartite of body, soul, and spirit. Moreover, theologians like Athanasius are considered to be "semitic" in their understandings, yet not Antiochene.

with their insights from Scripture. Both Alexandrian and Antiochene theologians were anxious to do justice to the Jesus of the Gospels. What, it seems, can be said is that the two approaches are not marked purely by a difference of philosophy. Nevertheless, with these provisos, the *logos-sarx* Alexandrian and *logos-anthropos* Antiochene Christologies remain useful focal points for what often becomes a complicated picture.

As for the analogies, Weinandy points out that the body-soul model is used in two different ways: first and legitimately, by simple analogy, early theologians recognize that just as the body-soul union illustrates how the distinctly different spiritual and material can be one by producing the one reality of the human being, the union between divinity and humanity also forms the one reality of Jesus; second, instead of simple analogy, most early theologians use the soul-body relationship as an exact model for how the union of divinity and humanity takes place.[10] This second approach seems deeply problematic, because seeing divinity and humanity as components means that when fused they result in a new third thing, neither fully God nor fully man, or that the divinity is diminished, or the humanity altered. In human beings, the spiritual and the material are aspects of the same person; in Christ, there is both full divinity and full humanity. Ironically, it is often those who are declared to be unorthodox, such as Paul of Samosata and Nestorius, who point to the weakness of the second approach.

Although Weinandy regards the second usage as "the most lamentable, unfortunate, and misconceived intellectual stratagem in the entire history of Christology," and he is correct in saying that there is no similarity between the way the soul is united to the body and the way divinity is united to humanity in Christ,[11] both usages, though inadequate, are most instructive regarding the human person. What perhaps is significant is that both the Platonic and Aristotelian approaches have resonance with some modern views of the human person because at times they see the person of Christ in terms of soul or mind or intellectual functions of judgment and consciousness.[12] This mirrors the way in

10. Weinandy, *Does God Suffer?*, 182.

11. Weinandy, "Zizioulas," 183.

12. John McGuckin describes these spiritual functions as "ancient psychology's realm of the soul." He points out that Cyril is often criticized for not developing a "soul-Christology"

which some bioethicists place emphasis on mental functions to establish personhood and so designate profoundly disabled people as nonpersons.

While the *logos-sarx* and *logos-anthropos* approaches consider the relation between the two natures in Jesus Christ, human and divine, and sometimes between body and soul, they remain inadequate accounts. In a radical shift from these Christologies, and in contrast to theologians who begin their reflection from human anthropology, Cyril of Alexandria begins by asking about the single, indivisible person, Jesus Christ. Cyril comes to realize that neither the soul nor the intellect nor the mind is the focus of the person in Christ. Rather, it is the Person of the Word who comes to be man. Cyril's insights focus on the person as the true self. In addition, application of Cyril's thought on *kenosis*,[13] the self-emptying of the person of Christ, further deepens the concept of the person by moving reflection beyond descriptive anthropology to theological anthropology that considers human persons in the light of the Word made flesh.

For Us and for Our Salvation

Locke formulates his influential notion that the person is "a thinking intelligent being, that has reason and reflection, and can consider itself as itself, the same thinking thing, in different times and places, which it does only by that consciousness which is inseparable from thinking" in the context of a discussion about the continuing identity of the person, especially in terms of the Last Judgment. Person as "a forensic term" is tied up with law and judgment and so is only applicable to "intelligent agents capable of a law, and happiness and misery."[14] Although this context specifically frames how he speaks of persons, Lockean bioethicists rarely allude to it.

(what many writers regard as the mark of Christological progress) and so is an antiquated thinker. McGuckin goes on to explain, however, that not only did Cyril speak of a soul in Christ, but he also came to realize that neither the soul nor the intellect was the focus of personhood in Christ; rather, it is the person of the Word who comes to be man. *St Cyril of Alexandria*, 206.

13. Augustine explains the patristic notion of *kenosis*, referring to Phil 2:6–7: the Word became man and "emptied himself not by losing the nature of God but by receiving the nature of man." *Letter* 219, 69–71.

14. Locke, *Essay Concerning Human Understanding*, II, XXVII, 9; II, XXVII, 26.

For the first Christians, the Person of the Word comes to be man for our salvation: Jesus is the Resurrection and the Life, and he calls human beings to share in his glory.[15] Notably, Locke has eternal life and theology in mind when he formulates his definition of the person that has become so influential for many secular bioethicists. Locke was not so much concerned about glory, however. He was more worried about the Last Judgment. Locke thinks that for a person to be rewarded or punished in the afterlife, the person who was accountable on earth must be the same as the person in heaven.[16] But Locke rules out both the body and the soul as principles of continuing identity: his commitment to the new scientific theory of the day, atomism, meant that the body as a mass of particles cannot be the same at the resurrection, for a change in body that inevitably happens as the body decayed would not make the same man. Nor can the soul alone be enough to make the same man, since a soul, united to a body, could be replaced or could replace another, thus making it difficult to reidentify it.[17]

Still, Locke was not the first thinker to have these worries. Although early Christological thinking on the resurrection of human beings does include consideration of judgment, it reflects more noticeably on resurrection as God's gracious act of salvation. Some tensions appear however: while Irenaeus and Tertullian speak of salvation and resurrection of whole persons[18] as embodied souls because the whole person matters to God, Origen offers resurrection of the rational soul in a spiritual body and seems to see the body as irrelevant. Origen's thought allows for the tendency to look to the rational aspect, what many consider to be most significant in the human being, as also the locus of the person, a tendency that reappears and is corrected in subsequent Christological discussion.

15. Jn 11:26; Rom 8.
16. Locke, *Essay Concerning Human Understanding*, II, XXVII, 16.
17. Locke, *Essay Concerning Human Understanding*, II, XXVII, 15.
18. See Briggman, *Irenaeus of Lyons*, 124. See Osborn, *Tertullian*, 237.

Irenaeus and Tertullian: Resurrection of the Whole Person, Body and Soul

In speaking about salvation of the whole human person, body and soul, Irenaeus and Tertullian use the analogy of body and soul to divine and human in Christ. Their starting points differ in that Irenaeus begins from his understanding of human beings made in the image of God, Tertullian from his understanding of human beings as body and soul colored by Stoic philosophy. Yet they both conclude that in order to save us, Christ had to be both true God and true man.

For Irenaeus, Christ's bodiliness was not incidental or in opposition to his divinity. Rather, it revealed his divinity: human beings are made in the image and likeness of God. Christ the perfect man reflects this completely. Just as the Word is perfect man, so too is the whole human being—soul, body, and spirit—made in the likeness of the Word.[19] Kelly indicates that it is not clear whether Irenaeus attributes a rational soul to Christ, something that later becomes contentious.[20] Given that Irenaeus insists that Christ's humanity must be identical with ours for the sake of salvation, however, Irenaeus probably does understand Christ to have a rational soul. To stress this identification, Irenaeus underscores Christ's experience of all stages of human life so that the Incarnation is seen as relevant for all humans. Christ "passed through every age," becoming an infant for infants, thus sanctifying infants; a child for children, thus sanctifying children; from the young to the old, and for Irenaeus old age set in after thirty, even to death, so that he is "the firstborn from the dead."[21] Moreover, alongside its sanctifying role, Irenaeus stresses the saving role of the flesh in the Incarnation through recapitulation, whereby what was lost in Adam is regained by Christ.[22] What is essential is that Jesus had to be both God and man, since for salvation both divine *and* human natures act to redeem.

19. Irenaeus, "Against Heresies," V, VI, 1..

20. J. N. D. Kelly thinks that Irenaeus probably accepts a soul in Christ, and he also explains that when Irenaeus was writing, this was not an issue. *Early Christian Doctrines*, 148.

21. Irenaeus (quoting Col 1:18), "Against Heresies," II, XXII, IV.

22. Irenaeus, "Against Heresies," III, XVIII, I.

Irenaeus adds that the Eucharist too offers salvation, as when our flesh is nourished by the body and blood of Christ, we can receive eternal life.[23] Against those who denied the importance of the body, Irenaeus explains that the essence of humanity is not spirit alone but "a united organization of soul and flesh who was formed after the likeness of God and molded by his hands, the Son and the Holy Spirit."[24] According to Irenaeus, the "heretics" were mistaken because they refused to allow the salvation of God's creation: the whole person. In this Irenaeus seems to be expressing ideas articulated more fully by Athanasius, that the Word "became man that we might become divine."[25]

Although Irenaeus insists that the Word and Jesus are one and the same, he does not seem concerned with how the union of divine and human takes place. He may be aware of the problems involved,[26] and perhaps he lacks the adequate terms to express the union,[27] or possibly he may think this is beyond human knowledge. Still, Irenaeus seems to be one who uses the simple analogy approved of by Weinandy that recognizes both the one reality of the human person and the one reality of Jesus Christ.

In contrast, Tertullian seems to present the body-soul unity as a model for the divine and human union in Christ, and perhaps this leads to problems for later thinkers. Like Irenaeus, Tertullian answers those who deny the reality of Christ's humanity because they mistrust all things material. As Tertullian explains, for these anti-materialists, the reality of Christ's humanity would imply his resurrection in the flesh and therefore the resurrection of the human body after death.[28] Tertullian agrees that it is foolish and unworthy of the Son to assume flesh. Nevertheless, Tertullian says, in this way God reforms our birth by a second birth from heaven and so restores our flesh,[29] for Christ's flesh is like our own.[30]

23. Irenaeus, "Against Heresies," V, II, III; see also Ignatius of Antioch, "Letter to the Ephesians," 20, 2.

24. Irenaeus, "Against Heresies," IV, Preface IV.

25. Athanasius, "On the Incarnation," 54, 13, 18.

26. Kelly, *Early Christian Doctrines*, 149.

27. Torrance, *Christian Doctrine of God*, 79.

28. Tertullian, "On the Flesh of Christ."

29. Tertullian, "On the Flesh of Christ," 4.

30. Tertullian, "On the Flesh of Christ," 9.

Beginning from a consideration of the union of human and divine as a union of distinct substances, Tertullian stresses that a *tertium quid*, third thing or composite essence, did not come about when the Son became man: silver plus gold may become an amalgam, but spirit remains spirit and flesh flesh; Christ's twofold state was not confused but joined in "one person Jesus God and man."[31] Although Tertullian does not accept many Stoic doctrines,[32] on the issue of this union in Christ, he does seem influenced by Stoic philosophy and its idea of *krasis*.[33] The mechanics of blending, *krasis* (κρασις) and mixture, *mixis* (μιγνυμι), from the Greek "to mingle," particularly seems to have interested ancient thinkers, and they debated what counted as a mixture.[34] They also discussed whether the embodied soul belonged to this debate, and the kind of language used surfaces in debates about the union of divine and human in Christ.

The notion of *krasis* seems to come from Aristotle, who thought that two things could be joined by *synthesis* (συνθεσις) or by *krasis*.[35] According to Aristotle, *synthesis* involved an external juxtaposition of two elements, for example, a mixture of two sorts of grain. *Krasis* meant that two substances interacted, and although they were changed into a third thing, they could also return to the original elements. For Aristotle, a mixture keeps the elements in some sort of balance. Certainly, there is a new thing, but the elements remain potentially what they were before the mixture. If one of the elements is completely dominated by another, then Aristotle says it is no longer a mixture. Rather, there is a confusion: *phythora* (φθορα), or destruction of one element, and *genesis* (γενεσις), arrival of the amalgam. The Stoics further refined Aristotle so that *parathe-*

31. Tertullian, "Against Praxeas," XXVII.

32. Tertullian was not entirely in agreement with the Stoics because, among other things, he does not believe that all bodies are of the same kind, nor does he believe in transmigration of souls. See MacDonald, *History of the Concept of the Mind*, 138–39.

33. See Colish, *Stoic Tradition*, 9–29, 202. Colish notes that there is some inconsistency in Tertullian's approach to philosophy: famous for his dictum "what has Athens to do with Jerusalem," on the one hand, Tertullian uses philosophy and in particular Stoicism to support his own arguments. On the other hand, he rejects it as an integral part of pagan culture (10–13).

34. MacDonald, *History of the Concept of the Mind*, 111.

35. Clayton, *Christology of Theodoret of Cyrus*, 238. Richard Sorabji gives a comprehensive account of ancient thinking on mixtures in *Philosophy of the Commentators*, 290–315.

sis (παραθεσις) referred to an external mixing of beans and wheat, for instance, corresponding to Aristotle's *synthesis*. In contrast to Aristotle, the Stoics thought that two bodies could be in the same place at the same time in a genuine *krasis*.[36] The Stoics took the notion of *krasis* and developed two forms of mixture: *synchysis* (συγχυσις), where the substances were altered and could not be returned to the original elements again, and *krasis di"holon* (Κρασις δι ολων), where the substances interpenetrated yet each retained its own properties. For the Stoics, neither *synchysis* nor *parathesis* was a fitting way to describe the union of soul, *pneuma* (πνευμα), with body. Instead, the Stoics opted for *krasis di"holon* as the form of mixture that describes the union of body and soul.

Tertullian seemingly takes up this Stoic idea that two things can be joined by a total blending, where the natures are preserved although they are united. Thus, like the union of divine and human in Jesus, Tertullian sees the union of body and soul in humans as a union of distinct substances that maintain their distinct properties.[37] Tertullian employs the same terse framework as used in his Trinitarian thinking: in the Trinity, the three persons have one substance; in Christ, the one person has two substances, *substantiae*.[38]

Although Tertullian uses the language of person for both the Trinity and Jesus Christ, he does not feel the need either to clarify or elaborate the term. But he details the relationship between body and soul, made clearer, he believes, by Christ's Incarnation and bodily Resurrection. Tertullian thinks that those who deny resurrection of the flesh also deny that Jesus is both Son of God and Son of man. Christ is "redeemer of the flesh," for whatever God promised to man is owed to the soul and flesh since the "entire" man is of "clay" and soul.[39] Tertullian uses the word "clay" in reference to the creation of man in Genesis 2, but he makes clear that this is not a "vessel" or "mere chattel" of the soul. Rather, the clay of the human being is the servant of the soul, and the soul is "incapacitated" without the body.[40] Tertullian continues, although the soul

36. Sorabji, *Philosophy of the Commentators*, 298.

37. Tertullian, "On the Flesh of Christ," 13. See Colish, *Stoic Tradition*, 23.

38. Tertullian, "Against Praxeas," XXVII.

39. Tertullian, "On the Resurrection of the Flesh," 2, 5.

40. Tertullian, "On the Resurrection of the Flesh," 16, 17.

is "more proximate in character" to God, the flesh is "co-heir" with the soul because they are in intimate union; moreover, it is only by means of the body that the soul gives service to God. Not only are the living acts of the soul the work of the flesh, but also the very act of dying is of the flesh.[41]

Although Tertullian does not speak about people with disabilities, it may be worthwhile applying Tertullian's thinking. Moss thinks that in early Church thinking, disability has no place in the coming Kingdom.[42] If continuing identity is significant for Tertullian, however, then presumably whatever marks out a person's identity will also continue in the afterlife, and that may include disability. In addition, the idea that the soul works out its service to God through the body has significance for the profoundly disabled and those whose worship appears to be primarily bodily. Simply because their worship seems lacking in the more traditional worship focused on mental prayer, it does not mean that it ceases to be effective worship. The profoundly disabled who come just as they are before God in worship come perhaps in a way less hindered by wants, needs, and desires. Tertullian's comment that the act of dying is an act of a united body and soul is significant for those bioethicists who claim that once a human being has lost the capacity for being a person, that individual is as good as dead.

Like Irenaeus, Tertullian explains through the sacraments how body and soul are united and so are owed the same recompense: resurrection,

> The flesh, then, is washed, so that the soul may be made clean.
> The flesh is anointed, so that the soul may be dedicated to holiness.
> The flesh is signed, so that the soul too may be fortified.
> The flesh is shaded by the imposition of hands, so that the soul too may be illuminated by the Spirit.
> The flesh feeds on the body and blood of Christ, so that the soul too may fatten on God. They cannot, then, be separated in their reward, when they are united in their works.[43]

41. Tertullian, "On the Resurrection of the Flesh," 7.
42. Moss, "Heavenly Healing," 991–1017.
43. Tertullian, "On the Resurrection of the Flesh," 8.

As "minister and servant of the soul," the flesh is "the hinge of salvation."[44] In notable contrast to Locke, Tertullian says that because a person's life is the cause of judgment, both soul and flesh are the subject of judicial examination, for "whatever is done in man's heart is done by the soul in the flesh, and with the flesh and through the flesh."[45] Tertullian argues that any censure of the flesh in Scripture is not criticism of its substance. Rather, censure is owed to misguided actions of the body and therefore of the soul, which compels the body to do its bidding.[46] Tertullian says that the entire man is lost, not just a part of him, through sin that takes place as much by the instigation of the soul as the body, so "he will be wholly saved, since he has by sinning been wholly lost."[47] Tertullian adds that wherever one locates thought, for instance, in the brain, "the flesh will still be the thinking place of the soul."[48] Tertullian makes the point that there must be identity of the risen body with the present flesh because it is only just that reward or punishment is given to the same person, and so he must be the same flesh and soul.[49] Unlike Locke, who dismissed the body as a point for continuity of identity because the body disintegrates,[50] Tertullian is not concerned with the practicalities of bodily resurrection because all is possible for God. But he is certain that "the flesh will rise again, wholly in every man, in its own identity, in its absolute integrity."[51]

While Tertullian specifies that the flesh is coheir with the soul to eternal life, and that judgment concerns the life of the whole person, it does not seem that free will and actual rationality are an essential aspect of ensouled beings. This may be because Tertullian is responding to a philosophical position, possibly that of Platonic Gnostics, which claimed that souls were joined to matter after evil done through their free will.[52] It may also be a reaction to the Stoic belief that only the souls of the wise

44. Tertullian, "On the Resurrection of the Flesh," 7, 8. See Osborn, *Tertullian*, 237.
45. Tertullian, "On the Resurrection of the Flesh," 14, 15.
46. Tertullian, "On the Resurrection of the Flesh," 10.
47. Tertullian, "On the Resurrection of the Flesh," 34.
48. Tertullian, "On the Resurrection of the Flesh," 15.
49. Tertullian, "On the Resurrection of the Flesh," 56.
50. Locke, *Essay Concerning Human Understanding*, II, XXVII, 3.
51. Tertullian, "On the Resurrection of the Flesh," 63.
52. See MacDonald, *History of the Concept of the Mind*, 139.

ascend to heaven.[53] Tertullian certainly believes in free will.[54] But he sees that there is an order to human life that does not consider embodiment a punishment: he says that the soul springs from divine breath,[55] and considering "from man's last moment of life we may get some idea of his first," since death is the "dissolution of body and soul," and then life begins when the soul begins.[56] A person has life when he or she has a soul. It is after that that the person is charged to live virtuously.[57]

Again, against the Gnostics, who divided bodily senses derived from the animal part of the human from intellectual faculties that arose from spiritual seeds, Tertullian counters that when a person is insane, out of his mind, the soul is demented not because the mind is absent but because the mind is a "fellow sufferer" with the soul, but when the soul leaves the body, the mind is also no longer left.[58] This marks a clear contrast to thinkers such as Apollinarius, who seem to think that an entity ceases to be when it loses its mind. Tertullian's view, that the body and soul are so closely united that each suffer together, is perhaps a useful interpretation for the situation of those who suffer from dementia. While some bioethicists may think that once the mind has gone, the person ceases to exist, Tertullian's comment reminds us that the person remains yet suffers in body, mind, and soul.

Tertullian also opposes those who believe that the Word only seemed to take flesh. Tertullian responds that if the Incarnation is a pretense, then so are his miracles, suffering, death, and Resurrection.[59] Tertullian is adamant that Christ took flesh and a soul like our own.[60] He received man "in his texture of flesh and soul," and "neither therefore of those

53. See Colish, *Stoic Tradition*, 16.

54. See Osborn, *Tertullian*, 167–70. Colish compares Tertullian's view of free will to that of the Stoics. *Stoic Tradition*, 25.

55. See Colish, *Stoic Tradition*, 20; Tertullian, "On the Soul," 22; idem, "Against Marcion," II.IX. The idea of the soul as divine breath seems similar to the view of the Stoic Chrysippus. In his critique of pagan philosophy, Tertullian makes frequent reference to Chrysippus. For Chrysippus on *krasis* and the soul, see Sorabji, *Philosophy of the Commentators*, 299–300.

56. Tertullian, "On the Soul," 27, 2–3.

57. Tertullian, "Against Marcion," II, VIII.

58. Tertullian, "On the Soul," 18, 9–10.

59. Tertullian, "On the Flesh of Christ," 3.

60. Tertullian, "On the Flesh of Christ," 9, 10.

parts which he has received will he allow to perish."[61] For those who are preoccupied with the novelty of the Incarnation, Tertullian replies that the only "novelty" is that the Word became flesh without the seed of a human father, which after all is what happened when Adam became flesh.[62]

For Tertullian, the blending of two substances—body and soul in humans, humanity and divinity in Christ—is possible through the *krasis* doctrine. Even though Tertullian seems to have offered a psychosomatic unity in the human being,[63] his presentation of body and a material soul as two substances, as opposed to the view of Irenaeus of the one reality of the human person, becomes problematic for later thinkers in terms of how two become one. One sees echoes of this problem as far as Locke, who developed his concept of the person out of the difficulty of identifying a stable unity out of two substances—body and soul—that for him were not intrinsically related (he believes in the transmigration of souls to various bodies).

On a different level, but equally problematic, is the widespread influence of Origen's Neoplatonic thinking. In contrast to Tertullian, Origenist understandings begin to see the soul as totally incorporeal and the body as no longer integral to the definition of a human being. Origen's Christology and his belief in the preexistence of rational minds that make use of the body allow the notion that the person resides solely in the rational part of humans.[64]

Origen: Resurrection of the Person, Rational Soul, and Spiritual Body

Origen agrees that human beings are "animals composed of a union of body and soul," though he also thinks that animal souls are different from rational souls.[65] Origen likewise believes that the whole man would not have been redeemed had Christ not assumed the whole

61. Tertullian, "On the Resurrection of the Flesh," 34.
62. Tertullian, "On the Flesh of Christ," 16, 21.
63. See Colish, *Stoic Tradition*, 24.
64. See Greer, "Introduction," in Origen, *Exhortation to Martyrdom*, 15.
65. Origen, "De Principiis," I, 6. Blosser, *Become Like the Angels*, 208.

man.[66] Yet in keeping with his preference for Platonism, he holds to the ancient classical notion of the higher part of the soul, *nous* (νους), as a preexistent reality.[67] Rufinus, one of Origen's translators, denotes this preexistent reality, this rational spiritual being, as *mens*, thus *nous*, corresponding to mind or spirit.[68] According to Origen, these beings lost their original state, fell, and "cooled down" to become souls.[69] Hence *psyche* (ψυχη), the word for "soul" that derives from *psychesthai*, means to grow cold.[70] The gravity of the fall corresponded to the nature of the body fallen into, be it stars, planets, angels, demons, or humans. Souls are thus imprisoned in bodies as a result of previous sin.[71] Origen says that, when purified, these souls rise until they attain the state in which they formerly were.[72] In one of the few patristic references to disability, Origen seems to account for "defects" in sight, hearing, and speech in terms of the gravity of the fall.[73] The link between sin and disability has always been considered problematic in disability studies.[74] Notably, Origen's theory of the fall of souls is later rejected.

From fragments of Origen's thought preserved by Methodius, Origen, along with Greek philosophers, seems concerned with the principle of continuity.[75] Responding to those who ask what happens at the Resurrection to flesh eaten by birds and animals when those creatures are eaten by humans, Origen seems to think that a better answer than Tertullian's "all is possible to God" is required.[76] Origen does not think the body provides personal continuity: it is in a state of flux. But the individual's inner life and experience seem to act as a stamp on the soul: real

66. Origen, "Dialogue with Heracleides."

67. For Origen's Platonism, see Greer, "Introduction," 6. Apparently, Origen had an "ambivalent attitude" toward the Platonic account of the soul and in some of his writing attempts to accommodate Platonism with Aristotelianism. MacDonald, *History of the Concept of the Mind*, 132–33.

68. Benjamin Blosser points out that although this preexistent "better" soul appears to equal man's, it is not absolutely clear in Origen's thinking. *Become Like the Angels*, 67–72.

69. Origen, "De Principiis," II, 8, 3.

70. See Origen, *Exhortation to Martyrdom*, 49n7.

71. Origen, "De Principiis," I, 8, 1.

72. Origen, "De Principiis," II, 8, 3.

73. Origen, "De Principiis," II, 9.3.

74. See Lewis, *Deaf Liberation Theology*, 61–68.

75. Methodius, "From the Discourse on the Resurrection," esp. Part 3.

76. See Daley, *Hope of the Early Church*, 53.

identity is in the individual's spiritual core.[77] This appears consonant with Origen's perpetual search for inner meaning, for real meaning, that he felt lay hidden, whether it be the inner man in the human being or a mysterious allegorical meaning in Scripture.[78]

It is unclear whether Origen thought that souls ever existed in a disembodied state, and it may be that the descent Origen describes is not so much falling into embodiment itself as falling into coarser forms of embodiment.[79] After all, Origen says that at the Restoration at the end of time, human rational natures do not remain altogether incorporeal, since he thinks only the Trinity can truly live without a body, so therefore these perfected souls will have a spiritual body.[80] But even if Origen thinks that souls do not exist disembodied, since souls are cooled-off minds that are immediately given bodies, this does not account for preexistent rational natures in the Beginning.[81] It seems clear for Origen that the fall of souls is part of their educative process: the Beginning involves innocence and instability; rational natures fell because they did not direct themselves to God. The body is both a sign of the state of the soul, since the kind of body the soul receives reflects its state, and the body also functions as a tool of God's providence: the rational mind's freedom may bring punishment, but God uses punishment to bring the sinner back.[82] On earth, the rational nature acquires experience and develops in attention to its divine teacher. The spiritual resurrected body, gained by the soul at the Restoration, still reflects the stamp of this earthly experience. Even though the Restoration is like the Beginning, it is on a higher level because rational natures reach perfection from which they cannot fall, and thus the Restoration is marked by stability.

77. See Williams, "Origen," 137. Blosser explains that, according to Origen, the divine image is impressed on the "inner man," nous. *Become Like the Angels*, 73.

78. For an explanation of the connection of Origen's thinking on creation to his theory of human nature and corresponding method of exegesis, see Williams, "Origen," 135–36.

79. See Blosser, *Become Like the Angels*, 200–201.

80. Origen, "De Principiis," II, 2, 2.

81. See Greer, "Introduction," 11–16.

82. See Blosser, *Become Like the Angels*, 203–4.

Christ and His Soul

According to Origen, just as the human rational nature uses the body as a sign of its fallen state, the Word uses a human soul and body to reveal God to fallen humanity in the only way fallen humans can understand.[83] For Origen, the Word (*Logos* and Son of God) was created at the very beginning[84] as the invisible image of the invisible Father, begotten from God's will and incorporeal.[85] Then everything else was made through him.[86] In this creative activity, the Word gives a share of himself to all rational creatures. But one soul was attached with "a warmer love" to the "author of its being" and inhered to the Word[87] in a real though mysterious unity.[88] The Word then put aside his glory and assumed flesh as an intermediate between God and flesh.[89] Moreover, as the God-man, Jesus Christ "truly possessed flesh so he truly possessed soul."[90]

Because Origen believes that all human beings are fallen souls, then his theory of one particular loving soul bears some similarity with Adoptionism, an early view that called Jesus a human being particularly inspired by God. Origen thinks the indwelling of the *Logos* in Christ is more than divine inspiration, however. For Origen, the *Logos* is completely in control of Christ, so he is incapable of sin.[91] Still, if from the very beginning this one soul of Jesus clung to the Word so that he is incapable of sin, it is difficult to see how this works with the idea that all human beings are fallen souls. Origen wishes to assert both that "the nature of his [Christ's] soul was indeed the same as that of all others; for otherwise, were it not truly a soul, it could not be called a soul" and that Christ's soul "so chose to love justice" that it clung to the Word.[92]

83. Greer, "Introduction," 15.
84. Origen, "De Principiis," I, 2, 3.
85. Origen, "De Principiis," I, 2, 6.
86. Origen, "De Principiis," I, 7, 1.
87. Origen, "De Principiis," II, 6, 3. See Blosser, *Become Like the Angels*, 235.
88. Origen, "De Principiis," IV, 4, 31.
89. Origen, "De Principiis," II, 6, 3.
90. Origen, "De Principiis," II, 8, 2.
91. Origen, "De Principiis," IV, 31.
92. Origen, "De Principiis," II, 6, 5.

Origen compares the unity in Christ with the one-in-flesh of man and wife and concludes that the Word is even more in one flesh with the soul of Christ because it is more becoming for this specific loving soul to be united with God.[93] By sharing in the divinity, Origen says that Christ's body and human soul were deified from the beginning.[94] According to Alois Grillmeier, by associating the higher part of the soul, or the controlling principle, *hegemonikon*[95] (ηγεμονικον), with the *Logos,* Origen "could ultimately be on the way to a metaphysical interpretation of the unity of Christ by means of the concept of 'person.'" Grillmeier adds, however, that "the lack of the concept of 'person' is a clear fact": Origen's belief that the *Logos* and the created soul of Christ are both centers of activity leads Origen to assume a "double personality" of Christ.[96] Nevertheless, Grillmeier seems to be associating the idea of person with center of consciousness, an association that patristic thinking goes on to reject. Moreover, later disputes clarify there are two operations, *energias* (ενεργεια), in Christ, indicating not a duality of subjects but the reality of two natures: all the actions of Christ are the actions of the one subject.

Origen's recognition that Christ had a created rational soul is excluded in subsequent patristic debate, possibly owing to Origen's problematic notion of the preexistence of souls and their fall into corruption.[97] After all, this conflicts with the biblical and patristic tradition on the goodness of creation. It contradicts also the idea of humanity bearing the image of God.[98] Still, even though Origen's thinking was later rejected, he left the legacy that a human being is essentially a rational soul or *nous*, mind, and the body is merely accidental.[99] Origen's view that the *Logos* is in complete control of Jesus remained highly influential and reemerged in later controversies. The corollary is that the inner man is the real person.

93. Origen, "De Principiis," II, 6, 3.

94. Origen, "Against Celsus," III, XL1.

95. *Hegemonikon* is a technical Stoic term for what centralizes and unifies the soul's functioning, its governing principle, and it was often associated with mind. Annas, *Hellenistic Philosophy of Mind*, 54, 29n36.

96. Grillmeier, *Christ in Christian Tradition*, 170.

97. Grillmeier, *Christ in Christian Tradition*, 177–79.

98. Gregory of Nyssa, "On the Making of Man," XXVIII.

99. Origen, "De Principiis," II, 8, 1.

The condemnation of Paul of Samosata gave even more reason to avoid speaking of Christ's created soul. At Paul's trial, however, Malchion, a presbyter at Antioch, who supposedly represented orthodoxy, freely uses the union of body and soul in human beings as an exact model for the union of the Word and body in Christ. And the unorthodox Paul points out that exact models do not hold. Even though the authenticity of the record of their debate is questionable, since it may in fact be a fourth-century Apollinarian forgery,[100] their verbal exchange sets out the lines for subsequent struggles where various anthropologies seem to have clouded early Christology, yet the early successes in Christology may illuminate modern anthropology.

Paul of Samosata and Malchion: The Emergence of the Inner Man

As with all those condemned, anything written by Paul of Samosata was destroyed, so accounts of his actual thinking remain uncertain. From alleged fragments, it seems that Paul of Samosata denies Christ's divinity. He says instead that Christ was "from below" and had a human soul and body.[101] Although later Christological thinking agrees that Christ had a human soul and body, Paul of Samosata seems to think that the *Logos*, who may have been an impersonal attribute of God, was conjoined to the man Jesus "according to friendship and not according to substance" in the form of an indwelling. Hence Paul of Samosata appears to fall in with the Adoptionists. Paul of Samosata's Christ appears to be an earthly man influenced by the divine in him to such an extent that he gives total obedience to those influences.[102]

Paul of Samosata was charged with heresy and examined, possibly at the Synod of Antioch. Malchion argues against Paul of Samosata's "conjunction according to friendship" and explains that the Word was born in a body and shares our nature. Malchion adds that the unity of the Word and the body corresponds to the "coming together of flesh and of

100. See Grillmeier, *Christ in Christian Tradition*, 177–78.
101. Paul of Samosata, "Fragments," 258–64.
102. See Prestige, *God in Patristic Thought*, 115.

something dwelling in the flesh" in human beings, the unity of the body and its "life principle": the *Logos* in Christ corresponds to the soul in man. Just as this unity makes us complete, so too does the unity of Word and flesh in Christ make him a complete person. In reply, Paul of Samosata is adamant that there can be no analogy between the constitution of a human being and the *Logos* to the flesh of Christ, so any discussion is irrelevant.

The fierce reaction against Paul of Samosata can be gauged by the kinds of accusations leveled against him: illegal financial dealings, fraud, pride, tyranny over his followers, "quackery" in church assemblies, and presiding over disordered and riotous liturgies.[103] While this reaction was certainly of its time, it also suggests that Paul of Samosata's contemporaries saw a serious threat to Gospel tradition. Anticipating the later thinking of Nestorius and Pelagius, the belief that a man, even one specially graced, could on his own accord follow God reduces the Gospel message to a form of self-salvation whereby Jesus acts as a model for other humans. Paul of Samosata thus speaks against biblical revelation and the tradition of the Church when he claims a mere moral union of the *Logos* to the man Jesus.

Still, it also seems that Paul of Samosata is correct in seeing the analogy of divine and human to soul and body as problematic. Although Malchion intends to present a unity in Christ, his suggestion that the union of body and soul in human beings corresponds to the union of divinity and humanity in Christ leaves open the possibility that the Word took the place of Christ's human soul. Moreover, once Origen's notion of a preexistent spirit in some way similar to ours taking on flesh had been rejected and talk of a human soul in Christ implied the thought of Paul of Samosata, some may have seen their only choice to be an identification of the *Logos* and the soul.[104]

Whereas only some of Origen's doctrines were criticized in the third century,[105] Paul of Samosata and his followers, the Paulianists, were condemned outright. The exchange between Paul of Samosata and Malchion

103. See Stevenson, *New Eusebius*, 258–60.
104. See Williams, *Arius*, 161.
105. Williams, *Arius*, 149.

seems to be the harbinger of both Arianism, which like Paul of Samosata denies full divinity to Jesus, and Apollinarianism, which denies Christ full humanity by substituting the *Logos* for the soul.

In response to Origen and to Paul of Samosata, two Christological tendencies developed, the *logos-sarx* model and the *logos-anthropos* model, and the tension between the two dominated Christology until the Council of Ephesus.[106] These tendencies are significant for anthropology because in their extremes, the *logos-sarx* approach veers toward seeing the person as soul or spirit with the body simply an extra, whereas the *logos-anthropos* approach gravitates toward the person as soul and body sometimes only loosely bolted together. These extremes bear similarities with some bioethical approaches to the concept of the person, especially the tendency to separate the person from the human being.

Logos-sarx and *Logos-anthropos* Christologies

Logos-sarx and *logos-anthropos* Christologies are commonly identified with the Alexandrian and the Antiochene schools of thought, since supposedly they centered on these locations. They are also recognized as having distinct methods of scriptural exegesis that seem to inform their Christological approaches. But this division into schools may be problematic, because research shows that these Christologies were not each confined to Alexandria or Antioch, nor were they the only Christologies.[107] Individual theologians may have followed their own paths or taken combined approaches rather than simply adopting a common purpose as suggested by the presence of a school of thought.[108] According to Weinandy, the "misconceived and artificial templates" of these two schools are often "capriciously imposed" on all patristic Christology, resulting in sometimes invalid inferences or discussion, for instance, whether Athanasius ascribed a human soul to Christ.[109] Weinandy has a point: the heretic Apollinarius appears to be the only thinker who can be consid-

106. Grillmeier, *Christ in Christian Tradition*, 175.
107. See Grillmeier, *Christ in Christian Tradition*, 175.
108. Herring, *Introduction to the History of Christianity*, 94.
109. Weinandy, *Athanasius*, 94.

ered to embrace fully the *logos-sarx* approach; the heretic Nestorius (and possibly Theodore of Mopsuestia) is the only one who takes up fully the *logos-anthropos* approach, yet other thinkers are described as being from the Alexandrian or Antiochene camp. Still, although bold distinctions between the approaches and the categorization of individual theologians may be problematic, the approaches serve as useful indicators of the kind of thinking and its tendencies that inform fourth-century Christology.

Having said that, there appears to be a measure of consistency in the method of biblical exegesis and the Christological tendency commonly associated with each of the two so-called schools.[110] The Alexandrian *logos-sarx* approach seems more accepting of Greek philosophy and more inclined to speculate beyond appearances to what is taken to be the truly real. As exemplified by the early theologian Clement, the Alexandrian cultural climate embraced Platonism, Greek classical literature, and allegory, so while not rejecting the literal meaning of Scripture, its tradition looks more to allegorical interpretation. Origen discerns three levels in Scripture that correspond to the Pauline (and Platonic) division of the person into body, soul, and spirit: the literal bodily level was helpful for ordinary people; the psychic level aided progress in perfection; the spiritual concerned the unspeakable mysteries. The theologian's task is to look behind the veil of words for their true meaning.[111] *Logos-sarx* Christology sees salvation as centering on the necessity for the Word to unite himself completely to humanity so that he makes it fully his own. It focuses on the divinity of Christ and is particularly opposed to Arianism, although Arianism ironically shares its features. In expressing this unity and influenced by an understanding of the human being as a body animated by a soul or spirit, however, it is tempted to reduce the humanity of Christ to mere passivity or to swallow up humanity, as Apollinarius seemingly believes.

110. Frances Young persuasively argues that Antiochene exegesis was grounded in the exegetical activities of the rhetorical schools. *Biblical Exegesis*, 171–75. Young also suggests that the difference between the Antiochene and Alexandrian approaches can be better interpreted by the terms "ikonic" and "symbolic." These terms express the different ways the text was interpreted (162, 210–11).

111. For further development of this view, see Young, "Alexandrian and Antiochene Exegesis," 335–37.

In contrast, the Antiochene *logos-anthropos* approach seems more committed to an Aristotelian pattern of thought and on concrete realities. The Antiochene method of exegesis seems to have been a reaction to Alexandrian allegorical exegesis.[112] Notably, the prominent biblical interpreter Theodore of Mopsuestia strongly attacked Origen's methods of interpretation.[113] The Antiochene approach focuses on literal and historical readings of Scripture.[114] Both Alexandrian and Antiochene approaches recognize that an exclusively literal interpretation of Scripture is impossible, particularly since theologians viewed the Old Testament in the light of Christ. Still, thinkers in the Antiochene tradition place emphasis on history, grammar, summary, and structure.[115] *Logos-anthropos* Christology sees salvation as principally brought about by the new obedience of Christ, the one who unites humanity and divinity in terms of the cooperation of the human with the divine. How to understand this union becomes problematic, however. The tendency is to see the *Logos* joined to a specific man, the "assumed man," which leads to the temptation to see the union purely in moral terms, as presented by Nestorius.

For Christology, both approaches offer essential aspects: for salvation, the *logos-sarx* insight that there is a complete union between the human and divine seems vital; yet equally vital is the *logos-anthropos* insight that Christ has a fully functioning humanity that is freely cooperative. Each approach also has something to say about the human person because, as with Trinitarian theology, the Christological discussion takes place alongside reflection on what it is to be a human person.

Alexandrian *Logos-sarx* Christology and the Real Person

The proclamation from John the Evangelist that "The *Logos*, Word became *sarx,* flesh and lived among us"[116] is the foundation of *logos-sarx*

112. Young sees this as principally a reaction to allegory associated with "Origen's 'playing' with the text." *Biblical Exegesis*, 296, 210.

113. McLeod, *Theodore of Mopsuestia*, 17–19, 23; McGrath, *Historical Theology*, 143.

114. It is said to be associated with Lucian, possibly the teacher of Arius, though according to McLeod the "real founder" is Diodore, teacher of Theodore. *Theodore of Mopsuestia,* 3.

115. See Young, *Biblical Exegesis*, 171–72. For an account of history as distinguished from modern historicism, see 166–67.

116. Jn 1:14.

Christology, where *sarx* denotes the reality of Christ's coming in human nature with all its frailty.[117] In John's Gospel, the unity of God with Jesus as Father and Son is critical for salvation. Reflection on Christ's "inner constitution"[118] or how the *Logos* is united to the flesh develops later. According to Grillmeier, this reflection appears to emerge out of the school of Alexandria and dates to early Arianism.[119] It also seems to have its roots in the debate between Paul of Samosata and Malchion. The fact that Paul of Samosata was bishop of Antioch, and Malchion a presbyter and head of the school of rhetoric there, seems to underscore the problem of making a rigid distinction between the two so-called schools.

Malchion's position that the *Logos* replaces Christ's soul to form a unity in the same way that body and soul are united in human beings appears to be the frame for *logos-sarx* Christology. For many early thinkers, the soul-body unity acts as a natural analogical resource since it illustrates how two seemingly incompatible elements, material and spiritual, can be united, and so it may help explain how the transcendent God renews his involvement with his creation without detracting from his transcendence.

The *logos-sarx* approach also develops in stages as a reaction against Arianism. Curiously, Arius closely follows Malchion yet also exploits his thought, so Arius appears to be one of the early proponents of *logos-sarx* Christology. Arius and his followers raise interesting questions about what it is to be a human person. These questions become more acute after the response of Athanasius to the Arian heresy, not least because Athansius leaves his position open to possible misinterpretation. Notably, Apollinarius thinks he is authentically developing the thought of Athanasius. Apollinarius's view resonates with some modern thinking that separates the person from the human being.

Arianism and Athanasius: Souls and Persons

Arius and Friends ❧ To piece together the Arian view of human persons, it is necessary to see how Arius develops his Christological ideas.

117. Vine, *Vine's Complete Expository Dictionary.*
118. Kasper, *Jesus the Christ*, 232–33.
119. Grillmeier, *Christ in Christian Tradition*, 175–77.

Heretical writings were usually destroyed, leaving only fragments, reports, or reconstructions, often set up by their opponents, making it difficult to piece together authentic thought. But Athanasius, the Syrian bishop Theodoret (ca. 393–460), and Epiphanius of Salamis (ca. 315–403), a writer noted for his list of heresies, preserved some of the works of Arius in their criticisms of him, and some of the letters of Arius are extant. Still, exploration of the Arian person inevitably involves some speculation.

Alexander, bishop of Alexandria (d. 328), who had placed Arius in charge of the church of Baucalis (it is unclear whether this refers to a place, church, or a person[120]) before their bitter doctrinal disagreement, claims that the roots of Arius's thinking lie in the error of Paul of Samosata and Lucian of Antioch (d. ca. 311).[121] Lucian himself was associated with Paul of Samosata and was excommunicated for it, even if Lucian did not share his views entirely. Lucian does appear to have had strong tendencies toward the subordination of the Son to the Father. Arius says he is a disciple of Lucian, though this may be a different Lucian.[122] By associating Arius with Paul of Samosata, Alexander may have been using a common technique of the time to tarnish his opponent. Rowan Williams may wish to dispel the notion that Paul was a direct influence on Arius, and Williams asserts that Arius is eager to avoid "crude adoptionism."[123] Arius is not an Adoptionist like Paul of Samosata, as Arius apparently believes that Christ is a heavenly being rather than a man in whom the *Logos* dwells.[124] For Alexander, however, any view of the Word as mutable entails that he is a creature who acquires merit and develops in perfection as human beings do, and such a view is rooted in Adoptionism whether the subject is a mere man (Paul of Samosata) or heavenly being (Arius). But Arius may be partly following Origen,[125] which is plausible

120. See Williams, *Arius*, 288n107.

121. Alexander of Alexandria, "Epistles on the Arian Heresy," 1, 9.

122. Arius, "Letter to Eusebius," 324–25. Preserved by Epiphanius in *Panarion of Epiphanius of Salamis*. Whether it was this Lucian that taught Arius is disputed; see Hanson, *Search for the Christian Doctrine of God*, 81–82.

123. Williams, *Arius*, 161–62.

124. See Arius, "Letter to Alexander of Alexandria," 277–78. Preserved by Epiphanius in *Panarion of Epiphanius of Salamis*. See also Bardy, *Recherches sur Saint Lucien d'Antioche et son école*, 217–95.

125. See Williams, *Arius*, 131–48, though as Williams points out, Origen's legacy to Arius may perhaps lie more in Origen's exegetical method (148).

given that the center of Origenism at Antioch seems to have been the school of Lucian, and Arius goes from Antioch to Alexandria.[126] For Arius, the Christological case is clear: God, the "unbegotten," "has no one His equal, nor like to Him, nor of equal glory," and the Son, although the "beginning of things created," "according to His own proper subsistence He has nothing that is proper to God. For He is neither equal nor is He consubstantial to Him."[127]

Presumably, Arius follows his avowed master Lucian in the way that he accounts for the Son. According to Epiphanius, Lucian claims the *Logos* takes flesh but not a soul, so that what happens in the flesh, such as hunger and thirst, can belong to him.[128] Up to this point, silence about Christ's soul may have been in keeping with the notion that, after Origen and Paul of Samosata, any idea of a human soul in Jesus was bound to attract criticism.[129] Grillmeier suggests that Christ's soul was "not yet a factor in theological discussion," and it was not a necessary principle for discussing the being or work of Christ in the third and fourth centuries.[130] Arius seems more explicit: according the unknown author Pseudo-Athanasius, Arius claims that the "inner man" or soul within us was taken by the *Logos* in Christ, his flesh being "a veil over the Godhead."[131] As Grillmeier points out, the use of the term "soul" may have been an interpolation used to taint Arius with overtones from Paul of Samosata and Origen. Nevertheless, Grillmeier thinks that the phrase "inner man" is a genuine Arian formula.

Although there may not have been an Arian school as such,[132] other Arians add to the picture. Eudoxius, bishop of Antioch (360–69), confesses that the Son became flesh but not man since he did not take a

126. See Wallace-Hadrill, *Christian Antioch*, 81.

127. Arius, "The Banquet," II, 1–4. See also Bardy, *Recherches sur Saint Lucien d'Antioche et son école*, 217–95.

128. Epiphanius, *Panarion of Epiphanius of Salamis*, I, 43.

129. According to Rowan Williams, the idea of a soul in Christ was therefore "doubly tainted." *Arius*, 161.

130. Grillmeier, *Christ in Christian Tradition*, 184–85.

131. Pseudo-Athanasius, "Contra Apollinarem," in Grillmeier, *Christ in Christian Tradition*, 185. Gregory of Nazianzus says that the Apollinarians use the notion of the flesh as a "veil" so that God can converse with human beings ("Epistle 101"); however, for the Apollinarians, the "inner man" is not the soul but the mind ("Epistle 101").

132. Williams, *Arius*, 173.

human soul, so that in Christ there is one composite nature.[133] Similarly, another Lucian, an Arian bishop of Alexandria (373–78), asserts that we know Christ as "one Person, one composite nature, like a man of body and soul."[134] The reason why this Lucian appears to refuse Christ a human soul lies in his understanding that the soul is, as Lucian puts it, the "self-determining agent." If Christ had a human soul, impulses from it and from God would necessarily conflict.[135] The flesh without the soul no longer has "any free motivating principle."[136]

The problem for the Arians appears twofold. On the one hand, the Incarnation demands that a real and substantial union of *Logos* and flesh takes place such that the *Logos* is the source of Christ's spiritual and psychical life. Within the *logos-sarx* framework, this would be a physical union so that one entity arises. Grillmeier terms the life-giving power the *Logos* gives to the soulless flesh in the Arian system "logos-vitalism."[137] On the other hand, for the Arians, it was unthinkable that the *Logos,* if he were God, could be joined to mere flesh. The Arian belief that the *Logos* took flesh without a rational soul resulted in the conclusion that the *Logos* was capable of suffering in his nature and so could not be divine.

Following strict *logos-sarx* union and anticipating Apollinarianism, Arian Christology seems to imply that if the *Logos* is the agent and subject of human experiences, then a body without a soul—that is, without a "self-determining agent"—is mere flesh. The Arian logic leads to the conclusion that it is the soul alone that is the person, even if Arians wish to present a composite in Christ as in human beings. This may be of special interest when considering whether, as some bioethicists suggest, the *real* person is found in rational self-conscious entities capable of making choices and having desires: truly "logos-vitalism" if *logos* is understood as word or reason. For the Arians, the fact that it is the *Logos* who suffers means that he is not divine; the flesh of Christ seems to be left out of the equation. Some bioethicists may claim that certain patients do not suf-

133. Grillmeier, *Christ in Christian Tradition*, 187.
134. Grillmeier, *Christ in Christian Tradition*, 189.
135. Grillmeier, *Christ in Christian Tradition*, 189.
136. As later pointed out by Theodore of Mopsuestia, *Commentary*, 5.
137. Grillmeier, *Christ in Christian Tradition*, 186.

fer because they only exist in biological life with no apparent conscious interaction. In theological terms, however, a patient who is not yet dead may still be suffering because he or she is not united with God.[138]

Athanasius The principal champion against the Arians, and apparently operating out of the *logos-sarx* framework, is Athanasius. Like Arius, he seems indebted to Origen, especially when he asserts the eternal generation of the Son as Wisdom.[139] In terms of human anthropology, however, the issue is the extent to which Athanasius sees the person principally as soul, though Athanasius repudiates the notion that souls fall into bodies.[140] After all, the Alexandrian *logos-sarx* approach risks seeing the human nature of Christ almost as an instrument or clothing for the use of the Son. Robert Doran suggests that Athanasius, "like most of his contemporaries," never thought of Jesus as having a human mind and soul. Doran accepts that Athanasius formally admits a soul in Christ. But Doran thinks that Athanasius did not integrate it into his vision of the Son.[141] Moreover, Roger Olson argues that while in the Antiochene school humanity was "never a passive instrument," for Athanasius, and Alexandrians in general, the human nature of Christ was "passive and impersonal," a "vehicle—almost nothing more than an animal shell" for "the use of" the Son of God.[142] Olson thus characterized the *logos-sarx* approach as presenting the reality of the flesh but without "its own center of consciousness and will distinct from the Son of God."[143] The charge that Alexandrian thinkers see the body as a "mere shell" may recall some bioethical viewpoints, notably, some views of patients in persistent vegetative state, whose nutrition and hydration are withdrawn in order to bring about death.[144] Key for Doran is that Athanasius does say that the Word makes the body his own as an "instrument," thereby indicating that Athanasius may see the body of Jesus as purely that.[145]

138. See Sulmasy, "End-of-Life Care Revisited," 194.

139. See Kannengeisser, "Origen's Doctrine," 889–99.

140. Athanasius, *Life of Antony and Letter to Marcellinus*, 74.

141. Doran, *Birth of a Worldview*, 101.

142. Olson, *Story of Christian Theology*, 205–6.

143. Olson, *Story of Christian Theology*, 206.

144. See in particular Brown's comment on Tony Bland's existence in persistent vegetative state in Airedale NHS Trust v. Bland, (1993) 2 W.L.R., 359, at 833.

145. David Gwynn argues that criticism suggesting that either Athanasius sees the

Notably, however, in the same passage, Athanasius also states that Jesus took a body no different from ours.[146] Nevertheless, exploration of two works by Athanasius, *On the Incarnation* and *Against the Heathens*, challenges this interpretation and illuminates what Athanasius could have meant by "instrument."

From his initial remarks, Athanasius realizes that there may be some confusion for the readers of *On the Incarnation*: although the title references the Incarnation, he begins by talking of human anthropology. He explains that in speaking of the appearance of the Savior among us, we must also speak of the origin of humankind.[147] The why of the Incarnation is to be understood in relation to the how of human beings. But this has not so much to do with the internal constitution of human beings, that is, the mechanics of how body and soul are united in one human being, or divine and human come to be one in Christ. Rather, it is a matter of theological anthropology: the "how" refers to human beings as created, fallen, and then redeemed by the God-man. In a similar fashion perhaps, many bioethicists are concerned with the separation of the human being and the (rational, self-conscious) person, almost the mechanical how of human beings: What are the grounds on which we are considered to be persons, when can it be said that a person begins to exist, and when does a person cease to exist? This perhaps mirrors the concerns of those to whom Athanasius addresses his *On the Incarnation*. His inquirers want to know how the divine and human relate in Christ. In contemporary bioethical thought, the how needs to be addressed because it carries such high stakes. Still, bioethics also asks what is and is not fitting to do in human biology and medicine, and what to make of perplexing situations at the margins of life. Doing justice to such complex issues requires more than easy definitions.

Returning to early theology, Athanasius continues, God the source of goodness makes all things out of nothing by the Word. Here it is important for Athanasius to stress the biblical and traditional understanding of the involvement of the *Logos* in creation because, against the Arians,

human body of Christ merely as a tool or Christ wears his body like a suit are "in part" reflecting Athanasius the controversies of the fifth century. *Athanasius of Alexandria*, 71–72.

146. Athanasius, "On the Incarnation," 8.

147. Athanasius, "On the Incarnation," 4.

Athanasius is arguing that the Word is consubstantial with the Father. God took "special pity" on the race of men and did not create them as the "irrational creatures." Instead, he made them in his own image, sharing with them the power of his Word so that, as a kind of reflection of the Word and being made rational, human beings are destined for eternal life.[148] As a race, humankind has a rational nature.[149]

For Athanasius, both nature and a special gift from God, grace, make up human beings. In keeping with the ascetic tradition,[150] Athanasius explains the fallen condition of humankind: the body has eyes to see the Creator's works, ears to listen to divine sayings, hands to pray, but the soul wanders away from contemplation of what is good and chooses lower things,[151] hence the necessity of the Incarnation to bring us back.

Only the Word of God could "bring what was corruptible back again to incorruption."[152] As when a portrait is ruined the sitter must return to renew it, so does salvation require the renovation of "the very image of God": "the Word of God came in his own person because it was he alone, the image of the Father, who could recreate man made after the image."[153] In the gift of a rational nature and in the act of salvation, Athanasius highlights the solidarity of humankind and the solidarity of Christ with the whole of humanity. "The Word became flesh" so that he could unite what is naturally man to what is naturally God,[154] for the Word "became a man and did not come into a man."[155] Answering Docetic and Gnostic notions, Athanasius states that Christ "took himself a body, and that not foreign to our own," "he did not wish simply to be in a body, nor did he wish merely to appear."[156] Christ was born of Mary, that is, naturally of her, not born in her.[157]

148. Athanasius, "On the Incarnation," 3.

149. Athanasius, "On the Incarnation," 3; idem, "Against the Heathens," 3.

150. For an account of the relationship of Athanasius to asceticism and in particular the monastic asceticism of Antony, see Gwynn, *Athanasius of Alexandria*, chap. 4.

151. Athanasius, "Against the Heathens," 4–5.

152. Athanasius, "On the Incarnation," 7.

153. Athanasius, "On the Incarnation," 13. Weinandy thinks that the move made by Athanasius is similar to that made later by Anselm in his *Cur Deus Homo*, though "less contrived and more biblical." *Athanasius*, 31.

154. Athanasius, "Against the Arians," II, 70.

155. Athanasius, "Against the Arians," III, 30–32.

156. Athanasius, "On the Incarnation," 8.

157. Athanasius, *Letter* 59, to Epictetus, 5.

To maintain the divinity of the Word, Athanasius must also defend his immutability and impassibility, and Athanasius introduces the body as instrument to achieve this. Athanasius explains that the incarnate Word does not undergo change: for, as the Arians note, if there is change, he is not divine. Rather, the Word "becomes" man, and this becoming is "taking," not change.[158] Athanasius understands that the Incarnation does not remove the Word from the universe, he was not "enclosed in the body," for "being the Word, he was not contained by anyone but rather himself contained everything."[159] The body of the Word incarnate, then, was not "a limitation." Rather, it was "an instrument," so that as man he was "living a human life" and as Word he was "sustaining the life of the universe... in constant union with the Father."[160] In confirmation, Athanasius offers the apparent paradox of the Word, "who suffered and yet suffered not,"[161] as he allocates passions to the human nature and miracles to the divine. An early example of the *communicatio idiomatum*,[162] where the divine is predicated of the man Christ and the human is predicated of the *Logos* while recognizing the unity of the person, Athanasius adds that "both these things and those are done by one,"[163] for "the body which ate and was born and suffered was no one else's but the Lord's" being a "true, not an unreal body."[164]

Although Athanasius claims a "true" body for Christ, "not foreign to our own,"[165] there is little mention of Christ's soul. This may be because Athanasius considers that Christ's soul is not a significant factor in his understanding of the being and work of Christ,[166] or more likely he thinks that after the affair of Paul of Samosata, a discussion of Christ's soul or intellect is a distraction.[167] Instead, Athanasius takes both soul and intellect for granted. Athanasius places the focus on the distinction

158. Athanasius, "Against the Arians," II, 47.
159. Athanasius, "On the Incarnation," 17.
160. Athanasius, "On the Incarnation," 17.
161. Athanasius, *Letter* 59, to Epictetus, 6.
162. See Gwynn, *Athanasius of Alexandria*, 71.
163. Athanasius, "Against the Arians," III, 35.
164. Athanasius, "On the Incarnation," 18.
165. Athanasius, *Letter* 59, to Epictetus, 7.
166. See Grillmeier, *Christ in Christian Tradition*, 194–96.
167. See Weinandy, *Athanasius*, 94.

between Creator and creature and on the instrumentality of the body as a means for the self-disclosure of the invisible God.[168] As Athanasius explains, the *Logos* "became man that we might become divine and he revealed himself through a body that we might receive an idea of the invisible Father."[169] What seems to be fundamental for Athanasius is that divinity attaches to Christ's human nature and humanity to his divine nature so that humankind can become divine. In this understanding, deification applies in principle to all human beings, but it is to be appropriated by the individual.[170]

Nevertheless, his *Tome to the People of Antioch* indicates that Athanasius did allow for a soul in Christ, though whether the crucial text about the soul is an interpolation remains at issue. This synodal letter deals with the acceptance in Antioch of the terms of the Nicene Creed. Athanasius says that Christ is not a body without a soul or without sense or intelligence; "for it was not possible, when the Lord had become man for us, that His body should be without intelligence: nor was the salvation effected in the Word Himself a salvation of body only, but of soul also."[171] Whereas Weinandy considers that this is a position Athanasius long held and not one he was persuaded to later,[172] Kelly argues that this is a "purely formal" acknowledgment of the human. Kelly continues, given Alexandrian Christology in general and the Alexandrian conception of the mind, *nous*, as image of God, for Athanasius, Christ's body could not be without intelligence because the Word as the archetype of mind or soul had united himself with flesh. He points out that this became the position of Apollinarius.[173] Yet if for Athanasius the Word became man so that we might become divine (as he says in his *Letter to Epictetus*), it seems that it is essential that the flesh the Word assumes is a full human nature, that is, with a rational soul, perhaps anticipating the

168. Khaled Anatolios suggests that Grillmeier's analytic approach is perhaps not appropriate because Grillmeier seeks to discover how Athanasius sees the body as an instrument, but for Athanasius the focus is on the distinction between Creator and creature. *Athanasius*, 70–72.

169. Athanasius, "On the Incarnation," 54.

170. See Russell, *Doctrine of Deification*, 177.

171. Athanasius, "Tomus ad Antiochenos," 7.

172. Weinandy, *Athanasius*, 95.

173. Kelly, *Early Christian Doctrines*, 288–89.

view of Gregory of Nazianzus that what "he has not assumed he has not healed."[174]

Athanasius seems to regard human beings as wholes, even if he speaks of the body as an instrument. As Athanasius explains, it is through physical activities like singing and reading that the soul is affected and grows;[175] a human being is like a "stringed instrument," the body, soul, emotions, and reason acting in harmony,[176] so the subject of deification is not merely the rational soul or *nous* of Origen.[177] The Christology of Athanasius is not so much concerned with the internal constitution of either human beings or Christ, however. Instead, Athanasius is more interested in the self-disclosure of the invisible God and what that means for humankind. Even though humankind has been given the gift of a rational nature, the frailty of human nature is such that humans tend toward lesser things in preference to orientating themselves toward God. Christ restores the image of God in humankind and—in keeping with the ascetic tradition—Athanasius urges a life of virtue where the body is servant to the soul and contributes to the conversion of the whole person to God.[178]

A colleague and close friend of Athanasius did, however, take the theologian's thinking and the *logos-sarx* approach in a more extreme direction: that of seeing *sarx*, the flesh taken up by the *Logos*, as empty flesh, and in terms of anthropology, of seeing the body as merely a shell. This colleague, Apollinarius (ca. 315–92), was the son of a presbyter and came from Laodicea in Syria. A successful teacher, rhetor, and Scripture scholar, he taught Jerome in Antioch. Eventually made bishop of Laodicea, Apollinarius gave Athanasius strong support during the Arian controversy, and Athanasius himself consulted Apollinarius on Christology. It would be easy to conclude that the two shared similar views.[179] But

174. Gregory of Nazianzus, "Epistle 101."

175. Athanasius, *Life of Antony and Letter to Marcellinus*, 111–14.

176. Athanasius, *Life of Antony and Letter to Marcellinus*, Interpretation of the Psalms Letter to Marcellinus, 123–25.

177. See Russell, *Doctrine of Deification*, 177.

178. Athanasius, *Life of Antony and Letter to Marcellinus*, Life of Antony, 64–65.

179. See Hall, *Doctrine and Practice in the Early Church*, 155. Olson claims that the Christ of Apollinarius is "nearly identical" to the presentation of Christ offered by Athanasius. *Story of Christian Theology*, 171.

Apollinarius operates out of a strict *logos-sarx* framework that looks not at the person of Christ or the why of the Incarnation but at how the internal constitution of human beings can act as a model for the God-man. Given that Apollinarius focuses on the human being, and that his views resemble the approach of those bioethicists who think that the human person is essentially mind, it is worthwhile to consider his views in some depth.

Apollinarius, Gregory of Nyssa, Gregory of Nazianzus: Minds and Persons

Apollinarius

Unusually, there are more than just fragments left from the writings of Apollinarius, though there is still some uncertainty about what he actually taught.[180] Some of his main Christological work, the *Apodeixis*, a proof, is quoted at length by Gregory of Nyssa in his *Antirrheticus*, and quotations can be found in the treatises of Gregory of Nazianzus. The followers of Apollinarius also saved many of his writings by falsely attributing them to orthodox writers. Cyril of Alexandria adopted one infamous Apollinarian formula, μίαν φύσιν του θεου λόγου σεσαρκωμένην "one incarnate nature of the divine Word," believing it to be from Athanasius. The *Anacephalaeosis*, a summary, can be found in the fifth pseudo-Athanasian dialogue, part of a collection of writings put together at the end of the fourth century. The *Detailed Confession of the Faith* of Apollinarius was attributed to the third-century bishop of Caesarea Gregory Thaumaturgos. Theodoret, fifth-century bishop of Cyrus, historian, and theologian, also quotes extensively in his dialogues from Apollinarius to show his opponents that even this heretic agrees with orthodoxy in maintaining both an unmixed humanity and divinity in Christ.

Whereas Arius uses the *logos-sarx* approach to claim that the *Logos* is not divine, Apollinarius uses it to explain the crucial theological principle that Christ had to be God for his redemptive work to be effi-

180. For a consideration and reconstruction of some of the texts from Apollinarius and their reception, see Carter, *Apollinarian Christologies*.

cacious. To safeguard Christ's divinity, Apollinarius repudiates any notion of Christ as simply a divinely inspired man.[181] Against, presumably, the Paulianists, Apollinarius claims they have introduced a division in Christ by making him a man conjoined, παραζευχθαι or συναφθεν, to God,[182] seeing Christ as no different from a prophet. Following Scripture, mere dwelling in man was insufficient. Instead, a perfect union of God and man was vital; otherwise, Christ's redemptive work would be frustrated: "the death of a man does not annul death."[183]

Apollinarius also confronted those who held that there are two persons in Christ, a completely self-existent man conjoined to the *Logos*. From preserved titles found in the fragments of his writings, Apollinarius seemingly writes against Eunomius, who thinks the Son, as begotten, is of a different nature to the Father; against Marcellus of Ancyra, whom he accuses of Sabellianism or, like Paulianists, of presenting a fully human Christ distinguished from the *Logos*; and against Diodore of Tarsus (d. ca. 390), who as teacher of Theodore of Mopsuestia was later linked to Nestorius, the disciple of Theodore. It seems that Diodore thinks that there are two sons in Christ: the Son of God and the Son of Man.

Apollinarius agrees with Nicaea and against Arius when he asserts that the Son (and Spirit) is consubstantial with the Father and that there is a real and eternal distinction between the Trinitarian Persons.[184] The patristic scholar Kelley McCarthy Spoerl thinks that Apollinarius tries to avoid a Sabellian interpretation of *prosopon* as a changeable mask that has no enduring ontological reality in order to affirm this eternal and real distinction.[185] Apollinarius then considers how the God-man can be consubstantial with the Father. Christians, he says, should not only adhere to orthodoxy, but they should also examine the faith well, "lest it should, in some part, fall in with the opinion of the Greeks or Jews."[186]

181. "Anacephalaeosis 1," in Carter, *Apollinarian Christologies*.

182. "Anacephalaeosis 29, 21," in Carter, *Apollinarian Christologies*. Charles Raven translates this as "yoke-fellow." *Apollinarianism*, 180.

183. Apollinarius, "Apodeixis," Frag. 94 in Carter, *Apollinarian Christologies*, 379. Gregory of Nyssa, *Antirrheticus*, 218.

184. Apollinarius, "Detailed Confession of the Faith," in Spoerl, "Apollinarius on the Holy Spirit," 571–72.

185. Spoerl, "Apollinarius," 584n65.

186. Apollinarius, "Apodeixis," Frag. 13, in Carter, *Apollinarian Christologies*, 340.

Apollinarius held differing views on the union of humanity and divinity in Christ, and this has been seen variously as simple inconsistency, oscillation, development over time, or complete change.[187] Nevertheless, the progression of the thinking of Apollinarius seems to move from a synthesis or mixture of human and divine, to an assumption of humanity by the divinity. Still, Apollinarius is consistent on one major point: Christ has no human conscious intellect or human will.

Apollinarius argues that since God is one, the unity in Christ also must be complete. So, Apollinarius offers a synthesis of parts, like the synthesis of body and soul. As Grillmeier explains, it is a *synthesis anthropoeides* (σύνθεσις ἀνθρωπειδης), synthesis of the human being,[188] and Apollinarius uses the *logos-sarx* framework to present this real union of divine and human. But Apollinarius believes that "the composite cannot be one."[189] Moreover, if the *Logos* became flesh, then there was a change in him, thus compromising his divinity. So, echoing Athanasius,[190] Apollinarius says the *Logos* assumed flesh; therefore he is not changed.[191] While Athanasius and Apollinarius agree on this point, for Athanasius, Christ remains a mystery, and for Apollinarius, the union of divine and human is a problem to be solved. And while Athanasius admits that it is "strange [a paradox], that the same one who was suffering was not suffering,"[192] for Apollinarius the solution is that Christ is *Logos* and flesh, "a human being according to the flesh, but God according to the spirit."[193] In the Apollinarian scheme, instead of there being a synthesis or mixture of parts, there is an assumption between the perfect divinity and incomplete humanity. To explain, Apollinarius looks to human beings.

Although he seems to believe that all the natural human characteristics, including the soul, are inherited,[194] Apollinarius teaches that human

187. As Carter points out, some think that Apollinarius changed his Christology, while others see inconsistencies where certain passages from Scripture forced Apollinarius to rework his ideas. *Apollinarian Christologies*, 40–50.

188. Grillmeier, *Christ in Christian Tradition*, 330–32.

189. Apollinarius, "Dialogue 1," 86.

190. Athanasius, "Against the Arians," II, 47.

191. Apollinarius, "Dialogue 1," 86.

192. Athanasius, "Letter to Epictetus," 6.

193. Apollinarius, "Dialogue 1," 87.

194. See Raven, *Apollinarianism*, 172; Carter, referring to the work of Henri de Riedmatten, *Apollinarian Christologies*, 18–19.

beings "are of the same substance as irrational animals in accordance with the irrational body" and that they "are of a different substance as rational beings."[195] In the same way, God, and presumably Apollinarius is here thinking of the *Logos*, who is "of the same substance as human beings in accordance with the flesh," is "of a different substance insofar as he is Word and God." If, reasons Apollinarius, a man has both soul and body, and these remain in unity, much more does the Christ who has Godhead and body keep both secure and unconfounded.[196]

But Apollinarius adds that if the divinity is simply united with mankind, then there are two Sons, one God by nature and the other God by adoption,[197] and "if he is from two complete (beings), he is not God in the one in which he is a man, nor is he a man in the one in which he is God."[198] Instead, he says that Christ is "one as each of us is one out of spirit and soul and body."[199] Just as the substantial unity of human beings is a synthesis of body and soul, so too is the "heavenly man" a compound unity in human form.[200] The difference between the flesh of Christ and real human flesh lies only in this union of the fleshly nature of Christ with the Godhead, so that Christ becomes divine: the Word gives life to the flesh.[201] Because two complete entities cannot become one,[202] however, Apollinarius sees Christ's human nature as incomplete, without *nous* or rational soul (or the intellectual aspect of the soul), so that only when the *Logos* takes flesh and takes the place of the rational soul does he become a totality.[203]

To understand this taking of flesh, Apollinarius uses the notion of *kenosis* from the letter of St. Paul to the Philippians. According to Apolli-

195. Apollinarius, "Dialogue 2," 173. See also Gregory of Nyssa, *Antirrheticus*; "Second Book against Diodore," Fr. 146, in Carter, *Apollinarian Christologies*, 310.

196. Apollinarius, "Dialogue 2," 173.

197. Apollinarius, "Apodeixis," 373.

198. Apollinarius, "Apodeixis," 377–78.

199. Apollinarius, "Apodeixis," 363.

200. Apollinarius, "Epistle Ad Dionysius," in Raven, *Apollinarianism*, 227; see also Carter, *Apollinarian Christologies*, 298–301.

201. Apollinarius, *Ad Serapionem*," 325.

202. Apollinarius, "Second Book against Diodore," Fr. 123, in Carter, *Apollinarian Christologies*, 311.

203. See Apollinarius, "Apodeixis," Fr. 89, and Carter's comment in *Apollinarian Christologies*, 377.

narius, "to be made flesh is to be made empty, but the being made empty declares not man, but the Son of man, who emptied himself, *kenosis,* not by undergoing change, but by investiture."[204] Here Theodoret is quoting Apollinarius in order to demonstrate that even this heretic confesses that the Word is immutable. Nevertheless, this saying implies that Christ takes on human flesh in the same way as he might put on a garment.[205]

Apollinarius thinks this also applies to human beings in general, in the sense that "man is a mind in flesh."[206] Ordinary man is made up of incomplete parts, body and soul (and spirit) that together make a totality, one *physis,*[207] though neither part loses its proper nature. It seems that Apollinarius has in mind the Stoic understandings of juxtaposition as parathesis or mixture as synchysis.[208] By *physis,* Apollinarius apparently means the self-determining being, though it seems that *physis* only became identified with abstract nature during later anti-Apollinarian disputes.[209] In his comprehensive analysis of the texts of Apollinarius, Timothy Carter notes that there is some ambiguity over whether this results in a *tertium quid.* Carter has pieced together the Apollinarian model of biological synthesis, and according to this model, the living human being has a body bereft of life that undergoes a qualitative change when animated or ensouled by an animating principle, possibly conveyed in spermatic matter. Carter notes that Apollinarius appears to hold to a traducian anthropology whereby the human father supplies the human animal soul, and since Christ does not have a human father, Apollinarius has difficulty introducing the notion of a human soul. According to Rufinus, Apollinarius was forced to admit that Christ had a human soul, and this may account for a change in the thinking of Apollinarius from a body-soul model to a model of body, soul, and mind.[210] Raven argues

204. Apollinarius, "Dialogue 1"; see also Apollinarius, "Second Book against Diodore," Fr. 124, in Carter, *Apollinarian Christologies*, 312. Carter translates thus, in order to bring out the distinction in the transformation, "enfleshment is an 'emptying,' σάρκωσις κένωσις. But emptying makes known not a man, but the Son of Man who emptied himself according to the outer form, περιβολην, and not according to (essential) transformation, μεταβολην."

205. See Apollinarius, "Apodeixis," Fr. 43.

206. Apollinarius, "Apodeixis," Fr. 72–73.

207. Apollinarius, "Apodeixis," Fr. 28.

208. See Carter, *Apollinarian Christologies*, 52–55.

209. See Grillmeier, *Christ in Christian Tradition*, 233.

210. Carter, *Apollinarian Christologies*, 40.

that because Apollinarius held to traducianism, he always kept to a trichotomy of body, soul, and spirit.[211] When it comes to Christ, according to Apollinarius, the flesh from Mary is divinely informed.[212] The Word, then, contributes the "energy part" to the whole so that the union provides a place for the "unity of subject (= person?) in Christ," the mind. Apollinarius appears to affirm Christ's unity as "the divine subject" in a composition that is either a possession or descent or interweaving in the body as a form or envelope.[213]

Perhaps Apollinarius adapts Origen's distinction between body (*soma*, *sarx*), soul (*psyche*), and spirit (*nous*).[214] Origen sees three levels of meaning in Scripture corresponding to body, soul, and spirit, each level being appropriate to different spiritual stages. Apollinarius, the onetime Scripture scholar, appears to connect this to his anthropology. For Apollinarius, the earthly elements are *soma*, the lowest bodily structure through which the invisible is expressed; *sarx*, both body and lower soul; and *psyche*, the nonmaterial part of personality belonging to all human beings by nature, such that it seems to be the irrational or animal soul. The highest element is *pneuma*, spirit, which apparently refers to the rational soul or mind and is the controlling determining principle and center of personality in human beings.[215] Just as Origen had regarded humanity as essentially soul, and soul as the purely rational and spiritual in man, therefore equating it with *nous*, mind,[216] Apollinarius also conceives of the human being as enfleshed mind, and he also attributes this thinking to St. Paul.[217] Moreover, Gregory of Nazianzus says that, like the Arians, the Apollinarians use the notion of the flesh as a veil so that God can converse with human beings.[218] Unlike the Arians, however, the Apollinarians claim that the inner man is not the soul. Rather, it seems to be the mind.

It is impossible to tell whether Apollinarius claims the *Logos* takes

211. Raven, *Apollinarianism*, 172.
212. Carter, *Apollinarian Christologies*, 67.
213. Carter, *Apollinarian Christologies*, 69–70.
214. See Raven, *Apollinarianism*, 196–99; also Johannes Quasten, *Patrology*, 382.
215. Apollinarius, "Apodeixis," Fr. 25.
216. Origen, "De Principiis," II, 8, 1.
217. Apollinarius, "Apodeixis," Frags. 186, 187, 190.
218. Gregory of Nazianzus, "Epistle 101."

the place of Christ's soul or the higher part of the soul, the mind. Moreover, what is meant by soul and mind is unclear. Donald McKim claims that the *Logos* replaces the mind, that is, "Jesus' normal human psychology or soul."[219] Guy Laurie says that, according to Apollinarius, souls are by nature fallible, and therefore Apollinarius denies a soul in Christ.[220] John Maquarrie thinks that for Apollinarius, the *Logos* takes only the "personal" part of the soul.[221] Based on evidence from Theodoret, David Wallace-Hadrill regards Platonist psychology used by Apollinarius as decisive for the claim that the *Logos* takes the "reasonable soul," the mind, in Christ.[222] But other writers point out that Apollinarius is concerned not only with mind but also with what vivifies.[223] As Kelly explains, "the Word was both the directive, intelligent principle in Jesus Christ, and also the vivifying principle of his flesh"; thus the Word is the "sole life" of the God-man, even, says Kelly, at the "purely physical and biological level," and not simply for the functions of the will and intellect.[224] Nevertheless, Apollinarius says that there are two souls in human beings, the vegetative soul and the rational soul.[225] He can then argue that in Christ the flesh is "not without a soul,"[226] since the Word seems to take the place of only the rational soul. It appears that the nonintellectual soul animates the body in an animalistic fashion and so is a second source of energy in the human being alongside the rational soul.[227] Having said that, in his first letter to Dionysius, Apollinarius says that "the body is not of itself a nature . . . since it is not life-giving according to itself," and in the case of Christ, "nor was the created body alive without

219. McKim, *Theological Turning Points*, 34.

220. Laurie, *Introducing Early Christianity*, 286.

221. Macquarrie, *Christology Revisited*, 51.

222. Wallace-Hadrill, *Christian Antioch*, 135.

223. See Ngaire Williams, *Divine Sense*, 86.

224. Kelly, *Early Christian Doctrines*, 292.

225. Apollinarius, "Dialogue 2," 173.

226. Apollinarius, "Apodeixis," Fr. 22.

227. See Carter, *Apollinarian Christologies*, 151. Later, the Council of Vienna (1311–12) condemned the doctrine of John Olieu, who had taught that the form of the body was not the spiritual soul. The council was faced with claims from the "spirituals" whose teaching tended to split human nature into the spiritual and the bodily reality. Instead, the council affirmed the unity of the person. The council clarifies that the rational soul, which is one with the sensitive and vegetative elements, is the form of the body. "General Council of Vienna," in Dupuis and Neuner, *Christian Faith in the Doctrinal Documents of the Catholic Church*, 164–65.

the divinity."[228] This is perhaps an illustration of the change or oscillation in his thinking.

Apollinarius is, however, consistent in thinking that, as with the different parts in human beings, in Christ the divine and human parts are not equivalent: preeminence goes to the divine *pneuma*. This becomes the life-giving spirit and animator of his fleshly nature, so much so that the *Logos* is in complete control not only on a spiritual or willing level but also of Christ's actual physical life,[229] the same kind of logos-vitalism found in the Arian system: in Christ, there is one life totally controlled by the Godhead. Similarly, Apollinarius calls the human mind the "sublime element" that does not participate in the flesh.[230] The mind is "autonomous, αὐτοκράτωρ, being moved by its own volition."[231] For Apollinarius, the mind supplies power to the flesh that is purely passive. Without this power of self-determination, mind ceases to be mind, for "it is the destruction of a self-determining creature to deprive it of its self-determination."[232]

Apollinarius reasons that the *Logos* unites with an incomplete, mindless body[233] on two accounts. First, he thinks two complete natures produce either a hybrid or two entities, and he wishes to assert a natural unity, a one, whose *physis* is the self-determining being. Second, Apollinarius is constrained by his notion of the workings of the human mind. Apollinarius explains that the rational soul, as center of self-determination, makes choices between good and evil and thus is liable to sin. But he also sees the operations of the human mind purely in terms of the power to choose, and inevitably sinful choice choosing sin over good.[234] God and man, then, are naturally opposites. For Apollinarius, there cannot be two minds operating in a single person without one

228. Apollinarius, "First Letter to Dionysius," in Carter, *Apollinarian Christologies*, 298–301, at 300.

229. Apollinarius, "First Letter to Dionysius," in Carter, *Apollinarian Christologies*, 298–301.

230. Apollinarius in Gregory of Nyssa, *Antirrheticus*.

231. Raven, *Apollinarianism*, 182; Apollinarius, "Letter to Julian," in Carter, *Apollinarian Christologies*, 328–29, at 328.

232. Apollinarius in Gregory of Nyssa, *Antirrheticus;* "Apodeixis," Fr. 87.

233. Apollinarius, "Apodeixis," Fr. 27.

234. Apollinarius in Gregory of Nyssa, *Antirrheticus*; "Apodeixis," Fr. 76.

striving against the other,[235] an argument employed later by the monothelites, who held that Christ had only one will. According to Apollinarius, those who think there are two minds in Christ fail to acknowledge this conflict: the presence of both a divine mind that is "self-moving and moved uniformly, ταυτοκίνητος, since immutable, ἄτρεπτος," and a human mind that is self-moving but not moved uniformly since it is mutable, and would create a being "at odds (with himself) torn apart by the opposing wills, θελήμασι, of which he consists."[236] Moreover, if Christ has a human mind, he cannot overthrow sin, and because of sin, redemption requires Christ to be God.[237] So, Apollinarius implies that the *Logos* replaces Christ's mind or spirit, and the energy of will and life-giving power of the *Logos* as the "life-giving spirit" completely fills the flesh to unite the two into a living functional unity.[238] Apollinarius concludes, "not one division of the Word and of his flesh is put forward in the divine scriptures, but he is one nature, one hypostasis, one energy, ἐνέργεια, one person, προσοπον, the same individual, ὁ αὐτός, wholly God and wholly man."[239] This implies that, for Apollinarius, *physis* is the self-determining being whose foundation lies in free will, decision, and thought. The person, the form in which the *physis* appears, is the *hegemonikon*, the inner man. There is one person in a shell of a body.

For Apollinarius, just as mind or the higher part of the soul governs and energizes the body, so too does the Word govern the flesh. In terms of anthropology, the position of Apollinarius implies that the *physis*, the reality of the human being, is its self-determining principle, the mind, perhaps recalling Cartesian and Lockean views of the person. Just as the *Logos* does not share in the suffering of the body, the enfleshed mind seems unmoved by the flesh. It appears that Apollinarius defines a living being by free will:[240] with the body merely the mind's instrument, once the mind is no longer functioning, the body is no longer properly alive.

235. Apollinarius, "Apodeixis," Fr. 22; see Carter, *Apollinarian Christologies*, 151.

236. Apollinarius, "Letter to Julian," Fr. 151, in Carter, *Apollinarian Christologies*, 328. Raven, *Apollinarianism*, 183–84.

237. Apollinarius, "Apodeixis," Fr. 93–97.

238. Apollinarius, "Apodeixis," Fr. 89–90.

239. Apollinarius, "On the Faith and the Incarnation," 6, in Carter, *Apollinarian Christologies*, 320; see also Raven, *Apollinarianism*, 211, 223.

240. Apollinarius, "Apodeixis," Fr. 87.

Although this is not a perfect parallel with some contemporary thought that separates the death of the person from the death of the human being, it perhaps has resonance with those who regard, for instance, a patient existing in a persistent vegetative state as "a living but unoccupied organism" with the same status as a dead organism.[241] In effect, Apollinarius has created a separation between the person and the human being.

Gregory of Nazianzus and Gregory of Nyssa

Gregory of Nazianzus and Gregory of Nyssa disagree with Apollinarius on one fundamental point, among other contentions: Apollinarius claims that the "man of the Lord," *kyriakos anthropos*, is Lord without a human mind.[242] Gregory of Nazianzus and Gregory of Nyssa explain that all human beings have a rational nature, so if Christ assumes true humanity, then he too has a human rational nature and so has a soul and mind.[243] Although Gregory of Nazianzus and Gregory of Nyssa refer their Christology to their Trinitarian theology, they do not seem to make full use of the understandings of nature and person that they had helped to forge in Trinitarian reflection. This may be because Apollinarius had already used *prosopon* for the man Jesus. Nevertheless, Andrew Hofer argues that certain philosophical and rhetorical words have been given "special treatment" such that they have been "used in scholarship to frame the entire history of Christology." Instead, Hofer thinks that Gregory of Nazianzus simply had "other ways of evoking the mystery of Christ."[244] In any case, the Christological concerns of Gregory of Nazianzus and Gregory of Nyssa lie more in the issue of salvation than in the "how" of the God-man.[245] Furthermore, Gregory of Nazianzus had already been attacked on his understanding of the coequality of the Spirit by those with subordinationist tendencies.[246] But Gregory of Na-

241. McMahan, *Ethics of Killing*, 446–47.

242. Gregory of Nazianzus, "Epistle 101," 216.

243. According to Andrew Hofer, both Gregories are adamant that Christ has a mind; however, Gregory of Nazianzus sees the mind as the mediating element in the Incarnation. *Christ in the Life and Teaching of Gregory of Nazianzus*, 114.

244. Hofer, *Christ in the Life and Teaching of Gregory of Nazianzus*, 93. Hofer also notes that Gregory of Nazianzus sometimes uses philosophical words in unexpected ways (93n6).

245. For Gregory of Nazianzus, see Beeley, *Gregory of Nazianzus*, 116, also chap. 2. For Gregory of Nyssa, see Daley, "Divine Transcendence and Human Transformation," 502.

246. John McGuckin argues that, in his two letters to Cledonius, Gregory of Nazianzus

zianzus and Gregory of Nyssa do engage with Apollinarius on his terms: using the analogy of body and soul in human beings.

Gregory of Nazianzus agrees with Apollinarius that the *Logos* assumes manhood for our salvation.[247] Gregory asserts that as soul and body are two natures, so too are God and man. As Weinandy points out, however, if body and soul are thought to be two natures rather than aspects of the one person, and then the divinity is factored in, there appears to be three natures.[248] Perhaps Gregory does realize the difficulties with the analogy of soul and body to divine and human in Jesus Christ. After all, Gregory says that the analogy is limited: as he explains, the human mind is "perfect and commanding" but only regarding the soul and body; it is "not absolutely perfect." The mind remains a servant and subject to God, not "a sharer of his princedom and honour."[249] Gregory nevertheless concedes that St. Paul speaks of an "inner and outer man." Still, he continues, since we do not talk of "two manhoods," in the Savior, the two natures are distinct from each other as invisible and visible, yet he is not two persons: both natures are one by the combination.[250] Gregory here is perhaps thinking of Diodore of Tarsus, who appears to take a view at the other extreme to Apollinarius in that Diodore suggests that in Christ there are two sons. To clarify, Gregory makes a further distinction: in Christ there is manhood and Godhead in one person, while in the one Godhead there are three different persons.[251]

Gregory claims that instead of the Apollinarian "Lord without a

deliberately chooses not to engage on a Trinitarian level because he had already been attacked on his understanding of the coequality of the Spirit by opponents with subordinationist tendencies, and he believed that these tendencies were shared by some of the Cappadocian hierarchs. *St Gregory of Nazianzus*, 389. McGuckin suggests that Gregory of Nazianzus is a "devotee of the 'middle way'" when it comes to Christology and becomes "bolder" in his Trinitarian theology during his mature years. But it appears that the dates given are 380 for the *Theological Orations* and 382 for the *Letters to Cledonius* (see the critical texts in Jurgens, *Faith of the Early Fathers*, 2:28, 2:40). Still, Gregory of Nazianzus prefers to place himself clearly within the orthodoxy of the Creed of Nicaea and its additional article on the Holy Spirit. "Epistle 101 and 102."

247. Gregory of Nazianzus, "Epistle 101," 216.

248. See Weinandy, *Does God Suffer?*, 184.

249. Gregory of Nazianzus, "Epistle 101," 220.

250. Hofer notes that Gregory may be adamant that Christ has a rational soul, but he does not detail its inner workings. *Christ in the Life and Teaching of Gregory of Nazianzus*, 95. Hofer also explores ancient mixture language in general (96–106).

251. Gregory of Nazianzus, "Epistle 101," 217.

mind," orthodoxy asserts the "unity and identity" of the person of Christ by not severing the man from the Godhead. The God-man is "passible in his flesh, impassible in his Godhead," "earthly and heavenly," "perfect man and also God."[252] Using the trichotomy of body, soul, and mind that Apollinarius presents, Gregory jokes that it is "mindless" nonsense to say that Christ has a soul but not a human mind because this does not reflect what man is: because of his rational human nature, "man is not a mindless animal."[253] This has nothing to do with whether a human being has the working faculty of a mind. Gregory is talking about the rational nature that all human beings have because of the kind of animal that they are. Gregory continues that divinity joined to flesh alone is not man, nor is it man if joined to the soul alone or to both apart from the intellect, "the most essential part of man."[254] For Gregory, the "Lord without a mind" is a mutilation.[255]

If Gregory's comment is applied to human beings, then it challenges those bioethicists who claim that human beings without a fully functioning mind are the equivalent of nonentities. Although we may wish to avoid the notion of mutilation, the idea that such a person is profoundly disabled rather than a nonentity perhaps better describes the situation. Moreover, Gregory's comment that the intellect is a major aspect of humanity allows us to acknowledge the severity of the situation of a brain-damaged person.

Again, in agreement with Apollinarius, Gregory says that Christ has to be fully human with a mind. But Gregory says this is a human mind since "that which he has not assumed he has not healed": for the salvation of the whole human, it matters that Christ is fully human.[256] Moreover, if as Apollinarius argues the mind tends toward sin, it is in even more need of healing,[257] and if Christ did not take on a mind, then God is the savior only of the flesh, the "less precious" part of man.[258]

252. Gregory of Nazianzus, "Epistle 101," 216.

253. Gregory of Nazianzus, "Epistle 101," 219. Apparently, Gregory frequently jokes about the "mindless" or "brainless" Christology. McGuckin, *St Gregory of Nazianzus*, 226.

254. Gregory of Nazianzus, "Epistle 101," 219.

255. Gregory of Nazianzus, "Epistle 101," 225.

256. Gregory of Nazianzus, "Epistle 101," 218.

257. Gregory of Nazianzus, "Epistle 101," 220.

258. Gregory of Nazianzus, "Epistle 101," 222.

In addition to the work done by Gregory of Nazianzus, Gregory of Nyssa examines further the belief of Apollinarius that because the human mind is "at enmity with God," Christ cannot have a human mind.[259] For Gregory of Nyssa, the mind does not consist of sin; it is what humans do with it that matters, and choice can be for the good. Moreover, just as Christ was not defiled through his birth in the flesh, neither is his mind corrupted. Gregory also questions how Apollinarius interprets St. Paul. Whereas Apollinarius splits human beings into three parts and places the mind at war with God by its inevitable turning toward evil choices, Gregory says St. Paul did not divide humans into three parts. Rather, the key point is that he "keeps man whole."[260] Significantly, discussions about human beings may focus on the mind or the person, soul, or body; however, they are not separate parts of a human being. In theological terms, as Gregory reads St. Paul, "no aspect of our human nature is unmindful of God"; indeed, we should have God in mind when engaged in eating, drinking, and in all our bodily activities, for "everything pertaining to the body, soul and spirit is intent upon sanctification."[261]

Although Gregory of Nyssa accepts a conceptual distinction in human beings as flesh, soul, and mind, he thinks that by actually splitting "man" up, by separating off mind, which is the "essential aspect," Apollinarius "defines the rest of man as a beast," possibly suggesting merely biological life, "a fact which" says Gregory "certainly is not true."[262] According to Gregory, Apollinarius identifies the mind with what belongs to the divinity even though Apollinarius also spurns the mind owing to its fallen and mutable nature. Apollinarius assumes that the human mind and the divine *Logos* fall in the same category as types of mind (notably, Swinburne makes the same move in his version of modern

259. Gregory of Nyssa, *Antirrheticus*.

260. Gregory of Nyssa, *Antirrheticus*. In his discussion of Gregory of Nyssa's "symbiotic unity" of body and soul in human beings, Peter Bouteneff in "Essential or Existential" explains that Gregory does not see the body either as given to human beings as a result of the Fall (415) or as simply an addition to human nature (417). While Gregory does not think the body is part of the image of God in itself, since "materiality is incongruous with the divine archetype," Gregory does regard the body as being the "image-by-association" (417).

261. Gregory of Nyssa, *Antirrheticus*, quoting 1 Cor 10:31.

262. Gregory of Nyssa, *Antirrheticus*.

Trinitarian theology).[263] Hence the minds are in competition. Gregory replies that neither mind nor body can be associated with the divine transcendent nature by reason of their essence. "Man," explains Gregory, is "a rational animal": he or she shares the nature of irrational animals yet is not dominated by instinct, the body, or the senses. Thought, reason, and the mind, which are "man's proper nature," distinguish humanity from irrational beasts. Humankind, then, has a rational nature, and this is attested to by the dominion over other animals, for anything that comes into existence in order to rule requires in its nature a "governing principle."[264]

While he accepts that some say mind resides in the brain, since injury to the brain affects reasoning,[265] Gregory argues that the mind is not simply in a part of the body because it is equally in touch with the whole human being.[266] He says that in human beings there are three specific faculties, one somatic, one sense related, and one concerned with reasoning. These are not three "souls" welded together, however. Rather, the "true and perfect soul is naturally one, intellectual and immaterial, which mingles with our material nature by agency of the senses."[267] As Gregory explains, the mind produces the "music of reason" by means of our "instrumental construction," so we are born rational. If we know how to play but are unable because the instrument is unfit, then we simply cannot demonstrate our skill.[268]

And the Human Being without a Mind?

Given this understanding of mind as the higher aspect of the soul, when Gregory of Nyssa argues that "man is necessarily rational and is not a man should he lack this capacity," it is precisely to underscore the point that rationality belongs to human nature. As Gregory's letter *On Not Three Gods* explains, "man" is not the individual man but what is in common. A human soul is a rational nature, so that a human being nec-

263. Swinburne, *Is There a God?*, 4–5.
264. Gregory of Nyssa, *Antirrheticus.*
265. Gregory of Nyssa, *On the Making of Man*, XII, 1.
266. Gregory of Nyssa, *On the Making of Man*, XIV, 1.
267. Gregory of Nyssa, *On the Making of Man*, XIV, 2.
268. Gregory of Nyssa, *On the Making of Man*, X, 1; XII, 8.

essarily shares in this rational nature, even if he or she does not actually have the use of this capacity. This means that Jesus is not a human being without a mind, the "Man-God" of Apollinarius, by analogy a "horse-deer" or "goat-stag," for "we do not have a half man."[269]

Gregory of Nyssa's discussion *On Infants' Early Deaths* further supports this idea. Some people were asking what to make of infants who died prematurely in terms of God's judgment: Are they to be treated as if they did not exist, or as one of the good ones who enjoy a life of blessedness? Gregory frames their question:

> A human being enters on the scene of life, draws in the air, beginning the process of living with a cry of pain, pays the tribute of a tear to nature, just tastes life's sorrows, before any of its sweets have been his, before his feelings have gained any strength; still loose in all his joints, tender, pulpy, unset; in a word before he is even human (if the gift of reason is man's peculiarity, and he has never had it in him) such a one with no advantage over the embryo in the womb except he has seen the air, so short-lived, dies and goes to pieces again.... [W]hat are we to think about him?

At first sight, with his questioners, Gregory takes the view that to be human, an entity must also actually be rational. In the context of this discussion, Locke's view that "person," as a forensic term, concerned with praise and blame, comes to mind. But Gregory argues that God gives existence to everything, including human nature, and that the design of "all that is being born" is to glorify God by means of their intellectual natures with their final eschatological end being to "look on God." This life of being "made friends with God" is not a reward. Rather, it is a hope in much the same way as one who is clear-sighted is not rewarded with the prize of being able to see but sight naturally follows. On the one hand, he says this future life of blessedness is in essence "a heritage of humanity"; on the other hand, it is also a reward, since by our actions we receive our just desserts. So, those who have been seized by the "plague of ignorance," that is, have willed and chosen things that move them away from God, but have taken the required treatment (been admitted to the sacraments and pursued a life of conversion and virtue)

269. Gregory of Nyssa, *Antirrheticus*.

and been purged receive their due reward. Those who refuse treatment become estranged from the "truly natural life." As for prematurely dead infants, they continue to exist in that natural life because they have not had the plague, that is, they have not personally sinned in the sense of deliberately moving away from God; thus their souls partake of that truly natural life according to their capacity. Gregory does not suggest that infants do not need to be saved by Christ. Certainly, the individual contributes toward his or her destiny, and so Gregory says that each receives a measure of blessedness though they also become capable of more through contemplation, for God can come into each of us as is appropriate to each. It seems, then, for Gregory, the embryo shares in the heritage of humanity, a life of blessedness, and thus he implies that even though fetuses are not functionally rational, they do each have a rational nature and share in the destiny of all human beings.[270] Augustine's view, though more cautious, is not dissimilar. Regarding fetuses who have died in the womb and babies who die shortly after birth, he says, "I do not venture either to affirm or deny that they will rise again. I do not, however, see why, if they are not excluded from the number of the dead, they should not share in the resurrection of the dead.... I do not see how I can say that even those who die in their mother's womb shall have no resurrection."[271]

Gregory takes issue with what he sees as the error of Apollinarius in defining a living being by free will, such that a person devoid of free will is not a living being. This, Gregory says, is plainly wrong. For instance, slaves do not have free will, they do not have minds of their own, says Gregory, because they are under the control of others, and following Apollinarian logic that a person without free will is not a living being, then all slaves are dead even if they have souls. Gregory adds that when the rational nature of human beings or any other aspect of human nature is denied, then the name "man" is destroyed.[272] Hans Boersma points out that, for Gregory of Nyssa, "the basic 'sameness' of human beings, based in their being 'of the same race,' ὁμόφυλος, implies a rad-

270. Gregory of Nyssa, "On Infants' Early Deaths."

271. Augustine, *City of God against the Pagans*, XXII.13. See International Theological Commission, "Hope of Salvation for Infants," 353–400.

272. Gregory of Nyssa, *Antirrheticus*.

ical equality." Boersma adds "with obvious social implications," as he is speaking in the context of slavery.[273] However, the same comment arises in the context of human beings with disabilities. In terms of Christology, Gregory says that just as the Good Shepherd carries the whole sheep, so too does Christ bear the whole man. For Gregory, this unity of body and soul is made even clearer beyond earthly life: since "death is the dissolution of body and soul, he who unites both to himself (body and soul) does not separate them" and unites both in the resurrection.[274] Thus the soul no longer suffers separation, and the result is total salvation for human nature.

Although Athanasius, Gregory of Nazianzus, and Gregory of Nyssa speak of the *Logos* assuming the whole human being, they talk of human nature, not human persons. In Christ there is only one divine person, though establishing two natures in Christ eventually leads some to the Nestorian position of asserting two persons. It seems that the issue between Gregory of Nazianzus, Gregory of Nyssa, and Apollinarius is that while the Gregories assert a rational nature, Apollinarius speaks of the significance of an entity being able to exercise rationality. For Apollinarius, the *Logos* is the vivifying element, the higher part of the soul, of the passive flesh of Christ. Therefore, according to Gregory of Nyssa, Apollinarius defines a living being by free will such that where there is not mind or free will, there is no longer life.[275] Bioethicists do comment on concrete entities, beings that do not have minds, people who are profoundly disabled like the anencephalic infant or the patient in persistent vegetative state. Following Apollinarius, it seems that flesh without a mind is lifeless, which implies that such patients are not human beings, never mind persons. Conversely, the Gregories recognize that human beings have rational natures, such that whatever a human being's capacities, he or she shares in all that belongs to humankind.

273. Boersma, *Embodiment and Virtue in Gregory of Nyssa*, 157.
274. Gregory of Nyssa, *Antirrheticus*.
275. Gregory of Nyssa, *Antirrheticus*.

Moving from *Logos-sarx* to *Logos-anthropos* Christology

While *logos-sarx* Christology stresses soteriological concerns and affirms that it is not merely an aspect but the whole human being that is healed and saved, *logos-anthropos* Christology also places focus on the whole person, yet it also centers more particularly on free will. Nestorius shares the same problem as Apollinarius but differently applied: Apollinarius thinks that if there are two natures in Christ, then there must be two persons, and he "mutilates" the human nature so that he can maintain a unity of one person, Jesus Christ. Nestorius assumes that if there are two natures, there must be two persons, and so he presents a conjunction in Jesus Christ instead of a true unity.

Antiochene *Logos-anthropos* Christology and the Joined-Up Person

How the union of two natures comes about in Christ is a general problem for Christology, even though it appears to be a particularly Eastern issue between Nestorius and Cyril of Alexandria. Nevertheless, a similar situation to that of Nestorius and Cyril had arisen in the West, with Leporius taking the part of Nestorius.

In about 418, a monk from Gaul called Leporius presented his version of the Incarnation. His version was regarded as problematic, and he took refuge with Augustine, who fortunately managed to resolve the situation before it became a crisis.[276] Leporius seems to think that it was improper for the transcendent God to be born as man, suffer, and die, so he sees Christ as the perfect man, with a human nature joined to the divine nature but not truly united to it. Leporius seems to be engaged in a form of pre-Nestorian thinking,[277] and he may have also had Pelagian tendencies.[278] Augustine was able to sway Leporius, and Leporius quickly ac-

276. Augustine, *Letter* 219. See also Lancel, *St Augustine*, 347–48. Augustine's letter is also from at least three other African bishops, and it asks the bishops of Gaul to accept back the now repentant Leporius. The letter is usually dated at 426, though it may have the earlier date of 418; see Teske's translation (69n1).

277. See Jurgens, *Faith of the Early Fathers*, 3:196.

278. Fairbairn, *Grace and Christology*, 169–70.

cepts that in Christ humanity and divinity are "united inseparably," not by conversion or change; rather, the Word becomes truly man.[279] Under Augustine's influence, Leporius sees that person and nature are distinct, and in the Incarnation, human nature is conjoined with the person of the Word, not with the divine nature. Thus there is one person in the Godhead and in manhood, so both human and divine properties can be predicated of this one person, the Word.

Augustine states that in Christ there are certainly two substances (meaning natures), God and man, but one single person, "God, soul and flesh,"[280] without addition or confusion, and without adding a fourth thing to the Trinity of Persons.[281] When Augustine speaks of "one person," he does not mean that the psychological human subject, Jesus, is either replaced or absorbed by the *Logos*. Instead, Augustine uses the analogy of body and soul to explain that "just as the soul is united to the body in the unity of the person in order that a human being might exist, so God is united to the man in the unity of the person in order that Christ might exist."[282] It is the very person of the Word who is Son of God and Son of man.[283] For Augustine, the union of divine and human in Christ is wonderful and indescribable,[284] though he also says that the union of body and soul, which "happens every day for the procreation of human beings," is equally surprising even if not beyond our experience.[285] Although Augustine has in mind that just as a human person has a psychosomatic unity of body and soul, Christ has this kind of unity insofar as he is truly man, Augustine also recognizes that Christ has a higher principle of unity since he is further integrated with the Word.[286]

Augustine appears to have easily dealt with Leporius. This is possibly

279. Leporius, "Libellus Emendationis," 197.

280. Augustine, *The Trinity*, XIII:22. Edmund Hill notes that Augustine "uses the word 'substance' in the same sense as Chalcedon was going to talk about 'nature'; the two terms are for him in fact practically synonymous, except that 'substance' could be said to be 'nature' in the concrete" ("Response," 364n50).

281. Augustine, *Sermon* 187:3, 4. The appendix to this volume (439–40) explains the complications surrounding the Latin texts. See also *Letter* 120:7.

282. Augustine, *Letter* 137:11.

283. Augustine, "Enchiridion on Faith, Hope and Charity," 36, 40; idem, *Letter* 137.

284. Augustine, "Enchiridion on Faith, Hope and Charity," 13, 41.

285. Augustine, *Letter* 137:11.

286. Augustine, *The Trinity*, XIII:22.

due to the personalities of the two, also perhaps because the Western language of the person was less problematic, notably given the work Augustine had already done on clarifying terms in his Trinitarian teaching. Augustine operates out of the Latin tradition based on Tertullian's "one person in two natures," even though he also brings in the newer strand that the union is a matter of grace.[287] Moreover, Augustine was not required to formulate his Christology in a battlefield of controversies. But it was a different story in the East with the angry clash between Nestorius and Cyril of Alexandria.

As a young man, Cyril of Alexandria had been present at the Synod of the Oak, which deposed John Chrysostom (ca. 345–407), the popular archbishop of Constantinople, in 403. In 412, Cyril was elected archbishop of Alexandria, succeeding his uncle, archbishop Theophilus. The election was not free from controversy, and his time as archbishop was marked by conflict between the Christians and both pagans and Jews. Although a political figure and a theologian, Cyril is perhaps best known as the opponent of Nestorius (ca. 381–452). Nestorius was a monk from Antioch and a disciple of Theodore of Mopsuestia. Nestorius became the archbishop of Constantinople in 428. But his negative attitude toward traditional piety made him unpopular and led to street riots. The controversy he stirred affected all the major Christian centers. Politics and personalities were certainly significant factors as the issue reached crisis point, even if the issue cannot be reduced to a clash of personalities.[288] Nevertheless, the roots of the Nestorian controversy seem to run more deeply in the East than in the West, which can be seen in the teaching tradition received by Nestorius.

Theodore of Mopsuestia, known as the Interpreter, was one of the main Antiochene biblical scholars and was highly respected in his lifetime. He was taught by Diodore of Tarsus (d. ca. 390), another of the great Syrian biblical interpreters who had also taught John Chrysostom. Diodore's theology was not without its critics: although his full work was destroyed, Apollinarius had already pointed out that Diodore presented

287. John McGuckin charts a development in Augustine's thinking, "Did Augustine's Christology Depend on Theodore of Mopsuestia?," 39–52. See also McWilliam, "Augustine at Ephesus?," 56–67.

288. See McGuckin, *St Cyril of Alexandria*, 21.

Christ as "two sons." Indeed, the anti-Apollinarian writings of Gregory of Nazianzus are as much concerned with the Apollinarian extreme of the divine swallowing up the human in Christ as they are with the other extreme of separating out Christ into two persons bolted together. Moreover, the relationship between Gregory of Nazianzus and Diodore had been tense ever since they clashed in 381 at the Council of Constantinople over who should succeed as president of the council after Meletius of Antioch's death. The teaching tradition of Diodore and Theodore came under the most scrutiny soon after Theodore's death, when Cyril of Alexandria accused the two teachers, now dead, essentially of being Nestorian before Nestorius.[289] Diodore was finally condemned at a synod in Constantinople in 499, and Theodore was condemned in the fifth ecumenical Council of Constantinople of 553. To explain this teaching tradition, the thinking of Theodore of Mopsuestia and responses to it are particularly instructive, not least because Theodore's use of anthropology to clarify his argument gives an interesting picture of the human person.

Theodore of Mopsuestia and Nemesius of Emesa: The God-in-Man and the God-Man; the Soul-in-a-Body-Bag and Embodied Soul

Theodore

From fragments of his work, Theodore appears concerned with defending what he regards as orthodoxy. Against the Paulianists, he argues that Christ was more than a mere man even though he had a "swifter growth." Christ was not born like human beings, either, since he was formed by the activity of the Spirit.[290] Against the Arians, Theodore asserts that the Word is fully divine,[291] but notably he refers specifically to the Word as opposed to Christ's humanity.[292] Against Apollinarius, Theodore claims that not only did "the assumed man," Christ, have a

289. Cyril of Alexandria, "Against Diodore of Tarsus and Theodore of Mopsuestia."
290. Theodore of Mopsuestia, "On the Incarnation," 126–47, 7.
291. Theodore of Mopsuestia, "Catechetical Homilies," 158–70, 5.
292. Theodore of Mopsuestia, "On the Incarnation," 6.

rational human soul and free will, but he also increased in moral wisdom. Moreover, he says that Christ had no separate operation apart from the Word, to which he was united from conception.[293] Theodore says it is "great madness" not to believe that Christ assumed a soul, since if the Godhead replaced the soul, then, against the evidence of Scripture, Christ would not have been hungry, thirsty, or tired. And anyone who thinks he did not assume a human mind would be "even madder," since such a person would be implying that he assumed an irrational soul like that of a beast. Besides, it was necessary for not only the body but also the rational soul to be assumed because Christ came to abolish sin first, and sin "has its origin in the will of the soul."[294]

Unlike Apollinarius, Theodore thinks that allowing Christ a human soul is unproblematic because Theodore preaches a clear distinction between the two natures in Christ. From his strong commitment to God's transcendence and impassibility, Theodore thinks that there cannot be a union between the uncreated, infinite, immutable, and the created, finite, mutable: any mixture is simply not fitting.[295] So, Theodore does not accept that the Word suffered, died, or was raised. Certainly, the impossibility of such a union is also part of the more extreme version of the *logos-sarx* framework that is resolved by swallowing up either the divinity (Arianism) or humanity (Apollinarianism) of Christ. Nevertheless, Theodore rejects Apollinarianism partly because it does not accord with his theological anthropology. For Theodore, it is vital that Christ takes "our very nature,"[296] is truly human, has a real physical human life, and exercises real freedom and moral responsibility so that his redeeming sacrifice is an act of his own human decision.[297] Theodore's reasoning that Christ grew in wisdom supports his view that human beings grow toward perfection through obedience until they become like God.[298] But

293. Theodore of Mopsuestia, "On the Incarnation," 7. See also McLeod, "Theodore of Mopsuestia Revisited," 447–80.

294. Theodore of Mopsuestia, "Catechetical Homilies," 5.

295. Theodore of Mopsuestia, "On the Incarnation," 8.

296. Theodore of Mopsuestia, "Catechetical Homilies," 7.

297. Theodore of Mopsuestia, "Catechetical Homilies," 15.

298. According to Norman Russell, for thinkers like Theodore, this becoming "like God" is more in title rather than adoption or full sonship; it may occur, but only as a remote eschatological event. *Doctrine of Deification*, 237.

it is unclear how he squares this with his view that Christ has no separate operation from the Word.[299]

To explain how two disparate elements, divine and human, can be united, Theodore uses anthropology. According to Theodore, human beings consist of body and soul, two natures—one mortal and one immortal—in one human unity, and he complains that Apollinarius introduces a third nature with his focus on mind.[300] Theodore thinks that the human soul differs from the animal soul by the fact that the animal does not have a distinct *hypostasis*,[301] which seems to mean real existence, of the soul apart from the material composition of the animal: the animal soul is not immortal. But the soul of a human being is "much higher" than the body, being immortal and incapable of injury, and because of its immortal nature, it is truly rational.[302] Apparently, Theodore also thinks that the soul becomes immortal at our resurrection, our "second spiritual birth," baptism being the first spiritual birth.[303] Because Theodore believes the soul to be incapable of injury yet united with a body, he can also say that the Word does not suffer physically but only metaphorically: when Christ's body is scourged, the Word suffers in love.[304]

In connection with the Trinity and the Old Testament, Theodore explains that *hypostasis* refers to what the Godhead really is, and it is therefore beyond comprehension. He adds that *prosopon* is linked to revelation and human apprehension, so we can come to recognize that God exists in three *prosopa*.[305] Using the analogy of body and soul for the union of divine and human in Christ, Theodore says that body and soul each have their own *hypostasis* and nature, yet the two natures are one. Similarly, each nature in Christ has a real existence, *hypostasis*, but "the

299. Theodore of Mopsuestia, "On the Incarnation," 7.

300. Theodore of Mopsuestia, "In Opposition to Apollinaris," 148–57, 4.

301. This seems to be translated as "person"; see, e.g., Alphonse Mingana *Commentary of Theodore of Mopsuestia*, 1–18), who regards the Syriac transliteration of *prosopon* as a probable translation of *hypostasis*. Mingana translates this as "person" or "personality, existence" to accord with what he sees as fourth-century terminology (58n3). McLeod, however, leaves *hypostasis* untranslated (Theodore of Mopsuestia, "Catechetical Homilies," 5).

302. Theodore of Mopsuestia, "Catechetical Homilies," 5.

303. See Russell, *Doctrine of Deification*, 237.

304. See McLeod, "Theodore of Mopsuestia Revisited."

305. Theodore of Mopsuestia, "Commentary on Haggai," 2.

person, *prosopon*, of the union is one."[306] Notably, Descartes asserts two substances in human beings;[307] they are so "tightly joined" that the person, the "thinking thing," has sensations of hunger, thirst, and pain as a result of "confused modes of thinking" rather than the "thinking thing" in fact being affected by sensations.[308]

To stress this oneness, Theodore uses the analogy of husband and wife, an analogy Origen previously used: that they are "one flesh" in marriage does not impede them from being two by nature.[309] Although it does not appear to be Theodore's intent, this analogy rather seems to emphasize the separateness of the two, just like his understanding of body and soul in human beings. In each case the two are joined together; still, there does not necessarily appear to be a deep unity, particularly since in the human being the soul does not seem to suffer with the body. As a result, Frederick McLeod calls Theodore the "father of Nestorianism" because in Theodore's Christology, the "one person" Jesus reflects the fragile union of the two natures.[310] McLeod also argues that Theodore, like the later Nestorius, rejects Mary as *Theotokos*, the title traditionally given to her: Mother of God.[311]

Theodore suggests that he does accept Mary as *Theotokos* when he discusses the question, "Is Mary Mother of Man or Mother of God?" His answer is "both": it was a man in her womb, and God was in the man who was born.[312] Nestorius asks the same question, but his answer is simply "mother of man."[313] Yet Cyril quotes Theodore as saying that the Word is not Mary's son, since what is mortal bears what is mortal by nature, a body like itself.[314] Cyril's seems an accurate interpretation

306. Theodore of Mopsuestia, "On the Incarnation," 8.

307. Descartes, "Principles of Philosophy," in *Philosophical Essays and Correspondence*, I, 48.

308. Descartes, "Meditations," in *Philosophical Essays and Correspondence*, Meditation VI, 81.

309. Theodore of Mopsuestia, "Catechetical Homilies," 8.

310. McLeod, "Theodore of Mopsuestia Revisited"; idem, *Roles of Christ's Humanity in Salvation*, 196–97.

311. Socrates, "Historia Ecclesiastica," in Stevenson, *Creeds, Councils and Controversies*, VII, 32.

312. Theodore of Mopsuestia, "On the Incarnation," 15.

313. Nestorius, "Fragment," 203.

314. Cyril of Alexandria, "Against Diodore of Tarsus and Theodore of Mopsuestia."

of what Theodore meant, so McLeod appears to be correct in his assessment, particularly if account is taken of how Theodore arrives at his conclusions.

Primarily a biblical scholar, Theodore looks to the New Testament and applies literal exegesis when formulating his Christology. Firmly in the Antiochene tradition,[315] he stresses concrete realities, and so he seems to regard each of the two natures in Christ as really existing and functioning in their own rights, just as he seems to see body and soul in human beings. His focus, then, is on each nature rather than on the person of the Word as the source for the activities of the Word and of the man. Theodore generally does not refer to Jesus but to the Word, the "one assuming" and to the "one assumed."[316] For Theodore, there is one common *prosopon* in Christ: the person of Jesus is the visible manifestation of the two separate natures, so, without this qualification, McLeod claims Theodore cannot hold that Mary is truly the mother of God.[317]

Theodore's insistence on two complete natures implies two sources of activity, and his descriptions of the "one assuming" and the "one assumed" make them into distinct agents, suggesting that he teaches two real persons in Christ. Twentieth-century scholarship[318] and the discovery of some of Theodore's original homilies propose that although Theodore concentrates on the distinction between the two natures, he does not thereby conclude that in Christ there are two persons, *prosopa*. Rather, Theodore claims to follow Nicaea by speaking of the natures while referring them to one *prosopon* on account of their "close union."[319] Indeed, Theodore says it would be "extreme folly" to speak of two Lords or two sons.[320] Perhaps somewhat obscurely, he explains that in Christ we distinguish the nature of God and that person, *prosopon*, is perfect. We also distinguish his human nature and that person, *prosopon*, is perfect. But when we look to their being conjoined, there is one person, *proso-*

315. See Clayton, *Christology of Theodoret of Cyrus*, 53–74.

316. Theodore of Mopsuestia, "Catechetical Homilies," 6, 7, 8.

317. McLeod, "Theodore of Mopsuestia Revisited."

318. As a background to the thinking of Theodoret of Cyrus, Clayton looks at the textual authenticity of the fragments from Theodore, and he gives an overview of recent scholarship on Theodore's Christology. *Christology of Theodoret of Cyrus*, 53–74.

319. Theodore of Mopsuestia, "Catechetical Homilies," 6.

320. Theodore of Mopsuestia, "Catechetical Homilies," 8.

pon.[321] Theodore then seems to accept that the one person of Christ expresses the inner reality of the two natures. But since for Theodore a nature inevitably has a *prosopon*, he cannot avoid the charge of presenting two persons (or possibly three) in Christ.

Theodore claims that in Christ "one Person is exhibited, indivisibly of both; and one will, and one operation, with one authority and dominion due to them," and this later seems to open the way to monothelitism, the belief that Christ only had one will.[322] But Theodore says this union is "according to the (divine) good pleasure."[323] Theodore thinks that God may be present to all, yet he only dwells in some human beings because he is pleased with those who are earnestly devoted to him. Since the Apostles and saints feared him, then those were the ones God chose to assist, a position that perhaps resembles some aspects of Pelagianism.[324] Theodore continues God's good pleasure and varies his mode of indwelling: he dwells in the Apostles and saints according to the mode of pleasure he has in the virtuous. But he dwells in Christ as in a son.

Cyril of Alexandria takes Theodore to task as part of his own polemic against Nestorius. In terms of comment on Theodore's anthropology, however, the insights of a relatively unknown bishop, Nemesius of Emesa, are worth exploring. Nemesius writes his treatise *On the Nature of Man* probably in the late 390s. Given that the treatise includes a description of the structure of human beings and specifically the workings of the brain, as well as comment on the medical thought of the time, Nemesius may have been a physician. His treatise was later wrongly ascribed to Gregory of Nyssa, though through that prestigious attribution it became known to scholastic thinkers like Albert the Great, Peter Lombard, and Thomas Aquinas.[325]

321. Theodore of Mopsuestia, "Catechetical Homilies," 8.

322. Theodore of Mopsuestia, "Fragment of a Letter to Domnus," 2:80.

323. Theodore of Mopsuestia, "On the Incarnation," 7.

324. See Wallace-Hadrill, *Christian Antioch*, 162. Clayton offers differing academic positions on this assertion. *Christology of Theodoret of Cyrus*, 61.

325. For the transmission and influence of the work of Nemesius, see Frampton, *Embodiments of Will*, 248–51.

Nemesius

Nemesius of Emesa composed his treatise *On the Nature of Man* over some time, and he also intended to revise and complete it, so it is not perhaps as polished and accurate as he would have wanted. Nemesius questions those who seem to offer merely a moral union of divine and human in Christ based on God's favor, and presumably he has the famous teacher Theodore in mind. Noting that for Theodore any suggestion that the Word undergoes change compromises his divine nature, Nemesius applies his understanding of the union of soul and body in human beings to the union of the Word and human in Christ to explain how one nature can act on the other without being changed by it. Nemesius dismisses any idea of a trichotomy in man, like the one promoted by his contemporary Apollinarius. He says that this creates a discontinuity between the higher faculty, the mind, and lower faculties, body and soul.[326] According to Nemesius, the human soul is "a real entity"; it is not unsubstantial, though it is not corporeal and, following the proper hierarchical order of created things, the body is the soul's instrument. However, the soul needs to take care of the body and render it fit for future life with God.[327] The soul is not in juxtaposition with the body, for any part not in contact with the soul would not be alive; nor is the union by mixture, for even wine and water can be separated by an oiled sponge; nor does the union entail change, for otherwise both soul and body would die together.[328] Nemesius thinks that the soul does not suffer change because it is immortal, though it is in a relationship of sympathy to its corporeal copartner.[329]

Nemesius nevertheless rejects the kind of argument, possibly put forward by Plato, that the soul uses the body as a garment:[330] it is not in the

326. Nemesius of Emesa, "Treatise on the Nature of Man," I, 1.

327. Nemesius of Emesa, "Treatise on the Nature of Man," II, 13, 14, 15.

328. Nemesius of Emesa, "Treatise on the Nature of Man," II, 20. For an account of the types of mixtures that Nemesius rejects as unsuitable for the union of body and soul, see Clayton, *Christology of Theodoret of Cyrus*, 240–41; also Sorabji, *Philosophy of the Commentators*, 204–5.

329. McLeod, *Image of God*, 102–4.

330. Sorabji, *Philosophy of the Commentators*, 204. Sorabji indicates that this nonspatial account of the soul may derive from Plotinus (205).

body "as in a bag." Instead, the soul is "bound by habit" to the body like the lover to the beloved.[331] Although he thinks that the relation of the soul to the body means that there is a community of feeling, in the union of divine and human, Nemesius thinks that this is something new, for the *Logos* is unaffected by the taking of manhood.[332]

As Nemesius surveys the workings of the body, he locates the source of voluntary movement and sensation in the brain. He also attributes different human functions to different parts of the brain.[333] In contrast, it seems to Galen (ca. 129–216), a physician from the Alexandrian medical school who may have located the soul in the substance of the brain,[334] that Nemesius concludes that the soul is involved in every part of life, even the vital processes divorced from consciousness. So, he clarifies his earlier statement and views the soul as a partner with the body rather than instrument.[335] Thus he says a human being is composed of soul and body; neither body by itself nor soul by itself is the living creature. Rather, expressing the common patristic theme, a human being is a "soul and body together."[336] As for death, Nemesius says that even if a creature should lose most of its sense organs, that is not fatal to life itself. When "feeling" goes, he says then the living creature also perishes. For Nemesius, "feeling" rests on a rational and irrational level so that it includes at the rational level sensations, and at the irrational level it concerns motions in the organic system.[337] Nemesius apparently sees death to occur when *all* activity in the organism has ceased.

Nemesius then counters Theodore's view that body and soul are distinct agents with their own activities and only loosely conjoined, or, as God dwells in Christ, the soul merely inhabits a body. Nemesius understands body and soul as two aspects of the same person, so the human being is "soul and body together." Although they exist in partnership, Nemesius still seems to present the human person as composite of body

331. Nemesius of Emesa, "Treatise on the Nature of Man," II, 21.
332. Nemesius of Emesa, "Treatise on the Nature of Man," III, 22.
333. See Frampton, *Embodiments of Will*, 251–56.
334. See Smith, "Beginnings," 3–4.
335. Nemesius of Emesa, "Treatise on the Nature of Man," XXVIII.
336. Nemesius of Emesa, "Treatise on the Nature of Man," XXX, III.
337. See Knuuttila, *Emotions in Ancient and Medieval Philosophy*, 106–7.

and soul. Theodore seems to offer a person who represents to the world the inner reality of two apparently complete natures, a separate soul and body. In both Nemesius and Theodore, there remains the common tendency to focus first on body plus soul and then try and work out the relationships between them that result in the person.[338] In Cyril of Alexandria's response to Nestorius, the focus falls on the person first.

Nestorius and Cyril of Alexandria: Emptying Persons

Nestorius

Although in his lifetime Nestorius was a prolific writer, little of his work remains after an edict in 435 called for all his writings to be burned. But near the end of his life and in exile, Nestorius had written his last book, which escaped destruction, possibly because Nestorius had it published under the pseudonym Heraclides. This *Book of Heraclides* is usually referred to as the *Bazaar of Heraclides*, but this appears to be a mistranslation of the original title. The book is written as if in dialogue with Sophronius, and Nestorius attacks Cyril of Alexandria and criticizes the decisions of the Council of Ephesus of 431. Nestorius declares that he himself follows the beliefs of the Pope Leo I the Great (reigned 440–61), who was highly influential in the Christological councils of Ephesus II (449) and Chalcedon (451), and the views of the patriarch Flavian of Constantinople (d. 449), who had tried to reach a reconciliation in Christology. Nestorius also adds a plea for charity and forgiveness.

As he explains in the *Book of Heraclides*, Nestorius sees a problem with the analogy that some writers make between soul and body and divinity and humanity in Christ. He correctly points out that this analogy can only be partial since the divine and human natures in Christ are each complete, whereas the soul and body are incomplete:[339] in human beings, the body and soul form a natural union and are created

338. McLeod notes that Nemesius also places stress on the role of free will in salvation, and to some extent this opens him to the charge of Pelagianism. But McLeod points out that the concern of Nemesius, as with the other Antiochenes, was to defend the will as good. *Image of God*, 105.

339. See Torrance, "Chemists or Terminologists?," 125.

one nature by God.[340] It would seem that, at least by the end of his life, Nestorius implicitly disowns this aspect of Theodore's teaching. In this discussion in his last book, Nestorius makes frequent reference to *prosopon*. When it comes to human beings, Nestorius says that soul and body are bound together, they do not exist apart from themselves, nor is man either body or soul, for "the union of these results in a nature and the *prosopon* of the nature."[341] Regarding God, God takes the likeness of a servant, not the *ousia* (shared human nature) of man, and he makes it his own likeness and *prosopon*. According to Nestorius, soul-body is a natural union combined through the power of God; in the divine-human union, the Word freely chooses to enter the union, so it is a voluntary union.[342]

At the time when Nestorius was writing, theological language was not set. Fortunately, however, Nestorius offers a guide to his Christological terminology.[343] Nestorius presents the example of a king dressed as a soldier.[344] In what Nestorius calls the *schema*, the external appearance of a soldier, the king acts as a soldier, not as a king, and he is dressed as other soldiers. He "lays aside his purple of royalty," although he remains the same in dignity, so that he can talk on equal terms with his men. Nestorius uses *ousia* to refer to the king's human nature, which he shares with other humans. His specific human nature as a king is his *physis*.[345] All his own characteristics making him into this specific king are his *hypostasis*, as Iain Torrance puts it, "an individualised *physis*."[346] *Prosopon* refers to how he appears, but not in the sense of *schema*, that is, not merely his external appearance. *Prosopon* seems to express the set of properties that shape the *hypostasis*,[347] or how a being's external appearance reveals his inner being:[348] as Grillmeier explains, for Nestori-

340. Nestorius, *Bazaar of Heracleides*, I, I, 47.

341. Nestorius, *Bazaar of Heracleides*, II, I.

342. Nestorius, *Bazaar of Heracleides*, II, I. See McLeod, *Image of God*, 176.

343. See McLeod, "Theodore of Mopsuestia Revisited."

344. Nestorius, *Bazaar of Heracleides*, I, I, 27–28.

345. According to Torrance, "to Nestorius: nature (φύσις, *physis*) and essence (οὐσία, *ousia*) mean the same thing." They denote reality. But nature is "qualified at different levels" of species and individual. "Chemists or Terminologists?," 125–26.

346. Torrance, "Chemists or Terminologists?," 126.

347. Torrance, "Chemists or Terminologists?," 126.

348. See McLeod, "Theodore of Mopsuestia Revisited."

us, *prosopon* (person) is the mode of appearance of a concrete nature.[349]

Nestorius says that the union in human beings of the incomplete natures of body and soul is a natural union creating one nature, and so one natural *prosopon*. Since the natures are incomplete, according to Nestorius, they do not have *prosopa* or their own.[350] In the case of Christ, however, each nature retains its set of properties, so there are two *prosopa*. This results in a union, not a mingling,[351] but the union in Christ of divinity and humanity is voluntary since "they are united for the use of the *prosopon* and not of the nature."[352] Nestorius clarifies that if the *Logos* became man in nature, then he would not have the *ousia* of God: he would be but "dust and ashes."[353] Moreover, since *Logos* and Father are of the same *ousia*, the Father and Spirit would be passible and created.[354] Nor, says Nestorius, perhaps in reference to Diodore, can there be "one Son and by Christ another Son," for "there are not two God the Words, or two Sons, or two only begottens."[355]

For Nestorius, *prosopon* is strongly tied to the doctrine of image of God.[356] Nestorius thinks that before the Fall, Adam had that image and "as the image of God, he [Adam] ought to have kept himself for God without spot and without blemish." This is achieved "by willing what God wills, since he had the *prosopon* of God. For (to have) the *prosopon* of God is to will what God wills, whose *prosopon* he has."[357] Christ then took the image up, and as perfect image he received the *prosopon* from conception and was unlike other men by virtue of his obedience.[358] So, Christ is "one *prosopon* without division" because he willed the will of God.[359] The Word as image of God and divine in nature becomes incar-

349. Grillmeier, *Christ in Christian Tradition*, 384.

350. Torrance, "Chemists or Terminologists?," 126.

351. Torrance, "Chemists or Terminologists?," 126.

352. Nestorius, *Bazaar of Heracleides*, I, I, 46.

353. Nestorius, *Bazaar of Heracleides*, I, I, 23.

354. Nestorius, *Bazaar of Heracleides*, I, I, 47.

355. Nestorius, *Bazaar of Heracleides*, I, I, 53.

356. McLeod argues that Nestorius makes this return to a biblical foundation either as a result of the influence of Theodore of Mopsuestia or as a conclusion from the implications of his own thought, rather than it being an original move or starting point. *Roles of Christ's Humanity in Salvation*, 167–68.

357. Nestorius, *Bazaar of Heracleides*, I, I, 63.

358. Nestorius, *Bazaar of Heracleides*, I, I, 64. See McLeod, *Image of God*, 76–77.

359. Nestorius, *Bazaar of Heracleides*, I, I, 72.

nate by taking the image of a servant, the *schema* of a human form, so that flesh is adopted for his *prosopon*.[360]

But Nestorius insists that there is no change or addition to the Trinity:[361] "the man is only man and God is only God."[362] Instead, referring to Philippians 2, Nestorius says that God uses "his own *prosopon* to condescend in poverty and shame even unto death."[363] This *kenosis*, emptying, appears to be on the part of the human element for, as Nestorius explains, the immutable God accepts a mortal and changeable *prosopon*[364] who "in exaltation" participates in "the likeness of God."[365] The Word appears to be joined to a man. It is a vital part of his thinking that Christ has a real human activity and wills what God wills, that he shows readiness to accept that he becomes *eikon* and *prosopon*.[366] This idea of Christ as *eikon* and *prosopon* seems to have echoes of image and likeness, in which case it may be that *prosopon* has to do with growing into the image of God through moral virtue and "willing what God wills."

According to Nestorius, there are two *prosopa* in Christ: the image of God, the *prosopon*, who by *kenosis* in the Incarnation is the likeness of a servant, and the image of God the *prosopon* of the man. Yet the *prosopon* is the same Lord Jesus Christ, the "one name which is more excellent than all names, (one) for both of them."[367] As McLeod explains, Nestorius thinks that the Word and Jesus can share in each other's *prosopon* because they are united in one common *prosopon*.[368] Nestorius then claims he follows Nicaea when he confesses two natures and one Lord Jesus Christ: "diverse are the natures which have come unto a true union, but from them both (there has resulted) one Christ and Son, not because the diversity in the natures has been abolished by reason of the union, but because they have perfected for us rather one Lord and Messiah and Son."[369]

To preserve divine impassibility, since it is unworthy of God to be

360. Nestorius, *Bazaar of Heracleides*, I, I, 57. See McLeod, *Image of God*, 77–78.
361. Nestorius, *Bazaar of Heracleides*, I, I, 34, 36.
362. Nestorius, *Bazaar of Heracleides*, I, I, 28.
363. Nestorius, *Bazaar of Heracleides*, I, I, 29.
364. Nestorius, *Bazaar of Heracleides*, I, I, 90.
365. Nestorius, *Bazaar of Heracleides*, I, I, 76.
366. Nestorius, *Bazaar of Heracleides*, I, I, 61.
367. Nestorius, *Bazaar of Heracleides*, I, I, 61.
368. McLeod, *Image of God*, 177.
369. Nestorius, *Bazaar of Heracleides*, II, I.

born, suffer, and die, and in order to preserve the voluntary element of Christ's will in the union, Nestorius proposes that Christ is the common title, the common *prosopon* of the "conjunction," *synapheia*, of Godhead and manhood.[370] Nevertheless, however close a conjunction Nestorius wishes to present, the term *synapheia* suggests a joining but not a real union. And Nestorius rejects as "barbaric impiety" the popular Christology of "God in the womb—God in the tomb."[371] This saying was first written down by Ephraim the Syrian (ca. 306–73), who was known as the Lyre of the Holy Spirit, in his *Homily on our Lord*.[372] Presumably, this saying had long been a part of the Christian tradition, as St. Ephraim was well known for collecting ancient liturgical hymns and poetry. Much more significantly, however, Nestorius rejected the extremely popular term *Theotokos*, recorded by Ephraim in a liturgical song of praise.[373] This term not only had huge theological significance, but also became a test of orthodoxy.[374]

Theotokos means "bearer of God," and although this title for the Mother of God was not generally in use until the fifth century, though it was used in hymns, the concept of Mary as Mother of God was very much alive in the Christian tradition: Irenaeus speaks naturally of Mary as the one who "would bear God,"[375] as does Alexander of Alexandria (d. 328).[376] Gregory of Nyssa calls Mary the Mother of God, and Theodore of Mopsuestia discussed the title. According to Gregory of Nazianzus, "if anyone does not agree that Holy Mary is the Mother of God, he is at odds with the Godhead."[377] Despite its provenance,[378] and clearly

370. Nestorius, "Letter 5, Second Letter to Cyril," 43–48. See Russell, *Cyril of Alexandria*, 44.

371. Gavrilyuk, *Suffering of the Impassible God*, 146.

372. Ephraim the Syrian, "Homily on Our Lord," 33.

373. Ephraim the Syrian, "Hymns of the Nativity," in Jurgens, *Faith of the Early Fathers*, 1:312, 1,1, 1,20.

374. See McLeod, *Image of God*, 178.

375. Irenaeus, "Against Heresies," V, XIX.

376. Alexander of Alexandria, "Encyclical Letter of Alexander of Alexandria to Another Bishop Alexander and to All Non-Egyptian Bishops," in Jurgens, *Faith of the Early Fathers*, 1:301.

377. Gregory of Nazianzus, "Epistle 101," 218.

378. As Clayton points out, Theodoret, a former friend of Nestorius, says that Nestorius innovates by his denial of Mary as *Theotokos*. *Christology of Theodoret of Cyrus*, 279–80.

against Gregory of Nazianzus, Nestorius says that *Theotokos* has Apollinarian connotations and, strictly speaking, Mary does not bear God. He says that another alternative, *anthropotokos*, bearer of man, is equally unsatisfactory, suggests Adoptionism, and Mary does not bear a mere man. For Nestorius, neither God nor man is born of Mary. Instead, Mary is *Christotokos*; she bears Christ,[379] the *prosopon* of both natures.

But Church *kerygma*, its confession in liturgy, worship, and practice, held that Mary is *Theotokos*, Mother of God, and that the Son of God was born, suffered, died, and rose again. As Cyril explains, "almost the whole of our contention for the faith has grown out of our affirmation that the holy Virgin is *Theotokos*."[380] Nestorius jeopardized this *kerygma*. Cyril claims that not only does Nestorius not "welcome tradition," but he also "innovates,"[381] and by such novelties the churches thrown into confusion and the laity is scandalized.[382]

Out of a concern to safeguard divine impassibility, Theodore and Nestorius make a clear division between the "one assuming" and the "one assumed." Their Christology appears to join the divine and human natures: Jesus Christ is the union of the *Logos* with a human being. This is a voluntary union brought about apparently by the goodwill of the man and aided by the indwelling of God, causing some to see Pelagianism as its foundation.[383] As Roberta Chestnut explains, through *kenosis*, the Son, who is the image of God, takes on the image of a servant, and in this likeness, the man Jesus must accept his task so that God's *prosopon* is his own *prosopon*: it is a union of wills.[384]

Following the reasoning of Nestorius, it seems that for a nature to be real it must exist, have an appearance as a *prosopon*. Nestorius understands that the *kerygma* teaches two real natures in Christ, God, and man, and if according to Nestorius and Theodore every nature has a

379. Nestorius, "Letter 5, Second Letter to Cyril."

380. Cyril of Alexandria, "Letter 39 to John of Antioch," in *St Cyril of Alexandria*. Frances Young argues that the belief that Mary is the antitype to Eve is crucial for Cyril's theology; hence his reaction to Nestorius. "*Theotokos*."

381. Cyril of Alexandria, *On the Unity of Christ*, 52.

382. Cyril, "Letter 17 to Nestorius," in *St Cyril of Alexandria*.

383. Grenz, *Theology for the Community of God*, 296. This appears to be the view of both Cyril and John Cassian; see Wessel, *Leo the Great*, 215, and Neil, *Leo the Great*, 37.

384. Chestnut, "Two *Prosopa*," 404.

prosopon, then the two natures in Christ entail two *prosopa*, persons. But Nestorius claims that the appearance presented by Christ is one person, where "person" expresses the concrete inner reality of two natures each with its own *prosopon*. For Nestorius, person appears to be the outward semblance of an inner reality, a mask over what is truly real. As for human beings, Nestorius correctly identifies that body and soul, unlike divinity and humanity in Christ, are incomplete. The human person remains a composite of body and soul, however, and the "natural union" he proposes appears to be as loose as his view of the conjunction of divinity and humanity in Christ, with "person" thrown over the body and soul reality.

Cyril of Alexandria

It seems that all patristic writers were committed to divine impassibility, and often reflection begins from considering how Jesus Christ can be both God and suffer.[385] But Cyril begins from reflection on the single, indivisible person, Christ, and so his starting point is not God's impassibility but the self-emptying of the *Logos*, following Philippians 2. So, Nestorius accuses Cyril of theopaschitism, the belief that God suffers and therefore changes.[386]

Nestorius sets out to solve what he sees is a problem of both God's impassibility and the suffering Son. But Cyril does not approach the union of *Logos* and man as if it is a puzzle that requires a solution. Instead, he reflects that how "flesh is united to the life giving Word" is a mystery beyond understanding,[387] and, in the context of his Commentary, "flesh" involves the whole man, body, soul, mind.[388] Moreover, the Word assumed all that belongs to a human nature, such as the possibility to grow, to have passions, and even to die.[389] As far as Cyril is concerned, however, though in the context of explaining the equality of the Father

385. Coakley, "Does Kenosis Rest on a Mistake?," 247.

386. Nestorius, *Bazaar of Heracleides*, I, II. See Gavrilyuk, "Theopatheia," 201–2.

387. Cyril of Alexandria, *Commentary on John*, IV, 3.

388. See van Loon, *Dyophysite Christology of Cyril of Alexandria*, 162–63. Norman Russell suggests that Cyril stressed the assumption of mind and soul once he became aware of the charge of Apollinarianism leveled against him. *Cyril of Alexandria*, 41.

389. Van Loon, *Dyophysite Christology of Cyril of Alexandria*, 165.

and Son, it is plainly true that "a man will neither be less than another man insofar as he is man, nor will he be greater insofar as he is man. That is because the principle of nature is seen to be equal in the case of all people."[390] It seems that, according to Cyril, the Word assumes a human nature that is common to all people. Because our common human nature is deified by the Incarnation, it affects the human nature of every single individual human being.[391]

For Cyril, those who split up the words and acts of Christ and attribute some to the Word and others to the man "have missed the straight and unerring way of knowing the mystery of Christ clearly."[392] Where Nestorius sees a contradiction or "fairy tale" in saying "that the same suffers and does not suffer,"[393] Cyril says in Christ there is a "strange and rare paradox of Lordship in servant's form and divine glory in human abasement."[394] Within this paradox, the two realities of divine and human nature remain, for the divine has the power to heal and transform the weakness of the human. This involves an understanding of *kenosis* as a paradox of strength in weakness.

According to Nestorius, the text of Philippians 2:6–11 and especially the *kenosis*, emptying, and "being obedient unto death," exclusively relates to the emptying of the human passible subject in Christ so that the *Logos* remains impassible,[395] though Nestorius does not explain how the human subject is able to empty himself when he starts empty. For Cyril, Nestorius merely offers a Christ who surpasses the prophets in the level of grace he has been given.[396] According to Cyril, the conjunction made by Nestorius necessarily implies a division,[397] and it is less about how the *Logos* self-emptied and more about how the assumed man is exalted.[398] The division of the "one true and natural Son" and the "son of David"

390. Cyril of Alexandria, *Commentary on John*, IV, I.

391. Van Loon, *Dyophysite Christology of Cyril of Alexandria*, 168.

392. Cyril of Alexandria, *On the Unity of Christ*, 106.

393. Cyril of Alexandria, *On the Unity of Christ*, 117.

394. Cyril of Alexandria, *On the Unity of Christ*, 101. See Gavrilyuk, "Theopatheia," 190–207.

395. Nestorius, "Letter 5, Second Letter to Cyril"; Cyril of Alexandria, *On the Unity of Christ*, 84–85.

396. Cyril of Alexandria, "Scholia on the Incarnation," 7.

397. Cyril of Alexandria, "Letter 4 Second Letter to Nestorius," in *St Cyril of Alexandria*.

398. Cyril of Alexandria, *On the Unity of Christ*, 70.

and their conjunction presents a joining that any other man could have with God if he is bonded with enough virtue and holiness.[399] Cyril says that the Nestorian notion that Christ is like any other man shares resemblance to previous heresy, which is presumably why Cyril brings up Nestorian thinking just after he deals with Arianism.[400] Conjunction by will is, he says, on a par with a disciple to his teacher or assisting another in a task,[401] and like any addition from outside or any moral union of will, the joining could be lost or broken by will.[402] Instead, Cyril says the Incarnation is not simply to be understood in terms of the amount of grace given. In the Incarnation, something new happened,[403] and the uniqueness of this event is not reflected in Nestorius's thinking.

Using Philippians 2:6–11 and the paradox of *kenosis*, Cyril explains that the *Logos* became flesh, not by undergoing change or conversion into flesh, or mixture or taking a soulless flesh. Rather, "he submitted himself to being emptied . . . and did not disdain the poverty of human nature."[404] The *Logos* in "an ineffable and inconceivable manner personally united to himself flesh animated with living soul, became man." Nevertheless, this did not eliminate the difference of the natures. Rather, "Godhead and Manhood completed for us the one Lord and Christ and Son" by this "true unity."[405] For Cyril, there is no change in the person of the *Logos*, the subject of *kenosis*. There is change in his condition, however: the unchanged Son becomes man.[406] Thus Cyril rejects any understanding of the person of Christ as soul or mind or flesh; rather, it is the divine *hypostasis* that comes as man.

Nestorius believes he follows Nicaea when he offers a prosopic union, a conjunction of the *prosopon* of the *Logos* and the *prosopon* of the assumed man to form one *prosopon*, Jesus Christ. Cyril understands by this that the name of Son and Godhead is "thrown over him (the assumed

399. Cyril of Alexandria, *On the Unity of Christ*, 74.
400. Cyril of Alexandria, *On the Unity of Christ*, 53.
401. Cyril of Alexandria, *On the Unity of Christ*, 74.
402. Cyril of Alexandria, *On the Unity of Christ*, 81.
403. Cyril of Alexandria, *On the Unity of Christ*, 98.
404. Cyril of Alexandria, *On the Unity of Christ*, 55.
405. Cyril of Alexandria, "Letter 4 Second Letter to Nestorius," in *St Cyril of Alexandria*.
406. See Weinandy, "Cyril and the Mystery of the Incarnation," 28.

man) like a mask or a cloak."[407] Cyril charges Nestorius with abandoning "union" in favor of a "conjunction" that seems to be an appearance and not the reality of a true union.[408] For Cyril, then, the Nestorian approach is problematic on two accounts: first, the person of Christ is merely an appearance or covering, and second, Nestorius seems to consider the human element in Christ as somehow able to stand alone and accept union with the *Logos* by human goodwill. Cyril argues that the person of Christ is the concrete reality of the *Logos* and that humanity needs the inbreaking of grace and the sacraments to heal human weaknesses.[409]

The problem of terminology is a principal source of confusion between Nestorius and Cyril:[410] by the *prosopa* of *Logos* and man, Nestorius may have meant two different roles that form the prosopic union, but Cyril reads this as implying two sons since he understands *prosopon* as *hypostasis*.[411] Later Nestorians would confess two separate subjects in Christ.[412] By *hypostasis*, Cyril describes the manner of the union in Christ, for he argues the *hypostasis* of the *Logos* is the subject of divinity and humanity in Christ. But Nestorius appears to regard *hypostasis* in terms of nature, so he hears Cyril suggesting something like material union that results in a third kind of nature. Nevertheless, the conflict between Nestorius and Cyril is not merely the result of language. While Nestorius argues that he follows Nicaea by asserting both the separate and distinct Godhead and manhood in the one Christ, Cyril claims he follows Nicaea, the Fathers, and Church tradition by confessing a single-subject Christology that acknowledges the *Logos* as subject of all the acts of Jesus Christ. Cyril describes the newness of the Incarnation as newness in the Son's existence in terms of a hypostatic union.[413]

Cyril may be reluctant to use *prosopon* because Nestorius overuses it in a superficial sense, and it still appears to be a fluid term. Instead, Cyril uses *physis*, essence of a thing, associated with *hypostasis*, real and

407. Cyril of Alexandria, *On the Unity of Christ*, 128.
408. Cyril of Alexandria, *On the Unity of Christ*, 73.
409. Cyril of Alexandria, *Commentary on John*, X.
410. For an overview of the confusion in terminology, see, Russell *Cyril of Alexandria*, 40.
411. E.g., in Cyril of Alexandria's "Tome, II, 1" and "Tome, III, 2, 5," in Russell, *Cyril of Alexandria*, 131–74.
412. Gavrilyuk, "Theopatheia," 194.
413. See Weinandy, "Cyril and the Mystery of the Incarnation," 42.

concrete substance, to indicate the hypostatic union. Cyril speaks of *mia physis*, one nature, in Christ, a formula he thinks is Athanasian but in fact is Apollinarian. Unlike Apollinarius, however, Cyril stresses that the *Logos* did not come into a man, but he truly became man while remaining God; he did not take soulless flesh, "but flesh animated with a rational soul and in all respects one factor, *prosopon*, with it."[414] Where for Apollinarius "one *physis*" refers to the *Logos* who takes the place of Christ's mind, for Cyril "one *physis*" refers to the *Logos* who comes to be man, one enfleshed nature of the Word.[415] The subject of the "becoming" is the *Logos*,[416] and this "becoming" does not mean change.[417] Nevertheless, as the difference between Apollinarius and Cyril demonstrates, there is some confusion where *physis*, understood as nature, stands also for personal subjectivity.[418] Because Cyril is wary of using *prosopon* and he wants to express concrete reality, hence his original choice of *physis*, he takes up *hypostasis* to convey the idea of personal subject. In this way, *prosopon* and *persona* came to be redefined as *hypostasis*, which was formalized in the Chalcedonian definition of faith.

On the hypostatic union, Cyril explains that with different natures there is not identity of essence, for "Godhead is one thing, manhood quite another."[419] Yet they are not separated in terms of individual distinctness so that they exist apart from one another; rather, "they are brought together into an indissoluble union."[420] This is a "true unity" of realities unlike one another even though it is one that "transcends speech and understanding."[421] Moreover, rejecting this "personal union" as "either impossible or unseemly" results in the error of claiming "two sons," "man in his own person," and "God in his own person."[422]

For Apollinarius, it is impossible for two complete natures to form a

414. Cyril of Alexandria, *On the Unity of Christ*, 109.

415. See McGuckin, *St Cyril of Alexandria*, 207–8.

416. Cyril of Alexandria, *On the Unity of Christ*, 109.

417. Cyril of Alexandria, *On the Unity of Christ*, 54.

418. The monophysites, some followers of Cyril's *mia physis* formula, continued to teach a union of natures, seeing in the decrees of Chalcedon a restatement of Nestorianism. See Grillmeier, *Christ in Christian Tradition*, 444.

419. Cyril of Alexandria, *On the Unity of Christ*, 77.

420. Cyril of Alexandria, *On the Unity of Christ*, 77.

421. Cyril of Alexandria, *On the Unity of Christ*, 83.

422. Cyril of Alexandria, "Letter 4 Second Letter to Nestorius," in *St Cyril of Alexandria*.

unity. Cyril believes that a union of complete natures is beyond understanding, but he finds something analogous in humans. Although also beyond full comprehension, a human being, he says, has a single nature but is composed of body and soul, two disparate things.[423] Together, soul and flesh "make up the person of a single man."[424] Distinguishing, as the Apostle St. Paul does, between the "inner" and "outer" man is "only theoretically conceivable."[425] On the one hand, Cyril explains, in making a distinction, the nature of each element is not lost in the union.[426] As Cyril points out, man is rational by nature: he may be a ship builder by will or infirm by accident, but he cannot become irrational even though he loses his ship-building experience or medicine cures his infirmity.[427] Cyril adds the Only Begotten is another nature: he is light while we need enlightening. For the economy of salvation, the *Logos* "entered our likeness" "while ever remaining what he was."[428] On the other hand, Cyril explains the unity: if the body is wounded, the soul "co-grieves," for "the soul makes its own the things of the body although in its own nature imparticipate of its sufferings." In the same way, Cyril says, "out of the perfect person of God the Word and of manhood perfect in its own mode, is one Christ, the same God and man. And the Word makes its own sufferings of his own flesh, because its own is the body and not another's."[429]

Nestorius rejects a strict unity because he believes that it necessarily entails that the *Logos* in his Godhead suffers. Yet Cyril is clear that "he did not suffer in the nature of the Godhead, but in his own flesh."[430] As God, he is entirely outside suffering:[431] tiredness and hunger, he says, are "not fitting to the Word if we considered him nakedly, as it were, not yet made flesh, or before he had descended into the self-emptying."[432] In the Incarnation, however, when he empties himself of glory and puts on the

423. Cyril of Alexandria, *On the Unity of Christ*, 78.
424. Cyril of Alexandria, "Against Diodore of Tarsus and Theodore of Mopsuestia."
425. Cyril of Alexandria, *On the Unity of Christ*, 78.
426. See Weinandy, "Cyril and the Mystery of the Incarnation," 28.
427. Cyril of Alexandria, *Commentary on John*, I, 8, 3.
428. Cyril of Alexandria, *On the Unity of Christ*, 61.
429. Cyril of Alexandria, "Scholia On the Incarnation," 8.
430. Cyril of Alexandria, *On the Unity of Christ*, 114. See Weinandy, "Cyril and the Mystery of the Incarnation," 48–49.
431. Cyril of Alexandria, *On the Unity of Christ*, 121.
432. Cyril of Alexandria, *On the Unity of Christ*, 103, 107.

"likeness of human littleness," "the Son possesses all things as God and receives as Man,"[433] for "there is only one Son, the Word who was made man for our sake" and "everything refers to him, words and deeds, both those that befit the deity, as well as those which are human."[434]

For Cyril, then, Christ cannot be separated into a man distinct from the *Logos*: he is "God made man," where "both the one and the other are this same reality for he did not cease to be God when he became man, nor did he regard the economy as unacceptable by disdaining the limitations involved in the self-emptying."[435] Thus Cyril confesses, "we believe that there is only one Son of God the Father.... our Lord Jesus Christ in one person, *prosopon*."[436] "The same one was at once God and man."[437] As to the manner of this union, the Word appropriates a human body to himself "in such an indissoluble union that it has to be considered his very own body" but "in a strange and most unusual manner."[438]

Following Athanasius, Cyril understands that the Word became human so that we might become divine; he descends so that we can rise with him. The Word made flesh is both the "wound and medicine," the "sick and physician,"[439] and the Incarnation restores the whole of human nature.[440] Moreover, by the Word's *kenosis*, we are re-formed to divine nature, we rise to a dignity that is above our nature and become adopted children of God, not like him in exactitude but "by grace in imitation of him."[441] This adoption is not merely a matter of external imitation of Christ. Rather, the Word roots grace in us again, and we become not "temples of ourselves" but "temples of God" because of the indwelling of the Holy Spirit.[442] The Spirit's sanctifying power begins in Baptism and is extended in the Eucharist, which, as partaking of Christ's body, is actual physical unity with Christ.[443]

433. Cyril of Alexandria, *Commentary on John*, XI, 3, 4.
434. Cyril of Alexandria, *On the Unity of Christ*, 107.
435. Cyril of Alexandria, *On the Unity of Christ*, 76.
436. Cyril of Alexandria, *On the Unity of Christ*, 133.
437. Cyril of Alexandria, *On the Unity of Christ*, 55.
438. Cyril of Alexandria, *On the Unity of Christ*, 63, 64.
439. Cyril of Alexandria, *Commentary on John*, I, 9.
440. Cyril of Alexandria, *Commentary on John*, II, 4.
441. Cyril of Alexandria, *Commentary on John*, I, 9.
442. Cyril of Alexandria, *Commentary on John*, II, 1.
443. Cyril of Alexandria, *Commentary on John*, XI, 11.

Cyril's premise is that the union of the divine and human in Christ is a mystery, a strange paradox, rather than a puzzle in search of a solution, and he applies this sense of mystery to the human person as well. His arguments demonstrate that once again in the tradition, and in contrast to some modern views, all human beings have a rational nature even if they cannot demonstrate rationality. Cyril offers a view of the human being as existing in a profound unity of the "inner" and "outer" man. Although in this unity the two elements are distinct, they cannot be broken apart: there cannot be a separation of the human being and his or her person, and so there cannot be a living human being who is not a person. Moreover, "person" is not merely an appearance or a covering or an attribution: persons are substantial and concrete entities. Cyril also speaks about the human need for the inbreaking of grace. This idea that human beings are in fact weak and in need of help in contrast to the Nestorian and Theodorian idea of the self-sufficient individual perhaps provides a point of reflection for those who today think of the person as essentially autonomous and self-sufficient. And Cyril's explanation of the *kenosis* of Christ as a change in his condition rather than a change in his person provides a powerful point of reflection on all human beings, particularly those with dementia.

In contrast to the Nestorian person that seems to be a cloak over the union of body and soul, Cyril sees the person as real and substantial, an indivisible union. Cyril also recognizes that a conceptual distinction can be made between body and soul. Eutyches, however, seems to deny a distinction altogether, and in contemporary bioethical terms his anthropology implies a vitalistic view of the human person.

Eutyches and Pope Leo the Great: Confused Persons

Eutyches

Concerned that there appeared to be a resurgence of Nestorianism after the death of Cyril in 444, Eutyches (378–454), archimandrite of a monastery outside Constantinople, decides to take Cyril's *mia physis*, one-nature formula, to its extreme. Few fragments from Eutyches remain, but his admission to a synod at Constantinople in 448 gives an indication of his thinking. Eutyches maintains that he follows in the Patristic tradition of Cyril and Athanasius by confessing that before the union the Lord was "of two natures," divine and human, but after the union "one nature."[444] Eutyches bases this on Cyril's assertion that "the Lord Jesus Christ is one, although we do not forget the difference of the natures, from which we affirm the ineffable union to have been formed."[445] Eutyches appears to think that affirming two natures inevitably means affirming two persons in Christ. So, he argues that after the union, the divine nature absorbs the human nature: Christ is *from* two natures rather than *in* two natures. Thus Eutyches misunderstands Cyril by thinking that Christ's human nature is assumed by the divine nature instead of the person of the Word. This intermingling of divine and human seems to produce precisely what Nestorius charged Cyril with advocating: a hybrid or divinized man. Moreover, Eutyches is adamant that the humanity of Christ, however it is viewed, is not consubstantial with us.[446]

Flavian, the Patriarch of Constantinople (d. 449), summoned Eutyches to appear before a council of bishops. When Eutyches refused to change his position, the council excommunicated him, and Eutyches appealed to Emperor Theodosius II (d. 450), to Dioscurus the Patriarch of Alexandria (d. 454), and to Pope Leo the Great.

Pope Leo the Great

Pope Leo, the first pope who did not die a martyr's death, saw both the crumbling of the Roman Empire before the barbarian invasions and the crystallization of the liturgical and disciplinary life of the Church.[447] Particularly concerned with the unity of the faith, Leo was keen to hear all sides and so was especially dismayed when at a synod in Ephesus in 449 the archbishop of Alexandria and Cyril's nephew, Dioscorus (d. 454), refused any bishop who opposed Eutyches to participate, refused the letters from Leo on the position of Eutyches to be read out,

444. Eutyches, "Admission of Eutyches," 335–36.

445. Cyril of Alexandria, *Letter 39*.

446. Eutyches, "Admission of Eutyches." See Clayton, *Christology of Theodoret of Cyrus*, 23–25; Davis, *First Seven Ecumenical Councils*, 170–73.

447. See Neil, *Leo the Great*, 1–2.

and refused any submission by the papal legates. It seems that Dioscorus wrongly believed that the position of Eutyches represented an accurate interpretation of Cyril's thinking.[448] Moreover, at the council, Flavian of Constantinople, who had originally condemned Eutyches, was beaten and then imprisoned before dying on his way into exile. The disgraceful events at Ephesus led Leo to declare the council the *latrocinium*, the Robber Council,[449] and the issue was eventually reviewed at a council at Chalcedon in 451.

Before the Robber Council, Leo had written a response to the Eutychean position in a widely circulated set of documents and a letter to Flavian, perhaps explaining his surprise that Dioscorus felt the matter still required resolution. As far as Leo is concerned, the position of Eutyches is the opposite of that of Nestorius, and both are contrary to the faith of the Church: with his focus on the humanity of Christ, Nestorius fails to acknowledge Christ's full divinity; with his stress on the divinity, Eutyches denies Christ's full humanity.[450] Moreover, if Eutyches is interpreted to suggest that only the divinity is born, suffered, and died—albeit, says Leo, "in a counterfeit appearance"—then Eutyches is guilty not only of docetism but also of patripassianism.[451] In response to Eutyches, Leo counters that the distinctive character of each nature remains unimpaired and comes "united in one person, *in unam coeunte personam*."[452] Yet he says that this union is a real unity: "one and the same, truly Son of God, and truly Son of Man."[453] By this unity of person, "the 'son of Man,' as we read, came down from heaven when the 'son of God' assumed flesh from that Virgin through whom he was born. And, again, the Son of God is said to have been crucified and buried," though he suffered not in his Godhead but in his human nature.[454] Moreover, the self-emptying of

448. Clayton sets out the political intrigue, power struggles, and rivalries that played a significant part in the events leading up to the Council of Chalcedon. *Christology of Theodoret of Cyrus*, 22–29.

449. Pope Leo I, "Letter 95 to Pulcheria," in *Letters*. For an account of events leading up to the Robber Council and the Council of Chalcedon, see Davis, *First Seven Ecumenical Councils*, 170–80.

450. See Neil, *Leo the Great*, 37.

451. Pope Leo I, *Sermons*, 28.5 (2). See also Wessel, *Leo the Great*, 216.

452. Pope Leo, "Letter 28 to Flavian, the Tome," in *Letters*.

453. Pope Leo, "Letter 28 to Flavian, the Tome," in *Letters*.

454. Pope Leo, "Letter 28 to Flavian, the Tome," in *Letters*.

the Son is not "a failure of power" but "an inclination to mercy."[455] In his critique of Eutyches, Leo says that Eutyches instead does not acknowledge human nature in the Son[456] and completely disregards Scripture.[457] For Leo, it was equally reprehensible to suggest that the Only Begotten was of two natures before the Incarnation, as if to say that he was one nature after.[458] In his admission, Eutyches states, "I confess that our Lord was of two natures before the union," that is, before the union of divinity and humanity in the Incarnation. Instead of the *Logos* coming to be man—that is, taking on a new mode of existence—Eutyches seems to think that the natures fuse together. His confession implies that the human nature somehow existed before the Incarnation. Moreover, his use of the title "Our Lord" before the union appears to deny the existence of the *Logos* as *Logos*.[459]

Even though Eutyches denies that Jesus is human like us, an anthropological view from his Christology can be extrapolated: whereas in Nestorianism body and soul appear to be loosely conjoined, in the Eutychean way of thinking, body and soul would be so mingled that the distinction between them is lost. This may parallel a vitalistic view of the human person. Vitalism originally emerged in the nineteenth century as thinkers began to challenge the mechanistic view of living things offered by philosophers like Descartes. These thinkers worked from the perspective that there is more to living things than mere chemistry or biology allows, and the search to find the vital force in living things began.[460] Of course, this neglects thinking earlier than Descartes. Nevertheless, vitalism has now grown beyond finding the spark of life, and in contemporary bioethical terms, vitalism represents the view that life should be preserved no matter the cost.[461] This view fails to appreciate that, al-

455. Pope Leo, "Letter 28 to Flavian, the Tome," in *Letters*.

456. Pope Leo, "Letter 28 to Flavian, the Tome," in *Letters*.

457. Pope Leo, "Letter 28 to Flavian, the Tome," in *Letters*.

458. Pope Leo, "Letter 28 to Flavian, the Tome," in *Letters*.

459. See Weinandy, *Does God Change?*, 62.

460. McLaughlin, "Vitalism and Emergence," 631.

461. Keown, *Euthanasia, Ethics and Public Policy*, 39–51. Keown draws the important distinction between vitalism, sanctity of life whereby life is recognized as limited but nevertheless cherished, and subjective quality of life. Keown stands as a useful contrast to philosophers like Peter Singer, who think that the sanctity of life principle is a form of vitalism. see Singer, *Rethinking Life and Death*, 1–6.

though life is a good, it is not the final good, for all temporal things are "subordinated to spiritual ends."[462] Allowing that there are limits to human earthly life means that a patient can both cherish his or her life and accept that certain treatments are extraordinary and so not obligatory. Extraordinary treatments involve means that are too burdensome, and as such the patient can legitimately decide to forgo such treatment.[463] This is important also for the profoundly disabled person. There are times when the limits of life are to be accepted, that life is cherished, but that the sanctity of life does not become idolatrous. The profoundly disabled, like the abled, are spiritual beings as well as being embodied. And, as with all human beings, the spiritual aspect has priority even if to the onlooker there is little evidence of spirituality.

Pope Leo's *Tome*, the *Nicene Creed*, Cyril's *Second Letter to Nestorius (Letter 4)*, and Cyril's *Letter to John of Antioch (Letter 39)* were all confirmed at the Council of Chalcedon (451). Chalcedon sought to counteract both Nestorianism and Eutychianism, to exclude Arianism and Apollinarianism, and to bring an end to the disputes that were causing bitterness in the Church. The Chalcedonian Fathers confirmed "person" as the key to the unity in Christ: they confessed that the Lord Jesus Christ is "one and the same Son," "the same perfect in Godhead, the same perfect in manhood, truly God and truly man." To underscore his full humanity, they added man "with a rational soul and a body," "*homoousios* with the Father," "*homoousios* with us as to his manhood." To emphasize that the unity occurs not on the level of the natures but on the level of the person, the Council Fathers explained that the Son is "made known in two natures (which exist) without confusion, without change, without division, without separation," and that the properties of each nature are preserved and "concurring into one person and one *hypostasis*" εις εν πρόσωπον καί μίαν ὑπόστασιν.[464]

Chalcedon's declaration of faith involved all the important Church centers: Alexandria, Antioch, Constantinople, and Rome. Moreover, rather than engage in speculative analysis or offer philosophical defini-

462. Pope Pius XII, "Address to an International Congress of Anesthesiologists."

463. See Pope John Paul II, *Evangelium Vitae*, 65.

464. "Chalcedon Definition of Faith," in Stevenson, *Creeds, Councils and Controversies*, 350–54. Bindley and Green, *Oecumenical Documents of the Faith*, 191–93.

tion, as Grillmeier explains, the Fathers opted for "listening to the proven witnesses of the Christian faith."[465] As "witnesses" rather than "scholars," Grillmeier admits that they left certain areas unclear; in particular, they did not define key concepts such as nature, *physis,* and person as *prosopon* and *hypostasis.* But since the *kerygma* remained the test for terminology, certain conclusions could be drawn so there was a clear sense of Church teaching, yet also possibility for further reflection and deepening of concepts.

The journey from the earliest Christological disputes, through *logos-sarx* and *logos-anthropos* Christologies, illustrates how reflection developed through struggle and refinement, argument and response, where each time a new question arises it is checked against the *kerygma.* Cyril makes a notable move for Christology and for the concept of the person. In contrast to Christologies that use anthropology as a strict model for the union of divine and human in Christ, Cyril says that analogy with body and soul in human beings is limited and can simply show how two disparate elements can be united. To express the coming of the Word as man, Cyril takes up the term *hypostasis,* signifying the person of the Word. From his struggles with Nestorius, Cyril sees it necessary to focus on the person of the incarnate Word in order to maintain the reality of both natures in one person and to clarify that it is not the Father or the Spirit who become incarnate.[466] Chalcedon's reluctance to provide neat definitions perhaps illustrates that this is not subject to easy solutions; rather, it concerns discerning a mystery that is always being deepened. Nevertheless, Cyril's Christology looks straight to the person as the place where the true self lies.[467] Instead of divine nature either swallowing up human nature or being bolted to it in some form of conjunction, the Person of the Word comes to be a human being.

465. Grillmeier, *Christ in Christian Tradition*, 483.

466. Cyril of Alexandria, *On the Unity of Christ*, 66; Pope Leo I, "Sermon 64, Passion of the Lord"; "Sermon 96, against Eutyches," in *Sermons*.

467. See McGuckin, *St Cyril of Alexandria*, 224.

Summary

Theologians like Athanasius and Cyril realize that both the issue of the union of the divine and human in Christ and the issue of the composition of human beings are complex and not the subject of easy definitions. Apollinarius and Nestorius go wrong perhaps because they see the person solely as an instance of nature, an entity to be explained and defined purely by specific characteristics. As a result, Apollinarianism suggests that the person is equated with soul or mind, while Nestorianism suggests that the person can be split from the human being.

Insights from early Christology endorse the bioethical view that mind and will are significant aspects of the human person. Yet equally significant is the insight that the human person is not merely mind or soul, nor is the mind or soul of the human person joined to the body in such a way that the bond can be broken, thus separating the person from the human being.

Moreover, the Christology of Cyril, repeated by Pope Leo and taken up in Chalcedon, supports the idea that the very being of Christ as perfect man restores the likeness to God in human beings: "human nature, by the very fact that it was assumed, not absorbed, in him, has been raised in us also to a dignity beyond compare."[468] Redemption, then, is in the very being of Christ and not merely in his acts. This may have implications for being a human person, particularly a human person unable to make and act on choices: the very being of a human being has dignity beyond compare. Furthermore, early Christology offers disability studies reflections on grace and *kenosis*, what it is to give of oneself to the point of dependence. These may challenge some people who see the person primarily as the autonomous individual who desires and wills, as opposed to dependent human beings who require assistance. For Cyril, in his understanding of *kenosis*, the person of the Word does not change. The change is in his condition, he becomes man. It is perhaps the ideas of *kenosis*, of emptying oneself while remaining the same person, and of persons as essentially dependent, that may be the key to deepening

468. Second Vatican Council, *Gaudium et Spes*, 22.

understandings of the profoundly disabled person and to the human person at the margins of life.

But the archetypal starting point for discussion on the person is found in the thinking of one writer: Boethius. Even if his interpretation of the person is finessed or developed, there is no avoiding the fact that Boethius offers a neat definition of the person and one that seems to fall conveniently into the modern bioethical idea of the person as possessing reason, self-consciousness, and autonomy—if, that is, his theological context is forgotten. It is problematic that such an interpretation bypasses the richness of early Christian thinking. Moreover, by ignoring the context in which Boethius writes, unwarranted conclusions are drawn from his definition.

Nevertheless, it is not only Boethius who is credited with influencing the overly individualistic and rationalistic modern notion of the person. Augustine is also charged with this, though not by bioethicists. Instead, it is some theologians who see Augustine as the author of the human person who is self-conscious, rational, and autonomous. And so discussion turns next to these two great thinkers on the concept of the person.

5. Defining Persons *Carefully Speaking about Boethius, Augustine, Rationality, and Persons in Context*

Introduction

Boethius provides what is at first glance a neat solution to the concept of the person: that "person" is an individual substance in a rational nature. For those who find the provenance for their view of the person in the definition from Locke, the Boethian definition seems to be an acceptable precursor to Locke's definition. Although it cannot be said with certainty whether Locke rejected this definition from Boethius as being too embedded in the scholastic system, he was certainly aware of its influence in debates on personal identity.[1] Nevertheless, it is possible that Locke interpreted "rational nature" as "soul," and Locke rejects the soul as the principle of personal continuity.[2] Whether intentionally or not, however, it seems that Locke expands (and arguably skews) this definition from Boethius so that the person becomes "a thinking intelligent being, that has reason and reflection, and can consider itself as itself, the same thinking thing, in different times and places, which it does only by that consciousness which is inseparable from thinking."[3]

Linked perhaps to Locke's nominalism and thus his dismissal of universals, "rational nature" for Locke becomes equated with the actual ability to reason and to be self-conscious. Once this move has been made, it is easy to see how it is speciesist to deny personhood to some

1. Galen Strawson says that Locke accepted the "widely accepted Boethian definition of person.'" *Locke on Personal Identity*, 12n10. Udo Thiel says that the Boethian definition "dominated" Scholastic thought and metaphysical disputes throughout the seventeenth century. *Early Modern Subject*, 28, 35–36.

2. Zachary Leader suggests that the Boethian definition of person is related to the soul. *Revision and Romantic Authorship*, 316.

3. Locke, *Essay Concerning Human Understanding*, II, XXVII, 9.

higher nonhuman animals, and how some human animals, notably the profoundly intellectually disabled, can fall below the threshold for personhood. The Boethian definition, supplemented by Locke, thus appeals to many modern thinkers because it seems to refer to the notion of rationality, and it allows writers like Cavalieri and Singer to interpret "rational nature" as the "capacity for reasoning."[4]

Yet Boethius himself says that he depends on Augustine,[5] and in some theological circles Augustine is challenged with presenting an overly isolated and rational account of human beings by his focus on the inner man.[6] This implies that Augustine is responsible for the rise of a reductive view of the person. On a different note, Augustine says that his contemporary the Pelagian Julian of Eclanum (ca. 386–454) accused him of Apollinarian tendencies.[7] Julian thus brings Pelagianism into the debate.

Because some secular and some theological thinkers claim that Boethius and Augustine lead to modern notions of the person as an isolated individual characterized by rationality, and Pelagianism bears some resemblance to notions of self-sufficiency and autonomy, it is worthwhile to explore more deeply the thinking of Boethius and Augustine in order to speak more carefully about the concept of the person. Significantly, the definition of Boethius seen in context clearly supports solidarity between all human beings. It demonstrates that denying personhood to the profoundly disabled is disablism. To explain this, it is necessary to see that Boethius writes squarely in the Christological tradition already outlined, and he formulates his frequently used definition specifically in response to Nestorius and Eutyches.

4. Cavalieri and Singer, "Great Ape Project," 286.

5. Boethius, "De Trinitate." See also Bowery, "Boethius," 108.

6. See, e.g., Zizioulas, *Being as Communion*, 40; Gunton, *Promise of Trinitarian Theology*, 42–43; Grenz, *The Social God and the Relational Self*, 67.

7. Augustine, "Answer to Julian," 5.55.

Boethius: The "Individual Substance of a Rational Nature" in Its Theological Context and Its Modern Legacy

Boethius against Eutyches and Nestorius

By the time Anicius Manlius Severinus Boethius was born in about 475, Rome had been overrun and so had lost its power and status though the old Roman public life continued. As a result of barbarian harassment, the Imperial Court moved from Rome to Milan and then to Ravenna. The Church was divided, with the pope in Rome and emperors in the West at Ravenna and in the East at Constantinople. As a child and after his father's death, Boethius was adopted by Quintus Symmachus, a Roman consul. Symmachus became a role model for the young Boethius; notably, Symmachus was interested intellectually in history and in the theological controversies of the time. Boethius wrote extensively on mathematical subjects, on translations and commentaries on logic and rhetoric, and on theology and philosophy. As well as being interested in rhetoric and philosophy, he was involved in politics, becoming a Roman consul in 510 and then later joining the court of the Arian Ostrogothic King Theodoric. As a result of political intrigue and accusations of treason, Boethius was tortured to death in about 525.[8]

The intellectual climate in Rome had looked to the city's venerable traditions, to Latin and Greek literature, particularly Neoplatonism, and to the seemingly unproblematic relationship of Greek culture and Christian belief. Keen to synthesize Christianity with ancient thought, Boethius set himself the task of translating some Greek sources into Latin.[9] His most famous work, aside from his definition of the person, is his *Consolation of Philosophy*, written when he was in prison for political reasons. Notably, Boethius translated Aristotle's work on logic and Porphyry's *Isagoge*. These texts became significant for medieval theologians and scholasticism, and through them, Boethius managed to bridge the gap between ancient Greek philosophy and the Latin of the Middle Ages. Alongside the synthesis of Christianity and ancient thinking, Boethius may have decided to apply himself to another synthesis: that of the hu-

8. See Marenbon, *Boethius*, 7–10.

9. For some of the influences on Boethius, see Marenbon, *Boethius*, 10–14.

man and divine in Christ and that of soul and body in human beings.

The West had accepted relatively easily the Christological formula hammered out at Chalcedon in 451, possibly because it confirmed Pope Leo's *Tome*.[10] But in the East, controversy had grown,[11] not least because the Council of Ephesus had been termed the Robber Council, and the Chalcedon definition itself was viewed with suspicion as being Nestorian. Although Nestorianism and monophysitism—the belief that in Christ there is one nature, a belief that developed from the thinking of Eutyches—had been condemned with the agreement of the Church in Constantinople, these heresies still had followers farther East. In the East, the monophysites in particular were influential, and while Acacius, Patriarch of Constantinople (471–89), did condemn Nestorius and Eutyches, he did not reaffirm the formula of Chalcedon, resulting in the Acacian schism that lasted until 519.[12] Various attempts were made to heal the schism, including an appeal from some Scythian monks. Boethius seemingly decided to step into the controversy after he had attended a meeting in about 512 or 513 with his spiritual mentor John the Deacon, later Pope John. At this meeting, a letter from an Eastern bishop was read out suggesting a possible interpretation of the Chalcedon formula that would be acceptable to all. In the ensuing debate, Boethius appears to be concerned that the discussion lacked sufficient rigor.[13] So, Boethius sets about remedying this by choosing the contrasting heresies of Nestorius and Eutyches as the subjects of his analysis.

According to Boethius, Nestorius and Eutyches make the same mistake: they treat "nature" and "person" as the same.[14] Nestorius thinks there are two persons in Christ since he believes that "person" can be predicated of every nature, and so he proposes a union of conjunction.[15] Eutyches thinks that there is only one nature in Christ since the "man" is so assumed that human nature does not remain, so while he correctly believes the person to be single, he wrongly considers that the nature

10. See Davis, *First Seven Ecumenical Councils*, 192–94.
11. Davis, *First Seven Ecumenical Councils*, 194–204.
12. See Marenbon, *Boethius*, 68–69.
13. See Hall, *Trinity*, 23–24.
14. Hall, *Trinity*, 24.
15. Boethius, "Against Eutyches and Nestorius," IV.

is also single.[16] In keeping with the distinction of nature and persons already made by Basil, Gregory of Nazianzus, Gregory of Nyssa, and Augustine in Trinitarian thinking, Boethius recognizes the need to define "persons" and "natures," since that is the heart of this Christological debate.[17] Although this treatise is directed toward Christology, Boethius uses it to discuss issues relevant for Trinitarian theology, perhaps indicating how both are inextricably linked.

Noting that there are different ways of defining "nature," and that the term is not always appropriate for Trinitarian theology,[18] Boethius indicates that "nature" points to a "special property of things"; it is generic, something shared, so, for instance, it is in the nature of wood to fall and fire to rise.[19] But the definition of "person" is, he admits, "a matter of great perplexity."[20] After much deliberation, he comes to define person as "the individual substance of a rational nature."[21]

Boethius thinks that a particular nature underlies the concept of person as a "substrate"; thus "person cannot exist apart from nature."[22] Moreover, person for Boethius is properly predicated of substances in the Aristotelian sense: person is not in the realm of changing characteristics, accidents such as color, for "person cannot consist in accidents," and there cannot be a "person of whiteness."[23] Cavalieri and Singer appear to think the opposite, though it is not clear. In Cavalieri's and Singer's discussion of person and its provenance through Boethius, they say that person is a "subject of relations," and they claim, at least from Aristotle, relation is accidental; that is, it is added to and not essentially connected to the substance of a thing.[24] If this is their reading, then it emphasizes the fact that for these two modern authors, the concept of the person is rather insubstantial and flimsy.

16. Boethius, "Against Eutyches and Nestorius," V.
17. Boethius, "Against Eutyches and Nestorius," introduction.
18. According to Boethius, "nature" can be predicated of all things that exist, including accidents and substances, but there are no accidents in God; "nature" can also be predicated of corporeal substances, but God is not corporeal. See Hall, *Trinity*, 24.
19. Boethius, "Against Eutyches and Nestorius," I.
20. Boethius, "Against Eutyches and Nestorius," II.
21. Boethius, "Against Eutyches and Nestorius," IV.
22. Boethius, "Against Eutyches and Nestorius," II.
23. Boethius, "Against Eutyches and Nestorius," II. See Hall, *Trinity*, 25.
24. Cavalieri and Singer, "Great Ape Project," 134.

Returning to the early sixth century, Boethius uses certain terms like "rational" within the framework of Greek philosophy.[25] This is significant given the modern tendency to see rationality as a necessary condition for experience, where rationality is thought of as a formal ability to reason, to process data provided from the outside, and to be neutral toward that data.[26] Michael Frede distinguishes this tendency from an older view, informed by Christianity, that reason has less to do with what allows human beings to form beliefs. Rather, it concerns what is in the human being to begin with: a rational soul[27] or rational nature. So, Boethius says, "person cannot be affirmed of bodies which have no life," for instance, stones; nor of "living things which lack sense," for instance, trees; nor "bereft of mind or reason," for instance, horses or oxen, since they do not have a rational nature, but we do say there is a person of human beings, of God and of angels.[28] For Boethius, then, "person" does not refer to inanimate objects or plant life or animals with an irrational nature: it only applies to beings of a rational nature, that is, beings of a particular kind. And this does not refer simply to those who can demonstrate reasoning.

Following the Greek differentiation between universals and particulars,[29] Boethius thinks that whereas some terms can be predicated of individuals universally, such as man or stone, in a generic way, person can only be applied to particulars, "for there is no person of a man if animal or general, only the single person of Cicero, Plato or other single individuals."[30] As Douglas Hall explains, for Boethius, the Latin *persona* means the same as the Greek *hypostasis*.[31] Thus according to Boethius, "nature is the specific property of any substance, and person the individual substance of a rational nature."[32] As John Marenbon ex-

25. See Grenz, *The Social God and the Relational Self*, 66.

26. See Camosy, *Peter Singer and Christian Ethics*, 125.

27. Frede and Striker, "Introduction," in *Rationality in Greek Thought*, 5–6.

28. Boethius, "Against Eutyches and Nestorius," II.

29. See Grenz, *The Social God and the Relational Self*, 66.

30. Boethius, "Against Eutyches and Nestorius," II. See Hall, *Trinity*, 24.

31. Hall, *Trinity*, 25. According to Marenbon, Boethius went "out of his way" to link his definition of person to an Aristotelian understanding of *hypostasis* (a substrata for accidents and a particular thing). Marenbon says that Boethius was "helped by a linguistic accident": the Latin *substantia* matches Aristotle's *ousia*. *Boethius*, 71.

32. Boethius, "Against Eutyches and Nestorius," IV.

plains, by linking person to *hypostasis*, Boethius indicates that a person is "an individual substance, the species of which has as a *differentia* endowed-with-reason."[33] According to Marenbon, Boethius follows Porphyry's categories as set out in the *Isagoge*: genus (as in "Man is an animal"); species (as in "Socrates is a man"); *differentia* (as in "Man is rational"); *proprium* (as in "Man is capable of laughter"); and accident (as in "Socrates is white").[34] Boethius then argues that God is a different substance from created things because he comes before all things. Furthermore, Boethius speaks of person in the Trinitarian context where he confirms that Persons do not indicate three individual gods, and in the context of the unique person of Christ. So, his notion of person as an individual implies not so much an individual instance of a human nature but rather a uniquely irreplaceable being, a Cicero or a Plato unlike any other of that name. John Crosby points out that Boethius takes Aristotle's notion of the human being as "*a* rational animal" and develops it further to an individual substance of rational nature precisely so that he can include incommunicability in contrast to Aristotle's individuality.[35] Notably, then, for Boethius, the person is not simply a rational nature or the soul.

In Trinitarian theology, the divine human analogy based on the general and particular is not adequate when applied to God since it tends toward tritheism. Nor perhaps is it adequate regarding human beings, since the reality of another is not fully grasped merely by ascertaining the species and then distinguishing the characteristics.[36] Nevertheless, the distinction of nature and person that began as a tool to distinguish orthodoxy from Sabellianism and Arianism in Trinitarian theology, and from Nestorianism and Eutychianism in Christology, seems to be reflected in the Lockean distinction of human being and person. But while the theological person cannot be reduced to nature yet is related to it and is a concrete reality, the Lockean bioethical person appears to be insubstantial and separated from, rather than merely distinguished from, the human being. Furthermore, instead of holding to the theological insight

33. Marenbon, *Boethius*, 71–72.
34. Marenbon, *Boethius*, 23–24.
35. Crosby, *Selfhood of the Human Person*, 59.
36. See Crosby, *Selfhood of the Human Person*, 47–48.

that persons are irreplaceable and incommunicable, some contemporary approaches to the person seem to resolve issues of personhood by separating rationality from animality, be it human or nonhuman, as if rationality is not an animal property but instead is a property that separates persons from non-persons. Once this bioethical human being is separated from the person, then it can be declared replaceable or redundant. In the case of the profoundly disabled human being, he or she is no longer seen as a unique individual or as a specific kind of animal, a human one, one with a rational nature. Instead, the intellectually disabled person is placed on "the other side of the gulf" between humans and animals, therefore receiving a lower status and thus worthy of lowered concern.[37]

A Legacy for Modern Human Persons

Although Boethius seems to focus on the uniqueness of the human person and on human rational nature, his definition is often mistakenly understood as an emphasis on individuality and actual rationality,[38] the interpretation taken up by Cavalieri and Singer. Similar charges of a focus on individualism and intellectualism are made against Augustine, on whom Boethius relies, though these charges are made in the theological arena.[39] Following the line of thinking that claims that focus on psychology or the inner man is rationalist, however, it could also be argued that Cyril of Alexandria is a party to this legacy, and perhaps even more so, since his Christology centers on the person of the *Logos* and the individual. According to McGuckin, Cyril's idea leads to seeing the person as a "dynamic agent of conscious action spiritually exemplified in the *hypostasis* of Christ."[40] Nevertheless, Cyril, Boethius, and Augustine check their arguments with the *kerygma*. For Cyril, the focus

37. Singer, *Practical Ethics*, 74–75.

38. Stanley Grenz argues that Boethius seems to share the Greek view that individuality lies principally in the soul rather than the body, which is subject to decay. *The Social God and the Relational Self*, 66. If this is correct, then this appears to support the view of Zachary Leader, who equates soul to Boethius's definition and the Cartesian cogito. *Revision and Romantic Authorship*, 317. Grenz adds that by highlighting uniqueness, Boethius began the modern trend of elevating individuality (67). But neither Leader nor Grenz seems to prove the case for saying that for Boethius the person is purely the soul.

39. See, e.g., Zizioulas, *Being as Communion*, 40.

40. McGuckin, *St Cyril of Alexandria*, 225.

of his Christology is not the person as an individual consciousness. Cyril concentrates on the concrete reality of the Person of Jesus Christ as God and man, and on the self-emptying of the *Logos*, not the autonomy and self-sufficiency of human nature.

In patristic theological anthropology, reflection on the self-sufficiency and autonomy of human persons occurs alongside Christology. The significance of human freedom and exercise of the will is clear and proved in the disputes with Apollinarius, who denies a human mind in Christ, and by the Antiochene insistence of a fully functioning human nature in Christ. But in patristic thinking, as also in reflection on the image of God in human beings, the concept of the human person is not reduced merely to an individual who is self-sufficient and has the capacity to exercise choice. A return to Augustine, on whom Boethius says he depends, seems to draw out a deeper understanding of the human person.

Augustine, Pelagius, and Julian: Beyond Autonomous and Self-Sufficient Persons

Augustine and Rational Human Nature

The definition from Boethius has been carried forward into bioethics perhaps because it seems precise and uncomplicated. Hall claims that the definition also stems from the desire of Boethius to "prove" dogmatic formulations,[41] and so it appears to be in keeping with the modern tendency toward definitions and answers. Even though Augustine allegedly holds a strongly rationalistic account of the person, however, his thinking does not appeal to authors like Singer and Cavalieri. The clearest reason for some to favor Boethius over Augustine is that Boethius is more popularly seen as a philosopher rather than a theologian; after all, Boethius is most famous for his treatise *The Consolation of Philosophy*. Still, there may be an additional reason. A cursory reading of Boethius that neglects the context and his theology and philosophy, and a reading that is in tune with anti-speciesism, may lead to the impression that animals can be thought of as persons if they are found to have some form of

41. Hall, *Trinity*, 25.

rationality. In contrast, Augustine responds unequivocally to those who want to make it unlawful to kill some nonhuman animals.[42] Augustine says that by their reasoning, plants also should be protected since they too have life. Augustine makes it explicit that "non-rational animals," nonhuman animals, do not have reason in common with human being, and "both their life and death are subject to our needs."[43] Augustine, and the Christian tradition, sees that a line can be drawn between human beings and the rest of creation and so privileges human beings, whatever their abilities, over nonhuman animals. According to Singer, "it is arbitrary to hold that only human beings are of intrinsic value"; however, he still thinks that a line needs to be drawn because it is impractical to give moral consideration to all living things. He (arbitrarily) chooses as a boundary not sentience but conscious interests.[44]

Augustine does not deny that nonhuman animals feel pain, and he sees that they have a place in God's harmony of the universe.[45] But he believes that God created human beings with a nature "in a manner intermediate between angels and beasts," and that human beings are destined for eternal fellowship with God.[46] Moreover, in the Creation story, Augustine notes that only in the case of human beings did God start with one individual, Adam, and then God creates another, Eve. In the case of nonhuman animals, God commanded many to come into existence at once. Augustine finds this particularly instructive. God's intention, he says, was so that "the unity of society and the bond of concord might be commended to him more forcefully" through their "similarity of nature" and "by the affection of kinship."[47]

Still, for Augustine, this bond cannot be reduced to sympathy or be merely a matter of concern for society, and he explains this in detail when it comes to all human beings, including the intellectually disabled. He says that in all cases, where reason or understanding appears to be

42. It appears that Augustine is referring to the Manichaean elect, who were vegetarian. See Harmless, *Augustine in His Own Words*, 204.

43. Augustine, *City of God*, I.20.

44. Singer, *Practical Ethics*, 274–80.

45. Augustine, *City of God*, XII.4.

46. Augustine, *City of God*, XII.22.

47. Augustine, *City of God*, XII.22.

"great" or "small" or "in a coma," "the human soul is never anything but rational and intellectual." Furthermore, this "image of God" is always there "from the moment this great and wonderful nature begins to be," and it remains "whether it is so worn away as to be almost nothing, or faint and distorted, or clear and beautiful."[48]

There is no remaining evidence to suggest that Pelagius considered the situation of the profoundly disabled person. His reasoning in general seems to create problems, however. According to Pelagius, Christ's redemption is simply a matter of instruction for human beings in contrast to Adam's bad example: what matters first is "being able" and then "choosing."[49] To be sure, reasoning and willing are significant characteristics of being human. Nevertheless, if, as it seems for Pelagius, human beings are essentially actually willing and choosing beings, this raises a question about those who are profoundly disabled and cannot choose. At first sight, it seems that the Pelagian controversy is primarily about human beings. Pelagius and his disciple Caelestius both appear to argue that human beings are able to keep the Commandments, that before the coming of Christ there were people who were without sin, and that people could obtain the kingdom of heaven without Christ's salvific action.[50] But for Augustine, the issue goes beyond what human beings are able to do. If, as Pelagius claims, Christ is merely an example, that his work is apparently not necessary for salvation, then the question arises: What need has humankind of Christ, and what difference did his coming as man really make? In terms of people with disability, if they are not able to choose or to be obedient to God's Commandments, this appears to mean either that their salvation is in question or that they have no need of Christ's saving action.

Augustine, Pelagius, and Self-Sufficient Persons

Although Augustine's Christology was not forged out of controversy, the bitter dispute with Pelagius seems to sharpen Augustine's thinking. There appear to be historical links between Nestorianism and Pela-

48. Augustine, *Trinity*, XIV:6.

49. Augustine, "The Grace of Christ and Original Sin," in *Answer to the Pelagians*, 1.3, 4.

50. Marius Mercator, "Admonitory Memorandum against the Heresy of Pelagius and Caelestius," in Jurgens, *Faith of the Early Fathers*, 3:185.

gianism. Theodore of Mopsuestia writes against Augustine's position on original sin, and he harbored refugee Pelagians, among them Caelestius and Julian of Eclanum.[51] Augustine corresponds with Cyril, and Cyril makes a connection between Pelagianism and Nestorianism.[52] Nestorius is interested in the Pelagian position, and he supports Caelestius, Julian, and other Pelagian fugitives,[53] although he apparently formally condemned Pelagianism.[54] Perhaps as a result of the Pelagian controversy, Augustine increasingly explains his Christology in terms of grace,[55] and the interaction of his anthropology and Christology is more evident.

Pelagius (ca. 350–425) was a British or possibly Irish monk. Renowned as a biblical commentator, he taught in Rome but left for Carthage before the Visigoths entered the city. In Carthage, his views were scrutinized, though at a synod held at Diospolis in 415, he was exonerated. Yet it seems that he either denied responsibility for the propositions that were being judged even though they had been taken from his own writings, or he replied so cleverly that their true intent was obscured, or he claimed that they came not from him but from Caelestius. Cyril of Alexandria sent Augustine a copy of the digest of proceedings that Pelagius had produced after the synod.[56] In this digest, Pelagius triumphantly boasts that "the statement in which I maintained that 'a person can be without sin and easily keep the commandments of God if he wishes' has been approved by the verdict of fourteen bishops."[57] After Augustine had read the digest, he set out the views and propositions of Pelagius alongside his own comments in his book *The Revisions* under the chapter "The Deeds of Pelagius" so that his readers could judge the proceedings for themselves.[58]

51. Brown, *Augustine of Hippo*, 384.

52. Wickham, "Pelagianism in the East," 210–11; see also Russell, *Cyril of Alexandria*, 215n25.

53. Neil and Allen , *Crisis Management in Late Antiquity*, 117.

54. See Wickham, "Pelagianism in the East," 208.

55. See McWilliam, "Augustine at Ephesus?," 56–67.

56. In his "Letter 4*" to Cyril, Augustine explains how he compiled his own deeds of Pelagius, 4.2. *Letters*, 4:245–47. This is one of twenty-nine letters discovered by Johannes Divjak in 1969.

57. As reported by Augustine, "Deeds of Pelagius," 30.54. See Harmless, *Augustine in His Own Words*, 379.

58. Roland Teske, "General Introduction" and "Introduction," in Augustine, *Answer to the Pelagians*.

Interested in moral reform, Pelagius is scandalized by those, like Augustine, who seem to suggest that human beings do not have sufficient moral willpower to be obedient to God's will. In contrast, Pelagius is certain that perseverance in prayer and in asceticism leads to a life free from the desire to sin.[59] According to Pelagius, human beings surpass nonhuman animals by their "intelligence and mental vigour," and, furthermore, human beings have human free will, that is, "the freedom to choose" from alternatives. Human beings also have a natural capacity to be able to choose good or evil. Pelagius adds that "the whole honour of our nature" consists in this freedom, and dignity is derived from it.[60] Indeed, Caelestius, a disciple of Pelagius and possibly an Italian lawyer, who became a lay monk and then was ordained a priest,[61] argues that if God assists an individual at every turn, then the power of choice would simply be in vain: "a will that needs the support of another is not a will at all."[62]

Pelagius asserts this radical importance of free will in response to those like Augustine who, in his view, engage in moral pessimism by suggesting that after the Fall human beings tend toward evil. Pelagius points out that many people living before Christ, and especially some pagan philosophers, lived good lives, so human beings have never been impelled toward evil and have always had freedom of choice. Yet, he says, much more can be expected of Christians because Christians have been instructed for the better by Christ and by the moral law.[63] Our moral obligations in turn stir our will, for "only one who has knowledge of the law can be without sin." As Augustine points out, it is entirely different to say, as he himself does, that a person is helped by knowledge of the law not to sin.[64]

At times, the thinking of Pelagius appears ambiguous and possibly inconsistent; indeed, in *The Deeds of Pelagius*, he is accused of redescrib-

59. B. R. Rees explains that the Pelagian heresy began as an ascetic movement. *Pelagius*, xi.

60. Pelagius, "Letter to Demetrias," 2.2–3.2. Rees points out that this letter survived because it was thought to be from Jerome, 33. It is listed under Jerome in J. P. Migne, *Patrologiae cursus completus: Series latina*, vol. 30 (Paris: 1846), 15–45.

61. Lamberigts, "Caelestius."

62. Caelestius, "Fragment," in Jurgens, *Faith of the Early Fathers*, 2:217.

63. Pelagius, "Letter to Demetrias," 3.2.

64. Augustine, "Deeds of Pelagius," 2.

ing his writings. But Augustine notes the assertion made by Pelagius, that human beings can be without sin if they want and they can keep the Commandments if they choose to do so.[65] Yet, as Augustine explains, some aids are indispensable: "no one sails without a ship"; without the grace of God, "no one lives rightly." Other aids, he says, render help: a man can thresh grain without a threshing sledge, but one helps. Nevertheless, it seems that for Pelagius, grace is natural human faculties, and it is knowledge of the law that enables human beings to live rightly.[66] Pelagius thinks the argument that human beings tend naturally toward sin is an excuse for those who find the moral struggle too hard: the only reason we find it difficult to choose the good is because of bad habits.[67] Moreover, God's law directs human freedom by its system of rewards and punishments, and to confirm God's goodness human beings must be endowed with reason and conscience.

What Pelagius sees as moral pessimism Augustine views as realism. Augustine agrees with Pelagius that freedom is God's gift to human beings so they can do what is right, and without freedom, human beings could not be morally responsible.[68] But Augustine also realizes that Pelagius claims that they are both of one mind. In response, Augustine writes in his *Revisions*, a critical reconsideration of his work, that in the past he has not dwelled on the topic of grace because at the time this was not an issue: he was, after all, addressing the problems posed by the Manichaeans.[69] With the advent of Pelagianism, the matter of grace has assumed importance, and he distinguishes his position from that of the Pelagians: the Pelagians, he says, "insist upon the free choice of will to such a degree that they leave no place for God's grace," further, they insist that grace is "bestowed according to our merits."[70] To clarify his position, Augustine affirms that freedom with goodwill is a "great good."[71] Augustine then points out that the will cannot be upright and virtuous

65. Augustine, "Deeds of Pelagius," 16.
66. Augustine, "Deeds of Pelagius," 3.
67. Pelagius, "Letter to Demetrias," 8.3.
68. Augustine, *Revisions*, I.9.3.
69. Augustine, *Revisions*, I.9.4.
70. Augustine, *Revisions*, I.9.3.
71. Augustine, *Revisions*, I.9.3.

unless it has been freed by God's grace.[72] To set the context, Augustine says that God provides us with minor-, middle-, and major-order goods. Using this framework, Augustine can then distinguish between two sorts of freedom: first, the middle-order good of free will, *liberum arbitrium captivatum*, as free will influenced by the tendency to sin. This is a middle-order good because we are able to use it badly. Second is the major good of graced free will, *liberum arbitrium liberatum*, as free will where, as Alister McGrath puts it, grace has removed the weights loading the scales toward sin.[73] *Liberum arbitrium liberatum* is the freedom to make the right choice. Good use of this freedom is a virtue, and so it is a major good.[74] Although both are good, free will matches free choice, the "freedom which makes men think they are free when they have no masters."[75] This distinction perhaps has resonance with some unrealistic accounts of the autonomy of strong independent individuals who forget that compromised vulnerability and dependence are also part of the human condition.

The problem, as Augustine sees it, is that as a result of Adam's sin we have a great interior struggle, and we cannot stand wholeheartedly with our will. We are engaged in combat within ourselves, and the conflict of desires we feel means that our wills are being torn apart.[76] Human beings are disabled by sin so that no one, Christian or pagan philosopher, can be master of himself, except through God's bounty.[77] Without grace, God's free gift, we are not able to know or do any good thing.[78] Clarifying this in his discussion of free will in heaven, Augustine explains that at creation, human beings had the ability not to sin combined with the possibility of sinning, *posse non peccare*, but in the future, heavenly life human will be freer because human beings will not be slaves to sin. Through God's grace, sinning will be impossible, *non posse peccare*,[79]

72. Augustine, *Revisions*, I.9.4.

73. McGrath, *Christian Theology*, 351–55.

74. Augustine, *Revisions*, I.9.6.

75. Augustine, "Free Choice of the Will," 72–242.

76. Augustine, *Confessions*, 8, 10.

77. Augustine, *Confessions*, 10, 31; idem, "Enchiridion on Faith, Hope and Charity," 30.

78. Augustine, "Enchiridion on Faith, Hope and Charity," 31–32.

79. Marcia Colish notes that Augustine is using a "weapon from the armory of Stoic logic": when a negative term—in this case, *non* is placed before the whole proposition rather

and human beings will not have the power to will evil because they will only want to do good and so they will be truly free.[80] As a modern illustration of what Augustine means, in playing the piano, the pianist can just simply hit any note, a freedom of indifference, *posse non peccare*, and playing just about any note is not truly music. But a pianist who has studied, learned the music, and wants to play well will only want to play the right notes, play the music.

Augustine thinks that not only will human beings be freer in the next life, but also every defect will be supplied, what is incomplete will be made complete, and what is injured will be renewed.[81] These beliefs seemingly extend to abortive conceptions, since, Augustine says, once a human being begins to live, then he or she is susceptible to death, and if he or she dies, then he or she will be resurrected.[82] Moreover, he says that conjoined twins will be restored to their normal shape each with their own complete body.[83]

The idea that people will be "remedied" in the next world has caused consternation for some modern authors who write on disability. Various models of disability, including the medical model that refers to an individual's physical condition and the social model that locates problems in social discriminatory structures and attitudes, challenge the different perceptions of disability.[84] Some point out that the very concept of normal is now disputed.[85] Others note the struggle to reconcile the reality

---

than simply before the verb—it is "negated more exhaustively." *Stoic Tradition*, 188. Augustine in fact means different things, not simply reinforcing a negative. Before the Fall, Adam was able not to sin, *posse non peccare*, and able to sin, *posse peccare*. But the first sin so permanently affected human beings that, after this first sin, human beings are under the power of sin and so are not able not to sin, *non posse non peccare*, without the aid of grace. In the Heavenly Kingdom, freed from the bondage of sin, the saints will have free will, but they will desire only the good and so they will not sin, *non posse peccare*. See Simon Gaine, *Will There Be Free Will in Heaven?*, 9–10, 21–25.

80. Augustine, *City of God*, XXII, 30. See also Gaine, *Will There Be Free Will in Heaven?*, 9–10, 21–25.

81. Augustine, "Enchiridion on Faith, Hope and Charity," 87, 91.

82. Augustine, "Enchiridion on Faith, Hope and Charity," 86; *City of God*, XXII, 13, 14. David Jones points out that Augustine is uncertain on when life does in fact begin. *Soul of the Embryo*, 118.

83. Augustine, "Enchiridion on Faith, Hope and Charity," 87.

84. See Messer, "Human Genome Project," 97–98.

85. See, e.g., Creamer, "Embracing Limits," 109.

of disability with a vision of perfection without appearing to devalue the person with disabilities.[86] Some people with disabilities believe that the disability is itself a part of their identity and not a defect to be made good, whether in this life or the next.[87] Some people with disabilities are now reframing their experience of disability: for many disabled people, the stereotypical notions of tragedy and suffering result more from their isolation in society; the disabled are beginning to respond to the view that they are afflicted with the social role assignment of a tragic, burdensome existence.[88] But Augustine's view is more nuanced than a simple suggestion that all will be restored to some sort of norm. According to Augustine, deformities will be removed in such a way that the total substance, the essential nature of that body, will remain intact; indeed, he says that the wounds of the martyrs may remain.[89] So, Augustine believes that each person will be recognizable in the next life even if deformities are remedied. God will arrange bodily resurrection even if the body has already been dissolved or eaten by animals or cannibals.[90] Augustine's conviction that although God can remove any defect disabled people retain their identity is therefore significant for some modern views of disability.

Nevertheless, for thinkers like Augustine, it is not disability that causes the problem. For Augustine, the problem is pride, and as far as he is concerned, the Pelagian view seems to follow the temptation to pride in us all. People, he argues, seek to "be light... in themselves"; their arrogance attempts to place them on a level with God.[91] Yet Augustine thinks that human beings are far away from God, so they need grace to bring them to conversion and God to raise them up to the truth. After all, says Augustine, "with him is the source of life, and in his light we shall see the light."[92]

86. See Patterson, "Redeemed Bodies," 123–43.

87. See Betcher, *Spirit and the Politics of Disablement*, ix; Lewis, *Deaf Liberation Theology*; Weiss Block, *Copious Healing*, 17–18; Eiesland, *Disabled God*.

88. Saxton, "Disability Rights and Selective Abortion," 107.

89. Augustine, *City of God*, XXII, 19. Kristi Upson-Saia explains how, for Augustine, wounds and physical disabilities may be signs of holiness. "Resurrecting Deformity," 93–122.

90. Augustine, "Enchiridion on Faith, Hope and Charity," 88–90; *City of God*, XXII, 20.

91. Augustine, *Confessions*, 8, 10.

92. Augustine, "The Spirit and the Letter," 11.

As for the remedy to pride, Augustine turns to Christology. Pride, Augustine says, may be "the cause of all human failings." But "God came humbly out of mercy, revealing his grace with wondrous clarity in the man whom he assumed," and it is this man who is our example of unmerited grace.[93] It is mistaken pride that thinks we can be restored through our own merits,[94] and it is also mistaken to think that the human nature assumed by the Word had earned some merit before its assumption.[95] Moreover, like Cyril, Augustine says that if union with God is achieved by an individual's own merit, then any human being could do it, and so there could theoretically be more than one Christ, which is plainly absurd.[96] Instead, Augustine explains that the Incarnation supremely manifests the grace of God; the Christological union is unique because it involves the exceptional grace of assuming human nature into a unity of the person with the Word.[97]

Pelagianism and the East

The Pelagian dispute did not have any lasting effects in the East,[98] possibly because the East always thought that human free will cooperates with divine grace. Some note an affinity between the Pelagian and Antiochene or at least Nestorian positions, while also acknowledging that there are differences.[99] McKim explains this in terms of East and West approaches to salvation.[100] According to McKim, the East sees sal-

93. Augustine, "Punishment and Forgiveness," 2, 27.

94. Augustine, "Enchiridion on Faith, Hope and Charity," 30.

95. Augustine, "Enchiridion on Faith, Hope and Charity," 36.

96. It has been suggested that Augustine's Christology depends on Theodore of Mopsuestia (for an analysis, see McGuckin, "Did Augustine's Christology Depend on Theodore of Mopsuestia?," 39–52. In words reminiscent of Theodore's, Augustine believes that God is present to all things, yet he dwells in beings that have volition and understanding but only insofar as they are oriented toward him (*Letter* 187). But whereas for Theodore, God dwells in those who are first devoted to him, for Augustine, those who are oriented toward God are those who are influenced by his grace. As McGuckin points out, there is no evidence that Theodore's work was circulating in Africa in a Latin translation and Augustine was not fluent in Greek. "Did Augustine's Christology Depend on Theodore of Mopsuestia?," 49.

97. Augustine, *Letter* 187.

98. See Wickham, "Pelagianism in the East," 210–11.

99. See McWilliam, "Augustine at Ephesus?," 66; Wallace-Hadrill, *Christian Antioch*, 162; Grenz, *Theology for the Community of God*, 296.

100. McKim, *Theological Turning Points*, 85.

vation as deification, where, through the Eastern ascetic tradition, the soul's union with God is a possibility even on earth, though deification is completed only in our future life. In the West, through the influence of Augustine, salvation is viewed as justification, though it is also linked to deification, since by justification humans become adopted children of God. Turcescu suggests that this difference of emphasis came about owing to differing historical circumstances: the West was confronting the fall of Rome, and so asking questions about the justice of God, the East was enjoying the rise of Byzantium.[101] McKim argues that Augustine stresses it is justification that effects the transformation of the human being, which takes place through grace. But it must be added that the Eastern tradition accepts that the "truly ascetic struggle" that requires our cooperation is impossible without grace.[102] As Russell points out, there was no formal definition of deification until the sixth century, and its usage before then was complex, encompassing both an ethical approach focusing on ascetic and philosophical endeavor and a realistic approach that saw human beings as being in some sense transformed either by participation in God or by relationship.[103] Nevertheless, there appears to be what Wallace-Hadrill calls a "wide gulf" between the optimism of Pelagius, that humans can reach their own perfection on earth, and Theodore, who sees it can ultimately only take place in the age to come.[104]

Still, the problem of Pelagianism brings with it discussion of ancestral or original sin. The East seems to accept the effects of Adam's sin in terms of death and corruption, and it holds to the view that human beings are born into a world where sin has dominion. But it also holds that humanity does not inherit Adam's sin. As Ware explains, the East tended toward a "less exalted idea" of the human state before the Fall, and so Adam was not judged too harshly for his error.[105] This state reflects the view of Irenaeus, who thinks that Adam and Eve were in a state of childlike simplicity.[106] Ware points out, on the one hand, that the East

101. Turcescu, "Soteriological Issues," 64–72.
102. Louth, "Place of Theosis in Orthodox Tradition," 37.
103. Russell, *Doctrine of Deification*, 1.
104. Wallace-Hadrill, *Christian Antioch*, 162.
105. Ware, *Orthodox Church*, 223.
106. Irenaeus, "Against Heresies," III, XXII, 4.

does not agree with the pessimism of later thinkers, like Calvin, who believe that after the Fall human beings were utterly depraved and incapable of good desires. Ware adds, on the other hand, the East does not agree with an Augustinian view that after the Fall human beings come to lack freedom.[107] This is based on the belief, strongly expressed by the Fathers, that while the image of God in human beings is distorted, it is never destroyed. Having been created in the image and likeness of God, human beings retain their natural orientation toward God; nevertheless, their vision is clouded, so they fail to recognize their true direction. Human beings do not need a special act of grace to orient themselves, though they do cooperate and respond freely in their salvation because salvation, as union with God, is relational.

The matter of original sin came to the fore with the conflict between Augustine and Julian, the Italian bishop of Eclanum (ca. 380–454). Along with eighteen other Italian bishops, Julian refused to sign a papal letter circulated in 418 that sanctioned the condemnation of Pelagius and Caelestius.[108] Moreover, Julian rejected the concept of original sin because he considered it an attack, along Manichaean lines, on the good of marriage.[109] Julian is one of the few Western thinkers who disagree with Augustine on the point of original sin, and he aligns himself with Theodore of Mopsuestia. Julian had taken refuge with Theodore in about 420–21; at this stage, Theodore was free from suspicion.[110] Julian also found Nestorius to be sympathetic to his cause.[111] Theodore of Mopsuestia speaks out against the "defenders of original sin": he says they are "preoccupied" with sin and that they introduce a novel teaching by suggesting sin is transmitted to all the descendants of Adam. As far as Theodore is concerned, although all humans sin, one man's sin is not visited on another.[112] Initially, Pelagius also seems to have agreed with Theodore of Mopsuestia in denying that the origin of death lay in the sin of

107. Ware, *Orthodox Church*, 223.

108. For the events leading up to the dispute between Julian and Augstine and their "dialogue of the deaf," see Lancel, *St Augustine*, 414–19.

109. See Hunter, *Marriage, Celibacy, and Heresy in Ancient Christianity*, 267–68.

110. Lancel, *St Augustine*, 417.

111. Wickham, "Pelagianism in the East," 201.

112. Theodore of Mopsuestia, "Fragment," in McLeod, *Theodore of Mopsuestia*, 25.

Adam. Pelagius later admits that death is transmitted to humankind, but not sin. Sin, he argues, occurs when human beings imitate Adam's disobedience. Although he is sympathetic to some aspects of Pelagianism, Nestorius does think that all human beings are involved in the condemnation of Adam, and equally all are freed by Christ.[113]

Julian also follows Pelagius in believing that all human beings have freedom of choice. This leads Julian to suggest that Augustine has Apollinarian tendencies, because Augustine says that Christ took on a sinless human nature. Julian says that Manichaean thinkers such as Augustine ascribe sin to an evil nature. In contrast, Julian calls himself a true "Catholic" and so ascribes sin to "an evil will."[114] Thus there can be no sin in an infant who has no will[115] and therefore no need for infant baptism. Julian passionately believes that it is a matter of justice that sin is not imputed unless the freedom to abstain from it is present.[116] Interestingly, however, according to Pelagius, an infant who dies unbaptized has eternal life but is excluded from the kingdom of God.[117]

Augustine refutes the charge of Apollinarianism by insisting that Christ took on the whole of human nature except for sin.[118] He repeats that just as any human being unites in one person a rational soul and a body, so Christ in one person unites the Word and man.[119] Equally passionately as Julian, however, Augustine pleads with Julian to allow infants, and those without a will, to come within the ambit of salvation and be rescued from the darkness by Christ. Augustine sees in Julian's rejection of original sin the possibility that human beings can be the authors of their own salvation. In his reply to Julian, Augustine systematically articulates the idea of original sin already current in theology from St. Paul and repeated at least since Tertullian.[120] Moreover, Augus-

113. See Wickham, "Pelagianism in the East," 209.

114. Julian of Eclanum, "To Florus," 1.24.

115. Julian of Eclanum in Augustine, *Answer to the Pelagians*, 2.24.

116. Julian of Eclanum in Augustine, *Answer to the Pelagians*, 2.39.

117. See Ronald Teske's introduction to Augustine, "Punishment and Forgiveness of Sins," 79.

118. Augustine, "Enchiridion on Faith, Hope and Charity," 34.

119. Augustine, "Enchiridion on Faith, Hope and Charity," 35.

120. See Rondet, *Original Sin*. It is commonly accepted that Augustine misread Rm 5:12, translating ἐφ ᾧ as *in quo*, in whom, instead of *quia*, because. Referring to Rondet's work, Philip Quin says that Julian of Eclanum, who knew Greek, translates the phrase correctly

tine finds texts from bishops from the East like Basil[121] and Gregory of Nazianzus[122] to support his position. Augustine points out that baptism is universally required for salvation, that baptism is for the remission of sins, and that in the tradition infants are baptized. This infant baptism suggests that infants need the remission of sins, so they must be guilty of sin, and since they are not guilty of personal sin, sin must be inherited.[123]

In response to those who take an overly high view of human freedom—notably the Pelagians and especially Julian, who claim that human beings need not sin and that human beings do not require divine assistance—Augustine explains that when we turn to God, he helps us. However, Augustine adds, our very turning to God is God's initiative.[124] By placing the initiative in God's grace, Augustine perhaps answers those who see his suggestion of human cooperation as semi-Pelagian. Augustine agrees that the human capacity for free will was not lost at the Fall. But he also recognizes that through ignorance and difficulty we no longer choose the right thing.[125] Grace for Augustine is divine enablement; it opens us up to God and brings forward the choice of the good, though it does not compel.[126]

The inclusion of grace into Christology may indicate the uniqueness of the Incarnation, but it also gives an opportunity for considering the operation of grace in the lives of human persons. Although Augustine is charged with introducing the modern notion of the person as an autonomous individual, his understanding of the need for grace, especially given the human tendency toward pride and self-sufficiency, does not bear this out. Moreover, Augustine's insistence that all human beings need grace, that all need to be saved by Christ, includes the profoundly

as "because." Nevertheless, Quin recognizes that even if Augustine mistranslates Rm 5:12, Augustine better understands the passage as a whole. Quin then goes on to explain how John Locke argues that it against God's justice to make a person guilty for the sins of another, and so Locke repudiates the idea of original sin. "Disputing the Augustinian Legacy," 238–42.

121. Augustine, *Answer to the Pelagians*, 1.5, 18.

122. Augustine, *Answer to the Pelagians*, 1.5, 15; 2.3, 7.

123. Augustine, "Punishment and Forgiveness of Sins," 1.

124. Augustine, "Punishment and Forgiveness of Sins," 2.2, 2.5.

125. Augustine, "Free Choice of the Will," 3, 18, 52.

126. Augustine, *Revisions*, 1, 22.

disabled person who does not have the capacity for willed choice. This approach emphasizes the significance of a spiritual life that all human beings have regardless of their condition because all human beings are in a relationship with God even if they cannot express that relationship, at least as far as other human beings are aware.

Summary

As Boethius explains, the problem of nature and persons goes to the heart of the Christological debates,[127] and although he attempts a definition, Boethius concedes that the concept of the person is complex. Nevertheless, in keeping with the tradition he inherits and building on it, Boethius emphasizes that person refers to a concrete reality and not to a mask or appearance. Person cannot exist apart from nature and that nature is rational, though not in the reductive sense of possessing rationality in terms of having the ability to reason. In this way, Boethius follows the early Christian view of the solidarity that binds all human beings: all human beings share in all that belongs to the humankind. Nevertheless, the concept of the person signifies not an individual instance of a particular nature but rather a unique and irreplaceable being.

By placing the definition of Boethius in its Trinitarian and Christological context, the understanding of the person as "an individual substance in a rational nature" does not exclude the profoundly intellectually disabled human being. Similarly, solidarity of all human beings as created, fallen, restored, and redeemed, and the subjects of salvation by Christ, extends to all human beings, whatever their condition. All are called to holiness, and as Augustine explains, God can break through all deafness and dispel all blindness.[128]

For some, Augustine's use of deafness and blindness to express apparent moral failure to listen to or see God are unfortunate analogies.[129] Indeed, many of the Fathers do compare blindness to spiritual lack of

127. Boethius, introduction to "Against Eutyches and Nestorius."

128. Augustine, *Confessions*, X, 27, 38.

129. For an account of how metaphor may be problematic in disability studies, see Koosed and Schumm, "Out of the Darkness," 77–92.

perception. In his book *City of God,* however, Augustine notes the difficulty of finding the right word, and he explains that the term "blindness" is a condition called in Greek *aorasia*, which means not physical blindness, *tuphlos*, but rather a failure to perceive. Augustine gives the example of the men of Sodom who were looking for the door of the righteous Lot and failed to find it.[130] As Augustine points out, if their condition was one of physical blindness or what he calls "true blindness, so that they could see nothing," then they would have looked for guides to lead them back home rather than for a door to give them entrance.[131] So, a different word for a different meaning, and, as Augustine adds, the problem is that the Latin uses *caecitas*, blindness, because there is no adequate Latin equivalent to the Greek term. Augustine uses this interpretive way of blindness and deafness to speak of human inability in general to see God as the source of love and goodness and to express God's activity that initiates and graces "sight." How, then, do these insights from theology bring light to the myopia that besets contemporary reductive notions of the person in bioethics?

130. Gn 19:11.
131. Augustine, *City of God*, XXII, 19.

6. Discerning Persons ◆ *Practically Speaking in Bioethics*

Introduction

The task of this book has been to take the concept of the person seriously. Current bioethical understandings of the "person" that rely on arbitrary lists of characteristics for a definition are confused and inconsistent; taking rationality and self-consciousness as the "two crucial characteristics" is reductive and does not do justice to the complexity of the concept, especially where it is aimed at a simple utilitarian adding up of apparent interests. Instead, this book returns the concept of the person to the theology of the early Church Fathers, where the concept originated and where it gained its content and force, in order to highlight some of the insights that have been neglected or overlooked by subsequent notions.

In particular, the patristic understanding of the person challenges the total separation rather than simple distinction of biological life from biographical life, and the association of "person" only with biographical life characterized by a level of rationality and self-consciousness. Initially, this separation seems only to allow for the abandonment of the distinction between human and nonhuman animals in order to counteract speciesism. But it also creates a tension between current and prominent concerns about speciesism as the "final frontier" of discrimination and the much less acknowledged and often implicitly accepted prejudice of disablism. As Singer's seminal work on animal rights shows, for many the acceptance of disablism becomes the price for countering speciesism, and it is a matter of justice,[1] but only to the nonhuman animal.

1. Singer, "All Animals Are Equal," 575.

In fact, this separation undermines the concept of the person altogether. Ultimately, as Singer hopes, it allows us to "refuse to adopt a distinction between persons and those who are not persons" and insist instead on a calculation of pain and pleasure in determining which individuals have a right to life.[2] In this line of thinking, the person no longer matters.

In this final chapter, the theology of the early Church Fathers on the person is put to work in bioethics in order to alleviate the implications of speciesism and to reject disablism, as well as to restore the connection between biological and biographical life. As a practical ethics dealing with real-life situations, bioethics links theory with practice, and it calls for critical reflection and moral reasoning that is carefully thought through. Taking a more reflective approach seems particularly apposite when the prejudice of disablism appears to be unchecked.

An overtly Christian approach may at times seem to be, to use the words of Pope John Paul II, a "sign of contradiction."[3] Nevertheless, insights gained from this theological thinking can rescue bioethical reasoning from disablism and can also clarify speciesism. Contemporary approaches seem to treat the concept of person as a problem that requires solving through definitions, and such approaches run into the dangers of reductionism, distortion, confusion, and ultimately irrelevance. Similarly, even if they did not eliminate the significance of the concept of the person, the struggles in early Trinitarian theology were marked by those, like Sabellius and Arius, who saw in the mystery of the Trinity a perceived problem, and the solutions they offered cut across the faith of the Church.

In taking up the term "person" and applying it to God, early theology demonstrates that the concept of the person requires discernment and profound reflection because in some sense it is part of a mystery. In patristic terms, a mystery is not a puzzle to be solved. The Greek μυστήριον (*musterion*) is derived from μύειν (*muein*), to have the mouth closed or to be silent.[4] It has the force of religious silence.[5] Analogized to human beings, even though such an analogy is admittedly limited, they also

2. Singer, *Rethinking Life and Death*, 222.
3. Wojtyla, *Sign of Contradiction*.
4. Vine, *Vine's Complete Expository Dictionary*.
5. Lampe, *Patristic Lexicon*, 893.

share in this mystery of being persons. Rather than coming to a clear definition of the person that in some cases leaves some human beings vulnerable to destruction or exploitation, an acceptance of the complexity of the "person" acknowledges and protects the unique and mysterious identity of the other. It takes the person seriously.

Discernment over Arbitrary Decisions

Theological reflection on God as one and as Trinity does not come about as a result of arbitrary decisions of the early Christian community. The early Christian *kerygma* and early liturgical practice proclaim that the one God is Father, Son, and Holy Spirit, and that this is revealed though hidden in the Old Testament and made manifest in the New Testament.[6] This revelation certainly challenged the early Fathers, and their struggles to express the Revelation of the Three and One unfold over the centuries. The term "person" is brought in precisely to aid in this struggle, not so that an easy answer can be found but so that a mystery can be deepened. Far from this enterprise is the search to identify an arbitrarily chosen set of characteristics that can define person so that certain human beings can be as readily identified as persons in the same way as, say, birds can be further specified as owls.[7]

Given that the roots of the concept of the person are deeply entwined with reflection on God and the God-man, theology inevitably takes the person seriously. It reflects on the person as a concrete and distinct reality in both strength and weakness. In its analogy of human and divine, it gives content to the notion of the person that goes beyond narrow or reductive definitions or easy solutions, to a concept that is always open to deepening reflection. Moreover, theological explorations of the person as image of God, of the Divine Persons of the Trinity, and of the Person of Christ each offer specific insights into contemporary bioethical questions. These insights appeal philosophically as well as theologically since anthropological issues run alongside theological ones. Rebounding from reflection on God and on Jesus Christ, the Son of God made man, early

6. See Col 1:26.
7. See O'Donovan, "Again: Who Is a Person?," 381.

Christian thinkers ask questions about what it means to be human; what are the relationships between body, soul, and mind; what is significant about human beings and about being a person; about the acting person and the person unable to act; and how we as personal beings relate to others, to the world, to other animals, and to God. Some of these insights seem to have been neglected in secular bioethical thought, perhaps owing to the perception that Christianity is merely concerned with reward and punishment in an afterlife.[8] Most particularly, some bioethical thought is myopic about the radically dependent person. Through these insights on the significance of using the language of the person, certain themes and concerns that have resonance with contemporary bioethical issues have emerged.

Language Matters

It has long been recognized that certain terms carry weight. This can be recognized, for instance, in the way in which Descartes and Locke, who began the trend toward separating the person from the human being, redescribed some disabled human beings as monsters, since these individuals did not fit with a certain view of humanity.[9] In part as a result of the naturalistic fallacy, that an ought cannot be derived from an is, some bioethicists claim that the "person" is merely descriptive, and they critique its use as a morally laden word.[10] Other bioethicists suggest that the status of person is not significant, and instead what becomes important are various characteristics that might ground a pain pleasure calculus or the calculation of interests,[11] and since these are associated with personhood, it appears that being a person counts as important. Yet as Singer says, the concept of the person is not merely descriptive.[12] In his own writing, Singer demonstrates only too clearly that the description of an entity as a person or nonperson is a normative enterprise. Such a description has significant ramifications.

8. See, e.g., Singer, *Practical Ethics*, 88–89.
9. Branson and Miller, *Damned for Their Difference*, chap. 1.
10. See Beauchamp, "Failure of Theories of Personhood."
11. Kuhse and Singer, *Bioethics*, 3.
12. Singer, *Rethinking Life and Death*, 182.

Trinitarian theological struggles were not simply arguments about words. Rather, they reflected deeper problems. The import of these struggles can be seen from the Arian use of nonpersonal language such as "unoriginate" to describe the Father in the context of the Arian denial of divinity to the Son; from Sabellian notions of person as "presentation" to avoid ideas of distinction in the Trinity; and from the Eunomian suppression of the names of Father, Son, and Spirit so that the persons seem to be mere appearances or fiction rather than persons who do properly exist. Orthodoxy recognized that this was not purely a matter of linguistics, and by taking the Divine Persons seriously, theology asserts that the Son as second Person of the Trinity is God and so can save us, that he became man so we can share in God's eternal life. The real distinction of persons means that the Father, Son, and Spirit are one, equal, incommunicable, and truly substantive.

Trinitarian debates took place alongside discussion of humans, and as images of God, human persons mirror in part the gravity of the theological concept of the person.[13] Even though these debates highlighted dissimilarity rather than similarity, still they seem to provide worthwhile points for reflection. Finding the appropriate language to fathom out the inexpressible involved taking up the concept of the person, and by association with the divinity, it gained immeasurable depth. Theology then reminds us that the language we use and whether we call a human being a person matters.

Language of a Person

The significance of calling human beings persons is borne out in bioethical language. If certain descriptions are denied, then the other entity is not seen as a human being, never mind as a person. Notably, this can be seen in relation to the human embryo. Like Eunomius, who distinguishes generation from essence and generation by will so that he can argue that the Son, as generated by the will, has subordinate status,[14] seeing the embryo as the result of the wills of scientists or parents, a product, useful yet disposable for the benefit of others, makes

13. See Zizioulas, *Being as Communion*, 27.
14. Eunomius, *Extant Works*, Apology 15.

it easier to think that it need not be regarded as "one of us." The desire to deny or lower the moral status of the human embryo, to distance it from "us," encourages the use of terms such as "tissue," "collection of cells,"[15] "experimental material,"[16] "products of conception" (a seemingly common medical term in obstetrics), "spare" or "doomed" embryos, "pre-embryo," or the "fertilised egg."[17] Similarly, people in a persistent vegetative state and people with end-stage dementia have been compared to house plants.[18] Although some object to the demeaning term "vegetative state" for post-comatose patients, there seems little inclination to replace the term,[19] and where once calling a human a vegetable might have shocked, it has now become part of official health care language.

This redescription of some humans allows discussion on, as Jeff McMahan puts it, the "reasonable justification" for killing those "at the margins" of life, where "at the margins" has not so much to do with nearness to life or death but perceived inferior moral status.[20] Redescription allows for the elimination of relationships, a central element for being a person, and this becomes part and parcel of only seeing the person in terms of insubstantial rationality.

Language of Relationship

All human beings, however small, are both unique and in relationship to other human beings. In the case of embryos, however, even their relationships are redefined, and children can have several mothers and fathers characterized as genetic, gestational, or social. An embryo's mother is the one who carries it, not the woman to whom it is genetically linked;[21] its father is not the donor but the other party to the marriage

15. See Warnock, *Warnock Report*, 11, 15; House of Lords Select Committee on Stem Cell Research, *Stem Cell Research*, 4, 14; 4, 24.

16. See Karen Dawson's approach ("Introduction," 3–13).

17. Warnock, *Warnock Report*, 11, 2, 3.

18. According to evidence presented at the petition case to remove Michael Schiavo as guardian of his wife, Michael Schiavo's attorney, George Felos, frequently used this language when speaking to the media about the case of Terri Schiavo. See also Brock, *Life and Death*, 363–64.

19. Jennett, *Vegetative State*, 5.

20. McMahan, *The Ethics of Killing*, vii.

21. Human Fertilisation and Embryology Act, 2008, Part 2, c. 33. http://www.legislation.gov.uk/ukpga/2008/22/contents.

so long as he consented to the procedure;[22] and a couple in a civil partnership, a couple of the same sex, are designated its parents.[23] Despite these redescriptions, whether the earliest of human life exists with its natural parents or even in isolation, in vitro, it is still in relationship with the human family. Moreover, the embryo cannot but exist in relationship, for even in vitro it is another's son or daughter in a real sense, not in the sense of a legal fiction. To borrow from Tertullian's Trinitarian theology, "a father makes a son and a son makes a father and they become what they are by relationship with one another."[24] Each human being, including the human embryo, exists in a personal relationship by virtue of the genealogical connection between us all.[25]

For the patristic thinkers, the language of three persons in the Trinitarian context is considered through relationship to the other persons: the names of Father and Son show they become what they are by relationship with one another;[26] whatever we can say about the Father we can say about the Son, yet Father is not Son and Son is not Father.[27] The three are distinct in their origin, as generating, being generated, and spirated, yet they have one nature and are in a divine life of *perichoresis*, mutual indwelling, and a communion of self-giving. Moreover, the three are real and substantial. Person then is substantial and describes uniqueness and relationship.

Although it may not be suitable to measure divine generation by human nature,[28] patristic writers found the relationship of Father and Son within the Trinity to be of great significance for Christians, such that they held out against using more impersonal terms as proposed by the Arians.[29] Furthermore, the endorsement of the phrase "begotten not made" at Nicaea expresses the idea of like coming from like.[30] As Oliver

22. Human Fertilisation and Embryology Act, 2008, Part 2, cc. 41, 35.

23. Human Fertilisation and Embryology Act, 2008, Part 2, c. 42.

24. Tertullian, "Against Praxeas," IX–X.

25. See Spaemann, *Persons*, 238.

26. Tertullian, "Against Praxeas," IX–X.

27. Athanasius, "Against the Arians," III, 23, 4.

28. Athanasius, "Against the Arians," I, 8, 26.

29. Athanasius, "Against the Arians," I, 9, 34.

30. Eusebius of Caesarea, "Letter of Eusebius of Caesarea to His Church on the Creed of Nicaea," in Stevenson, *New Eusebius Documents*, 344–47.

O'Donovan perceptively puts it, in an analogous way, human beings are begotten of other human beings though also made by God: "our human offspring are human beings, who share with us one common human nature, one common human experience and one common human destiny."[31] We are all related as entities of a particular kind, rational animals. It is this genealogical connection, not certain precise properties, that is part of the foundation of the community of human persons. Notably, this genealogical connection is a biographical connection because biography is not simply about what an individual makes of his or her life. Therefore all human beings are persons (though, as theology points out, not all persons are human beings). Given that "person" is not simply a descriptive term, however, the claim to commonality seems to fall into speciesism.

Alleviating the Implications of Speciesism; Rejecting the Prejudice of Disablism

Speciesism: A Specious Issue?

Many bioethicists query the special significance of human beings because of speciesism and the maltreatment of animals.[32] But at the outset, it is perhaps important to point out that the speciesist recognition that human beings have a special place in the created world does not thereby indicate that nonhuman animals either have no value or are of little or no concern to human beings. Similarly, greater concern for animals need not entail less concern for some human beings.[33] Nonetheless, those who challenge speciesism use the strategy of pointing out that the profoundly intellectually disabled are the weak point[34] since, they argue, these human beings do not exhibit some of the characteristics "we" value, while some nonhuman animals may. Such a strategy places the profoundly disabled human being in a precarious situation. As

31. O'Donovan, *Begotten or Made?*, 1–2, 3.

32. See, e.g., Singer, "Killing Humans and Killing Animals"; DeGrazia, *Taking Animals Seriously*; Bennett, "Chimera and the Continuum of Humanity," 347–87.

33. See Berkman, "From Theological Speciesism to a Theological Ethology," 11–34.

34. See Matthews, "Human Dignity and the Profoundly Disabled," 186.

Bernard Rollin explains in *A Companion to Ethics*, there are no morally relevant differences between intellectually disabled humans and many animals. Rollin notes, though not without a level of unease, R. G. Frey's argument that logically, instead of research on nonhuman animals, it is more beneficial to do research on "marginal humans" who have "lower qualities of life" than some animals since, being human, they are better research models.[35]

According to Singer, the value of different lives, human and nonhuman, can be compared, and he says that this ranking into "some hierarchical order" would "not necessarily be speciesist." It is not speciesist because, he says, while we may judge that the life of a "normal adult member of our species is more valuable than the life of a normal adult mouse," this judgment can be made from an "impartial standpoint." According to this standpoint, one that Singer attributes to the utilitarian philosopher John Stuart Mill, "in general it does seem that the more highly developed the conscious life of the being, the greater the degree of self-awareness and rationality and the broader range of possible experiences," so "the more one would prefer that kind of life." Singer and Mill conclude that the life of a normal human being has higher value than the life of an intellectually impaired one.[36] Furthermore, Singer can argue that the value of some profoundly intellectually disabled human beings falls below that of some nonhuman animals.

As his conversation with the disablist activist Johnson shows, Singer genuinely does not think that his logic amounts to disablism. Yet it seems that those who are anti-speciesist cannot avoid falling into some measure of disablism, since they claim that some human beings are inferior to some other human beings and also to some other animals. They argue against the speciesist worldview that gives these lesser human beings protection that is not afforded to other "more valuable" animals.

There are many arguments that rely solely on philosophy to defend giving special protection to human beings. These range from pointing to the solicitude that human beings naturally show for other human beings over and above their care for nonhuman animals, to appeals to human

35. Rollin, "Moral Status of Animals," 503.
36. Singer, *Practical Ethics*, 107–8.

dignity, and to the notion that human beings simply matter more.[37] But from a philosophical point of view, speciesism itself is a problematic notion. After all, if speciesism is the undue privileging of one species over another, then to privilege, say, higher apes, over other non-ape animals is speciesist. "Apeism"[38] is, it seems, a form of speciesism. Moreover, the views of some anti-speciesist philosophers are seemingly not only disablist but also speciesist, because they use characteristics of so-called normal *human* persons as the benchmark to raise the status of some nonhuman animals. Singer appears to make such a move when he links his notion of the person to certain human capacities. According to Singer, "the embryo, the later fetus, the profoundly intellectually disabled child, even the newborn infant" are all, as a biological fact, human beings. However, he thinks that they cannot be said to have "truly human qualities" because they are not "self-aware," they do not have "a sense of the future, or the capacity to relate to others." They are not persons.[39]

Singer does not find it problematic to rely on characteristics such as rationality; in fact, Singer does not seem to take the concept of the person seriously at all, since what appears to matter is a counting up of interests or weighing up of pains and pleasures.[40] Answering those who claim that animals do not have rights because they are not autonomous or members of a community, Singer counters that appeals to rights are not necessary. Rather, he says, the argument is about the principle of equality that requires suffering be counted with like suffering.[41] Singer adds, the "capacity to suffer and/or experience enjoyment is the only defensible boundary of concern for the interests of others. To mark this boundary by some other characteristic like intelligence or rationality would be to mark it in an arbitrary manner." In the case of human beings designated as nonpersons, they have no rights or interests to be protected, so they are vulnerable to being used—for instance, in research—or even killed. Following this thinking, since the profoundly intellectually

37. For a discussion of human dignity and human exceptionalism, see Calhoun, "Prospects for Human Dignity after Darwin," 172–98.

38. For a defense of apeism, see Machery, "Apeism and Racism," 53–66.

39. Singer, *Practical Ethics*, 86–87.

40. Singer, *Practical Ethics*, 69–70.

41. Singer, *Writings on an Ethical Life*, 35.

disabled human being is not a person, there is no real problem in terminating disabled fetuses; it may even be a duty, as in discarding disabled embryos, in conducting research, or in ending the life of any disabled human being—so long as it is done painlessly.[42]

And Disablism: Accommodating Nonhumans

In contrast, the theological approach is inevitably against disablism because patristic thinkers see human beings as the high point of material creation. Moreover, theology holds that all human beings are made in the image of God and as such are specially loved by God and destined for eternal friendship with him. But since theology and some philosophy single out human beings, they appear to fall into speciesism.

In his critique of speciesism, Singer may be right to point out the dangers of an aggressive anthropocentricism that has placed the world "under pressure" by seeing human interests as paramount. As a campaigner for animal rights, he uncovers perceived injustices perpetrated against (higher) nonhuman animals. Nevertheless, he may be further off the mark when he lays the blame squarely with the Christian concept of "dominion" in his interpretation of the Christian tradition that by its very theology, he says, exploits the natural world solely for human benefit.[43] The view of dominion as exploitation seems to come out of a seventeenth-century mechanistic view of the world, a view that had rejected earlier theological insights.[44] It was this mechanistic worldview that helped to form the Lockean notion of the person, which is taken up by thinkers like Singer. Bioethicists like Fletcher and Harris clearly offer an autonomy-centered and power-driven interpretation of dominion over creation that sees the material world as purely as raw material ready to be used.

For early theologians, it is precisely because human beings are created in the image of God that they are enjoined to exercise stewardship over creation, which involves the good use of the material world. Al-

42. Singer, *Rethinking Life and Death*, 219–22; Glover, *Causing Death and Saving Lives*, 190–202; McMahan, "Infanticide," 131–59.

43. Singer, *Practical Ethics*, 267–68.

44. See Wirzba, *Paradise of God*, chap. 4, 67–70, for the influence of nominalism and the crisis in meaning. See also Peter Harrison, "Subduing the Earth," 86–109.

though the rational nature of human beings is significant, early theologians resist the temptation to reduce the image of God to the actual possession of rationality. The call to exercise stewardship over creation certainly suggests a level of rationality. Yet early theologians also regard all human beings as unique individual worlds or microcosms, destined through grace to be deified *animals* by participating in the mystery of God. Human beings, as animals of a particular rational nature, then, are a part of the world, and the dominion they have is as royal rule in terms of justice that is related to God's justice.

The theological approach favors human beings: they are the only creatures on this earth that God wants for their own sakes.[45] Yet Singer's understanding that according to Christianity, the "dominant Western tradition," "God does not care" how human beings treat his creation because "nature has no intrinsic value"[46] is a misinterpretation of theology. The theological approach does go some way toward alleviating the implications of speciesism by seeing human beings as a midpoint between the material and spiritual, since human beings are concurrently material and spiritual beings. In the patristic tradition, then, human beings have a role to play: the material world was cursed as a result of the Fall, but "the whole creation is waiting with eagerness" and will be "freed from its slavery to corruption and brought into the same glorious freedom as the children of God"[47] with Christ, who is reconciling the world to himself.[48] The theological approach does not denigrate the material. Without deflecting from the significance of the place of human beings, the importance of biodiversity and interdependence within creation is a growing area of concern.[49] In his encyclical *Laudato Si*, Pope Francis points out that there can be no renewal of our relationship with nature without a renewal of humanity itself. If we mistreat our fellow creatures, then this will affect the treatment we give to fellow human beings.[50] But he also says that it is inconsistent to campaign against the

45. Second Vatican Council, *Gaudium et Spes*, 24.

46. Singer, *Practical Ethics*, 267–68.

47. Rm 8:19–21.

48. 2 Cor 5:19.

49. See Pontifical Council for Justice and Peace, *Compendium of the Social Doctrine of the Church*, 464–66.

50. Pope Francis, *Laudato Si*, 65–66; *Catechism of the Catholic Church*, §2418.

trafficking of endangered species while at the same time remaining indifferent to human trafficking, or to be unconcerned about the poor or to destroy a human being that is deemed unwanted.

The patristic idea of dominion then recognizes from the Genesis narrative that there are limits to human freedom. Moreover, in patristic writing, appreciation for the beauty and wonder of creation as well as its ordered harmony is always related to praise and worship of God as its designer, creator, and sustainer.[51] The theological approach is therefore also open to the beauty, mystery, and sacramentality of the universe. Respecting nature, then, is inevitably tied up with respect for the human body.

Body Matters: Beyond Instrumental Value, Beyond Price

As part of the material world, the body of the person matters, and this conviction challenges the current "technological culture," which thinks of all human activity in terms of products of the human will, when everything becomes "raw material, waiting to have something made out of it."[52]

When biological life is seen merely as a support system for biographical life, then the human body has only instrumental value, which seems to vary. The notion of value and the difficulty of seeing some human beings as others are perhaps most noticeable when it comes to the ambivalent views some have for the embryo. If persons are "thought of in the ordinary way as beings able to think, act and communicate,"[53] then embryos are not one of us, but then neither are some other human beings. If, as the *Warnock Report* states, embryos have "special status"[54]—the report recommends that there be no right of ownership in the human embryo yet gives a couple storing an embryo rights regarding its use and disposal;[55] it disapproves of drug testing on embryos purely because of

51. Basil, "On the Hexaemeron," 5, 9; 2, 6–7; Augustine, *Confessions*, 7, 13, 19; idem, *City of God against the Pagans*, XXII, 24. See Schaefer, "Appreciating the Beauty of the Earth," 23–52.

52. O'Donovan, *Begotten or Made?*, 1–2, 3.

53. House of Lords Select Committee on Stem Cell Research, *Stem Cell Research*, 4, 7.

54. Warnock, *Warnock Report*, 11, 17.

55. Warnock, *Warnock Report*, 10, 11.

the undesirability of the mass production of embryos;[56] and it sees a risk of commercial exploitation of embryos yet allows them to be sold where there is a license[57]—then embryos seem more like chattels than one of us.[58] According to the *Warnock Report*, embryos, as "potential persons," may be the first stage of the continuous process toward a new, unique human,[59] but as the "biological expression of human nature," embryos simply have some "value."[60] The "value" of different lives can then be ranked in "some hierarchical ordering,"[61] with human embryos some way down the list, where species boundaries are no longer relevant, and personhood merely has additional weight. To demonstrate Warnock's ambivalent yet "special status," the embryo is most wanted, so it has high value for those undergoing in vitro fertilization (IVF) treatment. The embryo is also prized by those who wish to use it in research. In IVF treatment, however, only "high-quality" healthy embryos are implanted; any "extra" high-quality embryos may be frozen for use later or donated to other couples. High-quality healthy embryos have value. Spare embryos left over from IVF, embryos that are not considered to be high quality, and those that are found to be abnormal or in other words disabled embryos are either discarded or used in research. Human embryos seem to be low on the list of value. Disabled embryos are lower still.

Not just embryos are ranked according to their value. McMahan suggests a "threshold of respect," the point measured on the scale of psychological capacity at which individuals not only merit consideration of their interests but also have "sufficient worth" or value to command respect.[62] The claim that certain human beings—fetuses, infants, the profoundly disabled—do not have interests or the capacity to be harmed is now "popular and empowering."[63] It is empowering because it seems to give permission to treat these human beings in ways that would otherwise be considered harmful. Ranking lives in terms of value means that

56. Warnock, *Warnock Report*, 12, 5.
57. Warnock, *Warnock Report*, 13, 13.
58. See Kennedy, *Treat Me Right*, chap. 6.
59. Warnock, *Warnock Report*, 11, 19.
60. Shannon, "Grounding Human Dignity," 116.
61. See Singer, *Practical Ethics*, 107–8.
62. McMahan, *Ethics of Killing*, 246.
63. Coope, *Worth and Welfare*, 198–99.

harm can be recategorized as merely apparent harm, as evident from the assertion concerning patients in vegetative state or end-stage dementia that starving only *appears* a harm and feeding only *appears* a benefit.[64]

Where lives are valued according to their apparent worth, even where it is claimed that a patient does have interests, it has been argued that death rather than continued life is in that patient's best interests.[65] Bodily life no longer seems to have any value. Pediatrician and ethicist Dominic Wilkinson thinks that infants have little interest in continued life, and disabled infants even less so. Although Wilkinson briefly notes some possibly positive impacts on the family of the birth of a disabled child, he takes considerable time to detail the negative consequences, burdens, and therefore the considerable harm to the family. In addition, he speaks of the harm of a continued life of negative experiences for the child. Notably, the only situation where the child's interests are stronger than its parents is where the child's "interests" favor the withdrawal of treatment.[66] According to Wilkinson, in many cases of severe disability, particularly the risk of future severe cognitive impairment, continued life is not in the child's best interests.[67]

The language of value also invites a language of trade-off, and not only in situations of killing in order to save in cases of fetal reduction in multiple pregnancies, for instance.[68] As Ronald Dworkin explains, by relying on notions of value, it becomes a matter of conflict whether, for instance, a deformed fetus should be allowed to be born when having such a child would "seriously depress" its mother's chance to make something "valuable" of her own life.[69] The bodily life of the disabled fetus is seen as disposable material.

The view that there is no interest or value in bodily life reduces the body to raw material to be used at will, and some bioethicists argue for a moral imperative to use this material. Harris, for one, thinks that we would "not only be crazy but wicked" to cut ourselves off from any po-

64. Coope, *Worth and Welfare*, 198–99.
65. See Bernat, *Ethical Issues in Neurology*, 318.
66. Wilkinson, *Death or Disability?*, 151.
67. Wilkinson, *Death or Disability?*, 248.
68. See Coope, *Worth and Welfare*, 60.
69. Dworkin, *Life's Dominion*, 151.

tential benefits of research on embryos.[70] Although there remains some unease about creating embryos specifically for research, "spare" embryos left over from IVF are often regarded as already doomed and so can be used.[71]

The unease surrounding the use of embryos has led many to look to more ethically appropriate research material, and notably for new sources of stem cells other than the stem cells harvested from embryos. While such new sources have been identified, many still regard the research on embryos as holding the most promise. But to bypass ethical concerns, entities have been created and redescribed so that they are no longer called embryos. Through the procedure of altered nuclear transfer, embryos can be genetically modified so that they do not grow beyond the blastocyst stage, or their development is deliberately halted, thus producing what are called "biological artifacts." Embryos for use in research have been created by research cloning, a technology that is not sufficiently developed to result in therapies. These embryos are not successful clones because their inherent anomalies are such that they would die if implanted; they are popularly known as "clonotes."[72] Human admixed embryos are perhaps the clearest cases of embryos that have been redescribed so that they are no longer considered embryos even though it is accepted they are technically embryos. According to the UK Human Fertilisation and Embryology Act of 2008, the term "embryo" does not include the "human admixed embryo."[73] The act goes on to describe the many ways in which the "human admixed embryo" is produced by either the addition of animal material to an existing embryo or the creation of an embryo from human and animal material.[74] If an embryo is modified so that it cannot develop, or if nonhuman material is added to it, then what has been created is arguably not a non-embryo but, possibly, a profoundly disabled embryo. Moreover, this misuse of nonhuman animal material should be of concern to anti-speciesists, especially where adult nonhuman animals are used to gestate modified embryos.

70. Harris, "Embryos and Hedgehogs," 79–80.
71. Edwards, "Ethics and Embryology," 49.
72. See George and Lee, "Acorns and Embryos," 90–100.
73. Human Fertilisation and Embryology Act, 2008, Part 1, c. 1, (2) (1.a).
74. Human Fertilisation and Embryology Act, 2008, Part 1, c. 4 (2, 6).

So, it seems that in the hierarchy of embryos, biological artifacts, clonotes, and human admixed embryos are among the least of the least, denied even the name embryo.

Sacramentality of Nature and the Body: A Matter of Justice

The most recent technologies that propose to create for research interspecies hybrids, entities that are deliberately created to belong to neither the human nor the nonhuman animal, come into conflict with ideas of justice and respect for the natural world. The concerns of justice here are broad and include the overstated claims of researchers[75] that have unduly swayed public opinion and raised false hopes, masked risks in potential therapies, done injustice to hybrids that may well be human embryos albeit radically disabled, raised concerns over the welfare of animals, and perhaps most significantly deliberately created an entity that does not belong.[76]

The sense of sacramentality of the natural world extends also to the human person as image of God, and so it questions any understanding of dominion as genetic or bodily manipulation that sees the body as "raw datum."[77] Many disabled people regard the medicalization of the body as a source of discrimination. The disabled body is made over into what appears to be the norm; the body is the problem. Such an attitude surfaces in recent technologies that researchers claim will alleviate disability and disease. Cloning, preimplantation diagnosis, and genetic engineering, whether embryos are sacrificed or not, reinforce the stereotypical view of disability as a condition to be avoided at all costs, rather than something to be treated and supported.[78] For many people with disabilities, this focus on technologies is taking away from the reality of their actual lived situations. Many disabled people point to the fact that they have unmet needs that can be satisfied with relatively uncontroversial technology and with no side effects, and that this can be done

75. See Submission from Christian Action, "Research and Education Memorandum 21.3."

76. For a comprehensive account of the ethical challenges involved in human-nonhuman experimentation, see MacKellar and Jones, *Chimera's Children*.

77. Pope John Paul II, *Veritatis Splendor*, 48.

78. See Reist, "Afterword," in *Defiant Birth*, 287–88.

now. In contrast, these new and as yet unproven technologies that offer promise a long time in the future come at great cost. Such technology is not seen or understood from the perspective of the disabled, and others make decisions on behalf of the disabled without proper consultation or appreciation.

Seeing the body as "raw datum" applies also to how parts of the body are used to relieve another's disability. It seems that the "Rubicon" of turning organs into commodities has long been crossed, as considering organs as "pieces of bodies," as "market goods," is well attested to in the debate about financial incentives for organ donation.[79] Similarly, in reproductive medicine, although egg donors are not paid in the United Kingdom, they can be "compensated" through reduction of IVF costs, and according to the *Warnock Report*, in the selection of embryos as tissue donors, such humans are seen as "useful sources of biological raw material for spare parts."[80]

There is also continuing debate on the permissibility of using live anencephalic neonates as donors of vital organs[81] and increasing the "donor pool" by inclusion of children with "isolated head injury." Nursing professional and ethicist Teresa Savage explains that "under certain conditions, children may have their moral status as persons questioned, as when disabilities are present or likely to evolve after illness or injury." Having looked at philosophical arguments that exclude newborns as persons, Savage calls anencephalic infants "nonpersons" because they are "those humans who never acquired the capacity to be a person." Consequently, she argues, the obligations are "different" than those to a person. She adds, "the language may offend some, but it reflects the harsh reality of allocation decisions."[82]

79. See Mahoney, "Should We Adopt a Market Strategy to Organ Donation?," in Shelton and Balint, *Advances in Bioethics*, 79, 86.

80. King, "Why We Should Not Permit Embryos to Be Selected as Tissue Donors," in Kuhse and Singer, *Bioethics*, 158–59.

81. For a robust argument against treating anencephalic neonates in ways that are dissimilar to any other neonate, see A. A. Howsepian, "Consciousness and Aesthetics in Decisions Concerning Organ Donation Using Anencephalic Neonates," in Jensen, *Ethics of Organ Transplantation*, 72–91.

82. Savage, "The Moral Status of Children," in DeWolf Bosek and Savage, *Ethical Component of Nursing Education*, 211–13.

Underestimating the mystery and sacramentality of the body as sharing in the image of God is also evidenced by those who regard seriously deformed infants as "monstrosities," as not "gifts of God,"[83] and therefore as fitting subjects for infanticide. It is also indicated by those who see patients in a persistent vegetative state as no longer imaging God, and therefore for all intents and purposes already dead,[84] or as existing merely in biological life since they can no longer respond to their God-given vocation.[85] These claims seem to mirror the notion that the image of God in human beings resides in the possession of intellect and free will; some bioethicists, like Thomas Shannon, make this explicit.[86] Shannon assumes that in the tradition, image of God refers to the intellect and will, and so he implicitly refers to Augustine.

The Fathers make much of the significance of the intellect and free will, and Augustine himself says that the image of God is in that aspect of the person that seeks to understand and behold God.[87] But the Fathers do not reduce their understandings of the image of God to the actual possession of a rational mind: the whole human being is made in the likeness of God, not merely a part of the person.[88] Furthermore, Augustine explains that all children, including those born with deformities, are God's creation.[89] Moreover, in his challenge to those presumably Neoplatonists who believed that a person's past sins committed in a former celestial body determined the grossness of his or her current body, Augustine argues that people then commonly called *moriones*, the intellectually disabled, are in fact Christian witnesses who show that God's grace and the Spirit do not pass over any kind of capacity. Indeed, he says, they may have a preference of grace over people with a keener intellect.[90]

In pedagogical research, there is a new emphasis on different ways of learning, and especially on the material, on sensory experiences. Com-

83. See Engelhardt, "Infanticide in a Post-Christian Age," 82–84.

84. Cranford, "The Case of Mr. Stevens," 199–211.

85. Biggar, *Aiming to Kill*, 47.

86. Shannon, "Grounding Human Dignity," 114. (His only named reference is to the medieval theologian Bonaventure.)

87. Augustine, *The Trinity*, XII, 7, 12.

88. Irenaeus, "Against Heresies," V, VI, I.

89. Augustine, *Answer to the Pelagians III*, 3, 16; 6, 43; 3, 4.

90. Augustine, "Punishment and Forgiveness of Sins," 1.32.

plementing cognitive learning, affective learning makes use of the material world, and this new understanding can be related to a renewed appreciation of the sacramentality of the created world: taking time to be with a person and to experience sights, sounds, taste, touch are profoundly human activities, albeit neglected in the busy-ness of life.[91] This appreciation of the stillness and receptiveness of human experience is a reminder that there is more to being human than the ability to make choices or express desires.

With both insights from the goodness of creation and from the fact that God in the Second Person of the Trinity assumed a truly human nature, the material and all of creation is brought under God's care. Significantly, in the earliest Christian iconography, the Christ child is depicted lying in the manger with the ox and ass standing by. The animals are not mentioned in the Gospel accounts of the birth of Christ, though they may be implied by the presence of the manger. Origen links their appearance in the tradition to the text of Isaiah 1:3, "the ox knows its owner and the donkey its master's crib."[92] As far as the early Church Fathers are concerned, nothing in the Old Testament is without significance for the New: the first witnesses to the Incarnation are nonhuman as well as human animals, and as the traditional matins responsory for the Christmas liturgy says, "O great mystery and wonderous sacrament, that animals should see the newborn Lord lying in a manger. O blessed Virgin, whose womb was worthy to bear the Lord, Christ Jesus. Alleluia!"

While theology can embrace the whole of creation, some philosophical attitudes seem to exclude the profoundly disabled. Professor of philosophy Licia Carlson notes the striking way in which some make much of the apparently close relationship between nonhuman animals and people with severe intellectual disability. She suggests that this perpetuates a view that some human beings are "qualitatively different" from "normal" human beings: it "obscures the distinctively *human* face of persons with intellectual disabilities."[93] Part of this discerning of humanity is to see the human being, disabled and abled, as an other.

91. See Matthews, "Communication Strategies and Intensive Interaction Therapy," 97–110.
92. Origen, *Homilies on Luke*, 13, 7.
93. Carlson, *Faces of Intellectual Disability*, 144–45.

The Human Person as an Other

Persons Count

In contemporary bioethical decision making, it seems that being a person, as opposed to being a human being, counts. On the one hand, who counts as a person appears to depend on which set of characteristics are valued by the person doing the counting. On the other hand, in some philosophical systems, even for designated persons, protection from killing is not always absolute, for personhood "counts" in the sense that it is weighed in the utilitarian balance so that "other things being equal,"[94] "almost always in practice,"[95] the ascription of personhood makes killing a person directly wrong.

In contrast to a utilitarian accounting, Christian theology (following the book of Genesis, particularly chapter 9) makes a link between human beings being made in the image of God and its moral implications: human beings count in the sense that they are both accountable to each other and to God for each other. This accountability and the respect owed to the other as a fellow human being can be recognized by all through reason, as evidenced by the outcomes following Cain's question in the Old Testament "Am I my brother's keeper?"[96] and the lawyer's question in the New Testament "And who is my neighbor?"[97] The answers to these questions readily admit that in not only family ties but also in the stranger we recognize an other, and that we do not merely regard the other as a possessor of interests. The dignity of human beings and the respect therefore owing to him or her are further elevated since, as images of God, human beings are called to share by grace in the divine nature. In both the human and divine dimensions, humans have "unassailable value," for they are manifestations of an other and of God in the world.[98]

Those who claim that analytic moral philosophy has a rigor that is lacking in theological thinking or who dismiss the theological approach

94. Singer, *Practical Ethics*, 94.

95. Glover, *Causing Death and Saving Lives*, 113, 139.

96. Gn 4:9.

97. Lk 10:29.

98. Congregation for the Doctrine of the Faith, *Dignitas Personae*, 8.

to human beings as outdated sectarianism overlook the profound philosophy of the other that has flourished, particularly in the twentieth century. Although a version of this philosophy of the other and a philosophy of relationship can be found in early Trinitarian thinking, this philosophy has perhaps come into its sharpest focus after the events of the Second World War and the Holocaust. The terrible fact of the Holocaust vividly challenged old conceptions: it became clear that the good are not rewarded, that the bad are not punished, and that duty-based ethics can fail or even be used to justify evil action. Philosophy moved away from concentration on the subject who thinks, the "I" that does the thinking. As a result, philosophy recognized in sharper relief the possibility of the dominion and exploitation of the other who is also another "I."[99] There is thus a shift away from a philosophy of power, where the other is seen in terms of what there is in common with other beings, the list of characteristics, reducing the other to the same. Instead, there emerges a philosophy of relationship that accepts the otherness of the other, his or her uniqueness, and this in turn leads to an ethics of responsibility for the other. For many modern thinkers, like the philosophers Martin Buber, Emmanuel Levinas, and Paul Ricoeur, to varying degrees, this is not an issue of reciprocity. Rather, I am responsible for the other without the other being responsible for me in turn.[100] As Paul Ricoeur explains, this is not an issue of equality. Solicitude, he says, "provides to the self another who is a face," and then "equality provides to the self another who is an *each*."[101] The language of the "face" and voice of the other represents the lived presence and "infinity" of another human being who comes to join me; the voice of the other is the call to responsibility.[102]

This strand of philosophy, then, is able to demonstrate that the other is an other, and it approaches the concept of the person from the right direction of mystery and infinity rather than from arbitrarily defined characteristics. Theology goes deeper than philosophy in seeing the other as an other, however. Theology asks us to follow the injunction found in the Golden Rule, "always treat others as you would like them to treat

99. See Matthews, *Pope John Paul II*, 51.
100. On this, see Matthews, "Participation and the Profoundly Disabled," 431–32.
101. Ricoeur, *Oneself as Another*, 202.
102. Levinas, *Totality and Infinity*, 213.

you,"[103] which chimes with philosophies of relationship as well as other world religions and ethical systems. Indicating perhaps that theology and philosophy do not inhabit precisely the same sphere, theology also goes beyond seeing the other as another. Following Christ entails "a new commandment: love one another just as I [Jesus] have loved you":[104] it calls us to see the other, and more so the small, the marginalized, the disabled, as another Christ.

When philosophy concentrates on relational personhood, however, it may lead to the conclusion that dignity and moral status are given to someone only through a relationship with another.[105] This appears to leave open the question of the very being of the disabled human or of human beings who are often not recognized as human persons. In part, this mirrors the theological positions that place their interpretation of the Trinity in either the relations between the Divine Persons or the unity of Persons instead of seeing the mystery of the Trinity as not either or, but both. Theology can offer further insights to help philosophy here, since theology places significance in the actual being, both the uniqueness and the bodiliness, of human beings as well as relationality.

The Human Person as Unique and Irreplaceable

If human beings merely share in a common nature, then it seems that there is nothing unique about each of them. Those who see human beings as replaceable do so apparently because they regard a human being as one among other human beings. The loss of one human being is not significant if another who shares his or her nature can take his or her place. Utilitarian-based bioethics calls for prenatal diagnosis followed by abortion in selected cases in order to avoid the birth of disabled beings and to replace them with the nondisabled, thus increasing the likelihood of happiness over misery in the world. Moreover, as Singer points out, since prenatal diagnosis cannot detect all disabilities, regarding infants

103. Mt 7:12.
104. Jn 13:34.
105. Elizabeth Purcell seems to make such a move in "Narrative Ethics and Vulnerability," 54.

in general as replaceable is advantageous.[106] Although McMahan does not find Singer's replaceability argument persuasive, as he argues that the harm done to an existing infant by killing it outweighs the reason to cause a better-off child to exist, he nevertheless believes in principle that infants are "sacrificeable" because they fall below the threshold of respect, having a weak interest in continuing to live.[107] But McMahan acknowledges that the implications of his and Singer's arguments are "intolerable" for most people, and he embraces them with "significant misgivings and considerable unease."[108] Similarly, Singer accepts that his views on infanticide may seem "too shocking to take seriously," but he counteracts that "our present absolute protection of the lives of infants is a distinctively Christian attitude rather than a universal ethical value."[109]

Even if we do not take into consideration Lisa Bortolotti and John Harris, who suggest that, having diagnosed disability in an embryo, there are "strong moral reasons" for not bringing "into existence" a child who is severely brain damaged,[110] the argument of replaceability in the context of prenatal diagnosis for disability masks the fact that we are dealing with human beings who do properly exist even if they do not yet possess the capacities that many say make them into persons.

But theology offers an understanding of reality that explains why replaceability of humans is as counterintuitive as even its proponents admit. Trinitarian theology asserts that God does not share his divinity, for there are not three gods. But God is three persons: the Father is not the Son or the Spirit, nor is the Son the Father or the Spirit. Yet each is God, for each person of the Trinity has the divine nature as if he were the only divine person. This incommunicability is each person being as if he were the only one.[111] But this distinction does not isolate each from the other since God is a community of persons. In their reflection on the Trinity, the Fathers spoke at the same time of the similarity and the more marked dissimilarity between God and humans. Whereas God does not

106. Singer, *Practical Ethics*, 186*ff.*, 190.
107. McMahan, *Ethics of Killing*, 358–61.
108. McMahan, *Ethics of Killing*, 360.
109. Singer, *Practical Ethics*, 172.
110. Bortolotti and Harris, "Disability, Enhancement and Harm Benefit Continuum," 35.
111. See Crosby, *Selfhood of the Human Person*, 49.

share his divinity, human beings do share their human nature. Nevertheless, as Boethius explains, a human being is not simply an instance of a nature or Aristotle's "a rational animal." Our humanity is common to all human beings, but as persons, individuals of a rational nature, our concrete reality is of a unique being, a Cicero or a Plato unlike any other of that name.[112]

Arguably, if every human is unique, then he or she is his or her own essence. As Augustine explains, humans share the nature of "man," but it is different for God because God is his essence.[113] Crosby points out, however, that an angel is traditionally its own species and so is a certain part of its essence; thus it can be said, though perhaps Crosby overstates this, that human persons may resemble God to the extent that each human being is an essential someone that no one else is.[114] One could respond that if every person is special, then no one is special, but this misunderstands special as a scale from ordinary to extraordinary, just as an approach that looks at the "value" of life thinks lives can be weighed and measured. But the common experience of many parents is that each of their children is special not simply because of their differing qualities or capacities—or disability—but because of who they are.

Following Gregory of Nyssa, God sets each human being on earth as a whole new world in this rather small world of ours. Each human being has greatness not because we are like the created world but because we are made in the image of the Creator.[115] What founds the dignity of each human being as a new and unique world is the call to participate in God's own life, and it is this that also expresses the incomparability and unmeasurability of every human being. Still, even on a purely philosophical level, an understanding of each human as a unique world has cogency: my perspective of the world, however limited, is unique, and when I die, that perspective is lost and cannot be replaced. It is seeing each human being not purely as a specimen of humanity but as this specific person.[116] Perhaps, as John Crosby suggests, if each exists as a

112. Boethius, "Against Eutyches and Nestorius," IV.
113. Augustine, *The Trinity*, VII, 6, 12.
114. Crosby, *Selfhood of the Human Person*, 64–65.
115. Gregory of Nyssa, "On the Making of Man," XVI, 1–2.
116. See Crosby, *Selfhood of the Human Person*, 65–66.

whole being in him- or herself, it may not be meaningful to speak of (or count) two persons.[117]

Seeing each human being as a unique world is perhaps most clearly demonstrated in the case of cloning, where initially it seems that a human being could be replaced by his or her clone. Cloning is a form of "biological slavery" since another person takes it upon him- or herself to determine arbitrarily the genetic characteristics of another person.[118] But those who support cloning also point out the uniqueness of every human being, however small. This point is made when they claim that each human being has his or her own specific perspective on the world, for in responding to philosophical challenges against cloning, they consistently argue that cloning is not a threat to uniqueness. As John Harris explains, it is impossible for a clone to be the same as the adult who supplied the genetic material for the procedure, since humans are not merely biologically determined.[119] It is perhaps noteworthy that this argument comes from a champion of reproductive choice who does not see replaceablity in a negative light.

The insight that each human being is a unique person, a microcosm, an irreplaceable world, does not depend on the capabilities it may have or it may develop. Rather, it focuses on shared common nature, solidarity with the other as an other. Although the Trinity does not share the divine nature, for each is God, as Basil explains, the three are not mere collections of properties making up individuals: it is the strong connection between the Divine Persons that makes them persons.[120] Gregory of Nyssa argues that the difference in substance proposed by Eunomius leads to alienation, subordination of Son to Father, and breaks the communion of relationship.[121] The real distinction lies, he says, not in the divine substance but in their manner of being, as three persons.

As early Christian theology shows, the manner of being a human being is as a person. Some philosophies of consciousness or thinking that separates biological life from biographical life reflect the Apollinarian

117. Crosby, *Selfhood of the Human Person*, 51.
118. See Congregation for the Doctrine of the Faith, *Dignitas Personae*, 29.
119. Harris, *Enhancing Evolution*, 127; Gillon, "Human Reproductive Cloning," 190.
120. Basil, *Letter* 38.
121. Gregory of Nyssa, "Answer to Eunomius," I, 19.

position that the person is located in the mind or soul, or this thinking has affinity with the Nestorian position that the person can be split from the human being. In Christian theology, however, the body and the soul, mind and consciousness, make up the human person. As a whole being, material and spiritual, the human being is an ensouled body or an embodied soul.

Person as a Unity

The unity of body and soul in Christian theology relates to the modern notion that only biographical life is crucial and that biographical life is "having a life" rather than simply "being alive." The term "biographical" normally relates to the facts or events in a person's life, in which case every human being has a biographical life because all human beings, including embryos, have a body and therefore a history, even if they are unaware of their life's story. Embryos have already been conceived from parents; infants have already been born. In contrast, the bioethical interpretation of "biographical" reduces a person's story to what he or she can make of his or her own life, to personal desires and interests, the life of the mind. Biographical life, associated with personhood, has become a disembodied notion related to rationality and autonomy but unrelated to the actual lived life of the individual. This disembodied notion of biographical life is perhaps most notable in the debates surrounding the definition of death as brain death. It also surfaces in cases of dementia and in one of the profoundest of disabilities, the persistent vegetative state. Here we find a blurring of distinctions, as some bioethicists begin to consider some profoundly disabled people to be as good as dead.

Defining Dead

In 1968, responding partly to fear of overtreatment and futile prolongation of life, the Ad Hoc Committee of the Harvard Medical School examined a new definition of death: brain death. The resulting report states that its "primary purpose is to define irreversible coma as a new criterion for death."[122] This report was recognized as authoritative, and

122. Ad Hoc Committee of the Harvard Medical School, "Definition of Irreversible Coma," 337–40.

brain death eventually became generally accepted as the definition of the death of a human being. Singer greeted the report as one of the "greatest achievements of bioethics" and the beginning of a dismantling of the sanctity of life ethic: the new definition meant that "warm, breathing, pulsating human beings" were now "excluded" from "the moral community."[123] The report coincided with pressing concerns of transplant technology. Organs deprived of oxygen rapidly deteriorate, so those harvested from a brain-dead donor with a beating heart are the most viable. How far redefining death and transplant surgery were linked remains contentious, but the danger for abuse of the new definition to serve transplant patients at the expense of severely disable patients is palpable.

Not everyone greeted the suggested redefinition of death as enthusiastically as Singer. The philosopher Hans Jonas was concerned that by redefining irreversible coma as death, the Harvard report endorsed a dualistic view of the human being: a body plus a brain. As Jonas pointed out, there were no grounds for saying that a patient diagnosed as brain-dead was a dead human being.[124] An additional problem was that the report's apparently clear-cut definition was ambiguous, and its reference to irreversible coma was sometimes interpreted as permanent loss of consciousness. This implied that the definition of brain death involved not loss of all brain functions but loss of higher functions, leading to another definition of death based on the higher-brain death criterion, which identifies certain attributes that a living being must have to be a person.[125]

Robert Veatch was an early proponent of the higher-brain death criterion. Veatch explains, "without really understanding what we were doing," we adopted "a new and radically different meaning of the word dead" that had little to do with biology, and "we chose to classify them [humans with dead brains] as dead."[126] He adds, these humans may retain many bodily functions and are "still living in the biological sense"; however, they are given a "radically different moral status": "the word

123. Singer, *Writings on an Ethical Life*, 170.

124. Jonas, "Against the Stream," 132–40.

125. President's Commission for the Study of Ethical Problems in Medicine and Biomedical and Behavioural Research, *Defining Death*, chap. 3.

126. Veatch, " Dead Donor Rule," 10–11.

dead has come to mean—for legal, ethical and public policy purposes—'having lost full moral standing as a member of the human community,'" losing "all the rights of living members such as the right not to be killed."

In its attempt to clarify some of the ambiguities surrounding brain death, the 1981 US President's Commission report *Defining Death: Medical, Legal and Ethical Issues in the Definition of Death* rejected the "philosophical" opinion of higher-brain death since there was no general agreement on what is essential to being a person, and since the issue of personal identity also remained unresolved. Moreover, the higher-brain criterion would place certain categories of patients, severely "retarded," senile, persistent vegetative state, outside personhood, and even dead.[127] Instead, the commission report endorsed the whole-brain definition of death as "sufficiently precise, concise and widely acceptable."[128]

The report recognized that there may still be cellular activity in a brain declared entirely dead, and this has been the focus of much criticism of the whole-brain criterion. Some suggest that the "dead donor rule" be abandoned altogether and the removal of vital organs be justified either on the utilitarian ground that the patient will die anyway or, where the patient has previously given informed consent, on the ground of autonomy.[129] But others justify the removal of organs on the grounds that certain patients lack personhood according to some definitions.

Some bioethicists suggest that some patients such as anencephalic infants or patients in persistent vegetative state should be considered *already dead* and are therefore suitable donors. Those like McMahan, who believe that we are "embodied minds" whose existence is supported by "the operations of our brains," and that "we begin to exist when our brains develop the capacity to generate consciousness and mental activity [... and] cease to exist when our brains lose that capacity," have no difficulty differentiating between two concepts of death: death of the organ-

127. President's Commission for the Study of Ethical Problems in Medicine and Biomedical and Behavioural Research, *Defining Death*, 40.

128. President's Commission for the Study of Ethical Problems in Medicine and Biomedical and Behavioural Research, *Defining Death*, 36.

129. Truog and Miller, "Dead Donor Rule and Organ Transplantation," 674–75; Rodriguez-Arias et al., "Donation after Circulatory Death," 36–43.

ism and death of the person or, more precisely, mind or self. According to McMahan, the death of a person often comes first, so there is "little reason to care about the exact timing of the death of the organism"[130]

Veatch disagrees with the kind of insubstantial "self" offered by those like McMahan, and Veatch is surely right in challenging "Manichaean" bioethicists who claim that to be alive we just need mental functions.[131] Veatch stresses that the human being is more than a body. Rather, he or she is an integration of mind (where, says Veatch, mind can also be equated with soul) and body.[132] According to Veatch, however, the relationship of body to soul or mind is a fragile one. Veatch claims that the classic Judeo-Christian idea that a human being is essentially an integration of mind and body entails that the existence of one without the other, of body without mind or mind without body, is not enough to constitute a living human being. Moreover, he believes that Christian thought and its "secular spin-offs" share the same outlook and hold "universal agreement" that "a human is not a mere body; it is a body combined with something else." That "something else," once called soul or spirit, is, he argues, essentially the same as the modern conception of mind or consciousness.[133] He adds, even though elements of this thinking come from "arcane" theological questions, Christian tradition and secular philosophical thought hold that the integration of mental function is critical: "when, and only when, this capacity for mental function is present is the minimal set of qualities present to treat the human as a living member of the moral community." Veatch asserts that this approach should have broad application since, he explains, where the tenets of Western religion and philosophical thought are held by a great many, any definitions should be allowed to reflect those tenets.[134] Instead, then, of somaticism, that human beings are just bodies, or mentalism, that human beings are minds, Veatch offers the "new defensible middle ground" of integrated mind and body, an "embodied capacity for consciousness" that grounds full moral standing.[135]

130. McMahan, *Ethics of Killing*, 439.
131. Veatch, "Dead Donor Rule."
132. Veatch, "Death of Whole-Brain Death," 353–78.
133. Veatch, "Death of Whole-Brain Death."
134. Veatch, "Death of Whole-Brain Death," 375n21.
135. Veatch, "Death of Whole-Brain Death."

While Veatch may reject some interpretations that make it possible for some living human beings to be nonpersons, his reasoning is not directed in favor of profoundly disabled human beings. In Veatch's controversial and problematic view, the word "living" is significant, since Veatch thinks there are no living nonpersons; rather, those who some claim to be nonpersons are, according to Veatch, in fact dead.[136] Personhood, he believes, is not a scientific question but an issue for moral, philosophical, and religious consideration.[137] Yet for Veatch, this integration of mind and body takes the form of the body plus the soul/spirit/mind/consciousness. There is a person only when the capacity for mental function is present: the existence of a body without a mind or mind without a body does not constitute a living human being.[138]

Although Veatch may suggest that notions of personhood are not scientific questions, the solution he offers is one verifiable only by the higher-brain criterion for death. The integration of body and mind seems to be a fragile one, one easily broken, rather than a deep unity. This may be where Veatch's association of mind with soul begins to break down. Although he acknowledges that the equation is not complete, he seems to accept it as near enough for the purposes of bioethical decision making, and he seems to be identifying mind with the principle of life.

Contemporary interpretations of what it is to be a living human being, particularly the emphasis placed on the requirement for a functioning brain and especially the quasi theological presentation from Veatch, find resonance in some of the earliest Christological disputes, notably the debate with Apollinarius. The differing approaches taken by thinkers to explain or respond to the *kerygma* of God-made flesh allowed for the emergence of a vital insight: that the person of Christ is not a biological problem to be solved but rather a mystery, albeit one about which we can still say something. The Christological disputes came to perceive that although Jesus Christ has two natures, he did not exist as two natures, the divine and human, existing side by side, or one nature swallowed up by the other, or the assumption of only a partial human nature by

136. Veatch, "Death of Whole-Brain Death."
137. Veatch, "Impending Collapse of the Whole-Brain Definition of Death," 18–24.
138. Veatch, "Death of Whole-Brain Death."

the Word. Instead, the Son of God personally came to exist as a human being. As they sought to explain this perception, early theologians made use of analogy with human beings, an analogy they accepted was limited but one they seem to view clearly: in the case of human beings, what exists is not a body plus a soul existing side by side or a body plus a soul that makes up a third thing, a human being. Rather, what exists is a human being. This unity in Christ, also in the person, is not a psychological unity of self-consciousness, for then Christ would be two persons. Instead, Christ is a unity of soul, body, and mind and divinity.

The modern notion that the person is essentially mind implicitly reflects the thinking of Plato and of Origen,[139] if mind is taken to mirror soul, and explicitly the thinking of Apollinarius on mind. For Apollinarius, human beings are of two different substances: an irrational animal body and a rational mind.[140] According to Gregory of Nyssa, Apollinarius defines a living being by the exercise of free will: for Apollinarius, the mind, the center of self-determination, seems to be the true person in both Christ and in human beings in general, with the body as purely passive, and when the mind is destroyed, so is the person.[141] The philosopher Michael Lockwood takes an Apollinarian view of the human being. Lockwood says he offers a "middle way" between protection of life from conception and permissibility of infanticide. He accepts that newborns and Alzheimer patients are not essentially persons in the Lockean sense, and that continued biological life is not enough for being a person. But he also says, "the essential me is the mental me, which resides in the brain"; the rest of the body is "merely a support system, toolbox, power pack and vehicle for getting about." Thus he can claim that we cease to exist when our brain structures can no longer sustain conscious mentality, and we come into existence at the onset of brain life.[142]

But both Gregory of Nazianzus and Gregory of Nyssa[143] see that this splitting up of the human being is highly problematic because it does not accord with the truth about us. We are neither souls without bodies nor

139. Origen, "*De Principiis, First Principles,*" 2, 8, 1.
140. Apollinarius, "Dialogue 2," 173, Eranistes.
141. Gregory of Nyssa, *Antirrheticus*.
142. Lockwood, "Moral Status of the Embryo," 17–20.
143. Gregory of Nazianzus, "Epistle 101"; Gregory of Nyssa, *Antirrheticus*.

bodies without souls but living animate beings.[144] Although Gregory of Nyssa agrees that rationality is an "essential aspect," human beings are rational animals; that is, they necessarily have a rational nature[145] even if they cannot at that moment exercise rational capacity.

Similarly, one of Cyril's difficulties with Nestorius is that Nestorius was offering a conjunction, more of an appearance of union rather than a true union, and one that could be easily broken when Nestorius speaks of the divine and human natures in Christ.[146] Instead, Cyril speaks of the deep and personal union in Christ, beyond our conception, whereby the Second Person of the Trinity comes to be man. By limited analogy with human beings, and in a manner also beyond our grasp, body and soul "make up the person of a single man,"[147] and since the human is a being of a rational nature, this is the kind of being he or she is; he or she cannot become irrational even though he or she loses his or her capabilities.[148] Instead, then, of the fragile union of body plus soul or mind that Veatch seems to suggest, traditional theology envisages the human person as a living whole.

Against those who locate the person exclusively in the soul or mind, early orthodox theologians instead offer a holistic anthropology, where not only does the *Logos* assume the whole man, but also the whole human being is the subject of resurrection and salvation.[149] Still, within this holistic anthropology, early theologians distinguish, though do not separate out, bodily and spiritual aspects of human beings. The body is often referred to as "instrument"[150] or as "minister and servant of the soul"[151] in order to express that even though the soul is incapacitated without the body[152] and the body and soul act together in harmony,[153] the rational nature of human beings has priority, for the soul is "more

144. Gregory of Nyssa, "On the Making of Man," XXX, 29.
145. Gregory of Nyssa, *Antirrheticus*.
146. Cyril of Alexandria, *On the Unity of Christ*, 73.
147. Cyril of Alexandria, "Against Diodore of Tarsus and Theodore of Mopsuestia," 9.22.
148. Cyril of Alexandria, *Commentary on John*, I, 8, 3.
149. Tertullian, "On the Flesh of Christ," 34; Gregory of Nazianzus, "Epistle 101."
150. Athanasius, *Life of Antony and Letter to Marcellinus*, 27, 8.
151. Tertullian, "On the Resurrection of the Flesh," 7.
152. Tertullian, "On the Resurrection of the Flesh," 16, 17.
153. Athanasius, *Life of Anthony and Letter to Marcellinus*, 27, 8.

proximate" to God.[154] In this way, theology attempts to do justice to the idea that a human being is "a rational animal,"[155] an animal of a specific nature who seeks to transcend him- or herself, and both these aspects are united in one person. Rather than the Apollinarian idea that a person ceases to exist once the mind has gone, the person continues to exist but with profound disability.[156]

Dead to the World: Profound Disability and Persistent Vegetative State

While many may resist the view that some profoundly disabled people—like anencephalic infants, people with dementia, or patients in persistent vegetative state—can be considered dead or at least have ceased to exist on the grounds that personhood has been lost, the view that these human beings are as good as dead is of equal concern. Both these views depend on interpreting personhood as essentially concerned with rationality and self-consciousness. But this view explicitly accepts that the human body is alive, but only as an outer shell or the remains of the inner person, and that continued existence is no longer in the patient's best interests.

The language of the body as merely an outer casing and the desirability of bringing about the death of this body were clearly expressed in the United Kingdom in the case of Tony Bland, a patient in persistent vegetative state. The High Court, then the Court of Appeal, and finally the House of Lords were asked to clarify whether artificial nutrition and hydration could legally be withdrawn from patients in persistent vegetative state. As Lord Browne-Wilkinson explained in the House of Lords ruling, "the whole purpose of stopping artificial feeding is to bring about the death of Anthony Bland."[157] Not only did the courts imply that certain lives are not worth living, the judgments also tended toward a dualistic view of the human being where the person is entirely separated from the living body of the patient. In the High Court, Sir

154. Tertullian, "On the Resurrection of the Flesh," 7.

155. Gregory of Nyssa, *Antirrheticus*.

156. Gregory of Nazianzus, "Epistle 101," 219.

157. Lord Browne-Wilkinson, in Airedale NHS Trust v. Bland, (1993) 2 W.L.R., 359; AC 789, at p. 876.

Stephen Brown declared that for all intents and purposes, Tony Bland was " 'dead.' His spirit has left him and all that remains is the shell of his body."[158] Lord Justice Hoffmann stated in the Court of Appeal, "his body is alive, but he has no life."[159]

The view that holds only a fragile and breakable union between the body and soul or mind seems problematic because human beings are psychosomatic wholes. Understandings of the body as a shell that is somehow filled up with the person or mind are reminiscent of the view of Apollinarius, whose thinking seems to be that the human body of Jesus is filled up and animated by the divinity in much the same way as the mind occupies and vivifies the body of a human being. According to Apollinarius, the self-emptying of the *Logos* involves the *Logos* clothing himself within a fleshly body. This interpretation of *kenosis* sees it as the kind of emptying that treats the body as a mere shell, either to be filled up with the divinity in the sense of Apollinarianism, whereby the *Logos* took the place of the mind or soul of Christ, or one that leaves a shell once the mind or soul or spirit has left. But the kind of *kenosis* offered by Cyril is an emptying that also raises up the human person.

Of course, most human beings would not choose to follow the path of emptying, of suffering, illness, disability, and the losses that old age brings. These are all part of the human condition (albeit not part of God's original plan), however, and we are encouraged to fight against sickness, to seek good health, to undertake ethical research into relieving suffering. When a human person takes on the condition of extreme and radical dependence through illness, disability, or trauma—or never moves beyond a state of radical dependence—he or she remains a human person with the dignity that that entails, even if his or her situation may seem to others to be undignified. A parallel may be found in the distinction made in Christology: for Nestorius, there cannot be an emptying on the part of the *Logos* since the *Logos* has to remain impassible, so Nestorius attributes *kenosis* to the human passible subject in Christ, even though he forgets that this subject starts empty. For Cyril, however, there is no change in the person of the *Logos*; there is simply a change in his

158. S. Brown, in Airedale NHS Trust v. Bland, (1993) 2 W.L.R., 804.

159. Lord Justice Hoffman, in Airedale NHS Trust v. Bland, (1993) 2 W.L.R., 825.

condition. The condition of profound disability is often seen in terms of a lack or emptiness, in part perhaps because many people find it difficult to relate to people in these conditions, especially where there are communication difficulties.

Incommunicability: A Way of Being

Incommunicability is sometimes misunderstood as being the impossibility of communicating with others, a form of isolation of the individual. Some people rely so much on words to discern other people that the inability to communicate in ways that some people think are normal becomes a source of discrimination. From evidence presented by Scope to the Joint Committee on Human Rights in 2007–8, it appears that nondisabled people continue to make assumptions about the mental capacity of disabled people who lack speech, and that it is all too often presumed that certain categories of patients cannot make choices or even have desires.[160] Moreover, the evidence from Scope shows that the rights of disabled people who cannot communicate by conventional means are being infringed.[161] Scope presents cases of patients who are not fed in hospital and do not receive equal treatment. In particular, it cites discrimination, especially regarding life and death decisions, where do-not-resuscitate orders are added to medical notes without patient consent, where treatment that ordinarily would be given to nondisabled patients is not administered, where patients are treated as though their lives are "less valuable," or where dying is considered to be in "their best interests." Lack of words seems to imply lack of personhood.

A better definition of incommunicability is something that cannot be conveyed from one person to another; pain, for instance, is said to be incommunicable, although one person can compare another's description of pain to one's own experience. But underneath that everyday sense of an incommunicable experience or concept is that each person has an interior life, and no one else can will or want for that person.[162] Also,

160. Scope, "Memorandum to the House of Lords," 79, 83.
161. Scope, "Memorandum to the House of Lords," 79–80.
162. Wojtyła, *Love and Responsibility*, 24; Matthews, *Pope John Paul II*, 78, 185.

no human being can fully grasp the mystery of another human being, whatever their capacity to express themselves. This fundamental incommunicability expresses the uniqueness of each person and the relationality experienced by discerning the other as unique:[163] it is uniqueness in solidarity.

Unique and in Solidarity

The ideas that a new world begins with each human being and human incommunicability do not imply that each human being has an isolated existence. Charles Taylor points out that what he calls "the voice of nature within us" reminds us of the importance of solidarity with others as part of our natural fulfilment and theirs.[164] John Crosby notes that the uniqueness of each human being allows the possibility of loving each one for him- or herself and that this is the beginnings of community.[165]

Early Christian reflection on the image of God in human beings speaks of the common origin and goal of all with Adam, the first man, as representative of all human beings, and Christ, the last man, in whom all things are reconciled. This unity of humankind is expressed theologically in relation to God, where "none of us lives for himself and none of us dies for himself," for we all "belong to the Lord."[166] It is also expressed in relation to the human community, where "if one part is hurt, all the parts share its pain":[167] the unity of humankind calls us to solidarity with all, and there can be no disablism. This uniqueness yet mutual dependence and relatedness are deepened again through reflection on the image of God as Trinity. Furthermore, the story of Christ offers a reversal in the understanding of lordship and dependence: while among the Gentiles, the rulers lord over them, for the followers of Jesus, the call is to be servant, not to be served but to serve.[168] In Christ there is lordship in weakness, as the Son puts on the "likeness of human littleness."[169] And

163. See Crosby, *Selfhood of the Human Person*, 41.
164. Taylor, *Sources of the Self*, 370.
165. Crosby, *Selfhood of the Human Person*, 66.
166. Rm 14:7, 14:9.
167. 1 Cor 12:26.
168. Mk 10:41–45; Mt 20:24–28; Lk 22:24–27.
169. Cyril of Alexandria, *Commentary on John*, XI, 3.

as Matthew's Gospel tells us, it is in the least, the sick, the hungry that Christ is found.[170]

Nevertheless, for many people, it is precisely the notion of human littleness and the possibility of a change in their condition that causes fear, that is, when it is a change from perceived autonomy to complete or even partial dependence and a life of disability. Fear of overtreatment, or of living a life of dependence, or of losing control, or of existing in a condition that may lead to being thought of as less than a person, has caused some to appeal to the principle of autonomy in order to claim not a right to life but a right to die.

The Tyranny of Autonomy

In tandem with the emphasis on rationality, self-consciousness, and the importance of biographical life for personhood, contemporary Western bioethics prizes autonomy and the active role of the patient. While freedom and choice are significant aspects of being human, some theologians like Hans Küng argue for a patient's right to "dignified dying" before he or she reaches "a vegetable existence" based on the God-given right to "utter self-determination" and as the most personal exercise of responsibility.[171] This suggests that there is something undignified about certain situations of disability. Margaret Battin, a bioethicist who champions the right of patient self-determination, also calls for an active, self-assertive, responsible role in death rather than an acceptant, obedient, and passive state.[172] According to Tom Beauchamp, the "right to die" has been a central and enduring topic in bioethics, but he argues that this is a discontinuity in the history of medicine: the history of bioethics in contrast to paternalistic medical ethics is one of "expanding commitments to autonomy."[173] Moreover, as part of the "logical extension of a primary commitment to patient autonomy," the actions of physicians in assisting in hastening death are a "legitimate interpretation" of the phy-

170. Mt 25:31–46.
171. Hans Küng, "A Dignified Dying," in Küng and Jens, *Dignified Dying*, 27, 30, 38.
172. Battin, *Ending Life*, 6.
173. Beauchamp, "Right to Die as the Triumph of Autonomy," 643–44.

sician's traditional commitment to the patient: "to care for and meet the needs and preferences of the patient in all stages of the patient's life."[174]

Still, the place of autonomy in bioethics remains disputed: despite language that sees the patient as client or customer and the health care worker as service provider, patients cannot demand treatment, and doctors act in what they consider to be the patient's best interests. Rather than being totally free, people are often paralyzed by the fear of a bleak future of dependence on others or by the fear that they will not be seen or treated as a person.[175] Yet calls for choice in determining the timing of one's death echo the radical importance of free will as freedom of indifference, freedom to choose whatever I want regardless, as "man's special character" that Pelagius defends[176] and the absolute autonomy Caelestius demands when he claims that "God has given me free will, and it is not free at all unless I do what I will."[177] This sense of freedom is considered by Augustine, who appreciates that freedom of choice is a good. Nevertheless, Augustine sees that genuine freedom, freedom to make the right choice, a freedom that is related to the truth, is an even greater good.[178]

The continuing complaint of Caelestius that "a will that needs support of another is not a will at all" encapsulates the modern fear that without the capacity for autonomy, we will be regarded as "vegetables," not as persons. This fear also seems to attend those who believe that any form of radical dependence is living in "a second-class existence," a view expressed by Daniel James, a young rugby player who was paralyzed in a rugby accident and ended his life by assisted suicide. It appears that a truly dignified death, like a truly dignified life, is linked to self-determination, and it is this kind of thinking that calls for assisted suicide and euthanasia. Ironically, as indicated by Caelestius about a will that needs support, neither assisted suicide nor euthanasia is a true exercise of autonomy: both require the help of another. Besides, denoting life in a disabled state as a "second-class existence" seems to say more about

174. Beauchamp, "Right to Die as the Triumph of Autonomy," 251.
175. See Matthews, "Right Rights, Authentic Autonomy."
176. Pelagius, "Letter to Demetrias," 35–70.
177. Caelestius, "Fragment," 217.
178. Augustine, *Revisions*, 1, 9, 5. P.

attitudes to disability and care of the disabled than about the state itself, and it may not simply be an issue of fear of loss of capacities. It is also an issue of pride, and pride associated with disablism—that I do not want to be like them.

By seeking to emphasize the "heavy weight" of responsibility of using free will, Pelagius correctly also wishes to stress that freedom is to be prized.[179] As Augustine explains, however, we think that freedom is concerned wholly with free choice when in fact the greater freedom is a graced free will that seeks to make the right choice.[180] According to Augustine, suicide is wrong because it is equivalent to self-murder,[181] and Augustine further points out that it signifies despair of God's mercy[182] as well as spiritual weakness and lack of courage in the face of adversity.[183] But above all, Augustine argues that God does not abandon a human being in his or her humiliation, so neither should that person despair and take his or her life; after all, God came down to us in true humility.[184]

In contrast to euthanasia's "death with dignity," studies by doctors involved in palliative care, notably by the psychiatrist Elisabeth Kübler-Ross, offer profound witness to the possibilities of dignified natural death for the terminally ill. This involves reaching, through various stages and over time, some sense of final acceptance and letting go of capacities, including rationality and life itself. Although these studies are invaluable for both patients and their friends, relatives, and staff treating them, it still must be acknowledged that not everyone reaches final acceptance, some do die in unresolved pain. Despite the advances in palliative care, it is the mental anguish that is often more difficult to treat.

For Battin and Quill, it is a "false dichotomy" to ask patients if they want either palliative care or physician-assisted death, as "we would choose palliative care and hospice every time." Instead, the more inclusive question should be whether we want palliative care (as the norm) or palliative care plus access to physician-assisted death when we choose

179. Pelagius, *Letter to Demetrias.*
180. Augustine, *Revisions*, 1, 9, 5.
181. Augustine, *City of God*, 1, 20; *Letter* 204, 5.
182. Augustine, *City of God*, 1, 18.
183. Augustine, *City of God*, 1, 22, 23.
184. Augustine, *City of God*, 1, 24.

the time is "right" for us.[185] Autonomy for the two authors is central,[186] but this appears to be at most an instance of Augustine's free choice versus the freedom to make the right choice. Arguably, the choice for death is not an exercise of autonomy at all, since it puts an end to all freedoms. As Battin and Quill say, assisted dying is a last resort if suffering becomes intolerable and you want an easier death, yet this is surely an example of action in extreme fear and duress, not an action of freedom. An action of last resort is not a choice since there are no alternatives.

In palliative care, work has been done to empower patients to deal with their fear of losing capacities and of death itself. Where at the surface level some situations appear intolerable and elicit the request for death, Michael Kearney, a hospice doctor, suggests going beyond this level and responding to soul pain with deep inner healing. He offers an approach that helps the patient die "metaphorically" without killing them.[187] Even though neither Kübler-Ross nor Kearney offers a specifically theological approach to dealing with patients at the end of life, we can see its foundations in a *kenosis* of letting go.

Terminally ill persons may then be active witnesses to the possibilities of a dignified dying. We can apply the insights of *kenosis* as a form of letting go to the "biographical life," the "sum of all we hold dear" that the ethicist James Rachels offers.[188] Both Kübler-Ross and Kearney see the stages of coming to terms with the loss of capacities and letting go as part of the patient's life story perhaps more accurately than Rachels, who places the end of a person's life story at the end of his or her mental life. Indeed, the medieval *ars moriendi*, the art of dying and dying well, encouraged dying to self and freeing oneself from unnecessary attachments long before one reached the final stages of earthly life.

Kenosis as letting go accepts that human life itself is limited and that treatments that are futile or burdensome need not be pursued. Vitalism, extending life no matter what, is a rejection of the reality of the human condition. But for those bioethicists who argue that patients cease to be persons if they can no longer take part in "humanly meaningful purposes

185. Battin and Quill, *Physician-Assisted Dying*, 1.
186. Battin and Quill, *Physician-Assisted Dying*, 6.
187. Kearney, *Mortally Wounded*, 94.
188. Rachels, *Created from Animals*, 199.

of life"[189] or if they can no longer respond to their God-given vocation,[190] it may be more constructive to consider further the vocation of every sick person, even those in extreme disability who, for some, are "more like the dead than the living."[191] Such patients, notably those in persistent vegetative state, are living witnesses to the fact that extreme suffering or disability does not deprive the patient of his or her dignity as a human person. In contrast to the view of those who think that the image of God rests only in the possession of rationality, in acts of intellect, will, and emotion, such that a patient who has lost these capacities no longer images God, unconscious patients still demonstrate relationship to their creator. Part of this vocation may be that God chooses "those who by human standards are weak to shame the strong. . . . those who count for nothing to reduce to nothing all those who do count for something, so that no human being might feel boastful before God."[192] Although extreme disability is not in itself wanted or desirable, as Pope John Paul points out in his 1984 encyclical *Salvifici Doloris*, it may express not so much the weakness of human beings but the power of God.[193]

This vocation can also manifest itself under the second aspect of *kenosis* as a call to solidarity, an "irreplaceable service" for the salvation of others.[194] It has long been the Christian tradition that if one member suffers in the Body of Christ, the Church, all members suffer with that member.[195] The paradigm for acting in solidarity, particularly in a health care setting, is the parable of the Good Samaritan.[196] The Good Samaritan sees the reality of the situation; he sees that the man is wounded, and he feels true compassion, a sharing of the pain of the other. He treats him and entrusts him to the competent care of others. He is completely generous both with his time and money, and he is continually solicitous. This forms part of Jesus's answer to the lawyer's question, "What must I do to inherit eternal life?"

189. Kelly, *Medical Care at the End of Life*, 106, 114.
190. Biggar, *Aiming to Kill*, 39.
191. Cranford and Smith, "Consciousness," 242.
192. 1 Cor 1:27–29.
193. Pope John Paul II, *Salvifici Doloris*, 26.
194. Pope John Paul II, *Salvifici Doloris*, 27.
195. 1 Cor 12:26..
196. Lk 10:25–37.

Although the lawyer's original question concerns how to inherit eternal life, the story moves away from personal salvation to questions about the other, "Who is my neighbor?" At first, the answer to this question is the wounded man: he is the neighbor we are to recognize and to love as an other. But there is a second answer to the question. Which of the passers-by proved themselves a neighbor? The answer is the Samaritan: he is the neighbor who shows recognition and compassion. As with all the parables, however, there is a third answer. The Good Samaritan ultimately in Jesus—the only one who can really bind up all our wounds whether physical pain or soul pain.

Concluding Thoughts: Discerning Persons in Bioethics

Discerning persons has two sides: on the one hand, a theological appreciation of the concept of person makes us aware that the person may not simply be the subject of definition, of setting out the boundary of who does and who does not qualify, and this may perhaps better express the original vision of bioethics: to be attentive to the patient as person. We can say some things about human persons: as a kind, they are rational animals and have the capacity to transcend themselves; furthermore, both of these aspects are profoundly united in the one human being. Even as we reflect on these in order to discern persons, we cannot say all there is to say about human persons and the human family. In contrast to providing definitions, the nature of discernment requires constant deepening and reflection. But we are called to be discerning persons. We may reflect on what it is to be a particular kind of animal; nevertheless, our own self becomes real for others, and the self of others becomes real for us: we see the other as an other. The exhortation from John the Evangelist's first letter may be appropriate here, and not just in a theological context: "let us love, then, because he first loved us"[197] reminds us that we are a community of persons. Discernment also requires us to use practical wisdom in coming to bioethical decisions.

Following in the tradition of Augustine, Basil, Gregory of Nazianzus, and Gregory of Nyssa, Boethius makes a distinction but not a separation

197. 1 Jn 4:19.

between nature and person, and he takes nature to be a "substrate" of person such that "person cannot exist apart from nature."[198] Moreover, unlike Cavalieri and Singer, who speak of person in terms of "a subject of relations," where relation is "something added to, and thus accidentally and not essentially connected to, the substance of the thing,"[199] in Trinitarian theology, there is priority of neither persons nor substances, because the one God is a Trinity of Persons. Person, then, does not belong to qualities or changing characteristics—it does not come and go like, as Elizabeth Anscombe puts it, the magnetized iron of modern personhood.[200] There is no such entity as a live human being who is not a person. Moreover, because theology reminds us to have regard for *this* particular person and not merely qualities that can also be found in others, as Crosby explains, it offers a view of the person that is on a "vastly deeper level" than the level at which a person has rights: it is a level of dignity, of "ontological nobility."[201]

Bioethicists may be right to affirm that human beings have both a biographical and biological life. But it is not merely a one-sided story of autonomous life decisions; it is a whole life story. All human beings, from the embryo, even in vitro, to the human being in persistent vegetative state, have a biographical story: just as I have been, am, and will be reliant on others and indebted to them since they help to make my life story, so too am I summoned to responsibility for them. This is not to say that I act out of self-interest when I care for others on the understanding that they will care for me when the time comes. Nor is it to say that when I care for others it is for my own benefit or reward since I may perhaps become a better person. Rather, I care for others because it is the appropriate response.

Attempting to do justice to all the aspects of human life, biographical and biological, in its independence and dependence, is not a new undertaking. Taking account of the transcendent aspect of human beings and the aspect that considers them as a particular kind of animal and unifying both aspects in the same person is something with which

198. Boethius, "Against Eutyches and Nestorius," II.
199. Cavalieri and Singer, "Great Ape Project," 134.
200. Anscombe, "Murder and the Morality of Euthanasia," 267.
201. Crosby, *Selfhood of the Human Person*, 71.

theology has long struggled. Perhaps we may agree with Boethius that the definition of "person" is a "matter of great perplexity."[202] The theological concept of person expresses a sense of solidarity, a community of persons in relationship, yet also an idea of uniqueness; it reflects a unity of being in each person yet also accepts the losses and letting go that inevitably follow from the human condition. It can accept human *kenosis* because hope in the Resurrection means that suffering and death do not mark the end of the human person. Moreover, while it celebrates the possibilities of human freedom and the capacity of the acting person to make and shape his or her life, it also is prepared to embrace an issue that is more difficult to face and one that bioethics in particular seems to be myopic about: the really human issue of dependence and need. These theological insights are not merely commentaries on how we view human beings in certain perplexing situations. They present a perspective on how we rise to the challenge of difficult cases, on how we are to discern persons. But they also offer exhortation on what we are to become, a prophetic voice urging us to be discerning persons.

202. Boethius, "Against Eutyches and Nestorius," II.

Bibliography

Ancient Primary Sources

Alexander of Alexandria. "Epistles on the Arian Heresy." In *Fathers of the Third Century Ante-Nicene Fathers*. Vol. VI, edited by A. Roberts and J. Donaldson. Grand Rapids: Eerdmans, 1971. J. P. Migne, *Patrologiae cursus completus: Series graeca*. Vol. 18. Paris: 1857, 547–72.

Ambrose. "Exposition of the Christian Faith." In *Ambrose: Select Works and Letters Nicene and Post Nicene Fathers*. Series II, Vol. X, edited by A. Roberts and J. Donaldson. Grand Rapids: Eerdmans, 1997. J. P. Migne, *Patrologiae cursus completus: Series latina*. Vol. 16. Paris: 1845, 527–698.

Antony of Egypt. "The Letters of St Antony." In *Monasticism and the Making of a Saint*, translated and edited by S. Rubenson. Minneapolis: Fortress Press, 1995.

Apollinarius. *Ad Serapionem* Fragment 161. Fourth-Century Christianity, accessed January 17, 2013. http://www.fourthcentury.com/ad-serapionem/. T. J. Carter, "Ep. Ad Serapionem." In *Apollinarian Christologies: A Study of the Writings of Apollinarius of Laodicea*, 325. London: Hamley King, 2011. H. Lietzmann, *Apollinaris von Laodicea und seine Schule, Texte und Untersuchungen*. Tubingen: 1904.

Apollinarius. "Apodeixis." In *St. Gregory of Nyssa: Anti-Apollinarian Writings*, translated by R. Orton, 41–58. Vol.131 of The Fathers of the Church. Washington, DC: Catholic University of America Press, 2015. T. J. Carter, "Commentary upon the Fragments of Apollinarius' Apodeixis." In *Apollinarian Christologies: A Study of the Writings of Apollinarius of Laodicea*, 339–84. London: Hamley King, 2011. H. Lietzmann, *Apollinaris von Laodicea und seine Schule, Texte und Untersuchungen*. Tubingen: 1904.

Apollinarius. "Dialogues." In Theodoret. *Eranistes*, translated by G. H. Ettinger. Vol. 106 of *The Fathers of the Church*. Washington, DC: Catholic University of America Press, 2003. H. Lietzmann, *Apollinaris von Laodicea und seine Schule, Texte und Untersuchungen*. Tubingen: 1904.

Arius. "The Banquet." In *Faith of the Early Fathers*. Vol. 1, edited by W. Jurgens. Collegeville, MN: Liturgical Press, 1970. Fragments preserved by Epiphanius. In *Panarion of Epiphanius of Salamis*. Translated by F. Williams. Leiden: Brill, 1994. K. Holl, *Die griechischen christlichen Schriftsteller der ersten Jahrhunderte*. Vol. 37. Leipzig: 1933.

Arius. "Letter to Alexander." In *A New Eusebius: Documents Illustrating the History of the Church to AD 337*, edited by J. Stevenson. London: SPCK, 1995.

Arius. "Letter to Eusebius of Nicomedia." In *Faith of the Early Fathers*. Vol. 1, edited by W. Jurgens. Collegeville, MN: Liturgical Press, 1970.

Athanasius. "Ad Afros Epistola Synodica." In *Athanasius: Select Writings and Letters,* edited by P. Schaff and H. Wace. Series II, Vol. IV of *The Nicene and Post Nicene Fathers.* Grand Rapids, MI: Eerdmans, 1980. J. P. Migne, *Patrologiae cursus completus: Series graeca.* Vol. 26. Paris: 1887, 1028–48.

Athanasius. "Against the Arians." In *Athanasius: Select Writings and Letters,* edited by P. Schaff and H. Wace. Series II, Vol. IV of *The Nicene and Post Nicene Fathers.* Grand Rapids, MI: Eerdmans, 1980. J. P. Migne, *Patrologiae cursus completus: Series graeca.* Vol. 26. Paris: 1887, 11–468.

Athanasius. "Against the Heathens." In *Athanasius: Select Writings and Letters,* edited by P. Schaff and H. Wace. Series II, Vol. IV of *The Nicene and Post Nicene Fathers.* Grand Rapids, MI: Eerdmans, 1980. J. P. Migne, *Patrologiae cursus completus: Series graeca.* Vol. 25. Paris: 1857, 3–97.

Athanasius. "De Synodis." In *Athanasius: Select Writings and Letters,* edited by P. Schaff and H. Wace. Series II, Vol. IV of *The Nicene and Post Nicene Fathers.* Grand Rapids, MI: Eerdmans, 1980. J. P. Migne, *Patrologiae cursus completus: Series graeca.* Vol. 26. Paris: 1857, 681–794.

Athanasius. "Letter to Epictetus." In *Athanasius: Select Writings and Letters,* edited by P. Schaff and H. Wace. Series II, Vol. IV of *The Nicene and Post Nicene Fathers.* Grand Rapids, MI: Eerdmans, 1980. J. P. Migne, *Patrologiae cursus completus: Series graeca.* Vol. 26. Paris: 1857, 1049–70.

Athanasius. *The Letters of Saint Athanasius Concerning the Holy Spirit (To Serapion).* Translated by C. R. B. Shapland. London: Epworth Press, 1951. J. P. Migne, *Patrologiae cursus completus: Series graeca.* Vol. 26. Paris: 1857.

Athanasius. *Life of Antony and Letter to Marcellinus.* Translated by R. Gregg. Mahwah, NJ: Paulist Press, 1980. *Life of Antony,* J. P. Migne, *Patrologiae cursus completus: Series graeca.* Vol. 26. Paris: 1857, 835–978; *Letter to Marcellinus,* J. P. Migne, *Patrologiae cursus completus: Series graeca.* Vol. 27 Paris: 1857, 12–45.

Athanasius. "On the Incarnation." In *Athanasius: Select Writings and Letters,* edited by P. Schaff and H. Wace. Series II, Vol. IV of *The Nicene and Post Nicene Fathers.* Grand Rapids, MI: Eerdmans, 1980. J. P. Migne, *Patrologiae cursus completus: Series graeca.* Vol. 26. Paris: 1857, 983–1028.

Athanasius. "Tomus Ad Antiochenos." In *Athanasius: Select Writings and Letters,* edited by P. Schaff and H. Wace. Series II, Vol. IV of *The Nicene and Post Nicene Fathers.* Grand Rapids, MI: Eerdmans, 1980. J. P. Migne, *Patrologiae cursus completus: Series graeca.* Vol. 26. Paris: 1857, 794–810.

Augustine. "Answer to Julian." In *Answer to the Pelagians II,* translated by R. Teske, edited by J. Rotelle, 268–536. New York: New City Press, 1998. J. P. Migne, *Patrologiae cursus completus: Series latina.* Vol. 44. Paris: 1865, 641–874.

Augustine. *Answer to the Pelagians III* [Unfinished work in answer to Julian]. Translated by R. Teske. Edited by J. Rotelle. New York: New City Press, 1999. J. P. Migne, *Patrologiae cursus completus: Series latina.* Vol. 45. Paris: 1865, 1050–608.

Augustine. *The City of God against the Pagans.* Edited and translated by R. W. Dyson. Cambridge: Cambridge University Press, 1998. E. Hoffmann, *Corpus scriptorium ecclesiasticorum latinorum.* Vol. 40, Part 1 (Books 1–13). Vienna: 1899; Vol. 40, Part 2 (Books 14–22). Vienna: 1900.

Augustine. *Confessions*. Translated by M. Boulding. Edited by J. Rotelle. New York: New City Press, 1997. P. Knöll, *Corpus scriptorium ecclesiasticorum latinorum*. Vol. 33. Vienna: 1896.

Augustine. "Deeds of Pelagius." In *Answer to the Pelagians*, translated by R. Teske, edited by J. Rotelle, 336–81. New York: New City Press, 1997. C. F. Urba and J. Zycha, *Corpus scriptorium ecclesiasticorum latinorum*. Vol. 42. Vienna: 1902, 51–122.

Augustine. The De Haeresibus of St. Augustine. Translated by L. G. Muller. Washington, DC: Catholic University of America Press, 1956.

Augustine. "The Enchiridion on Faith, Hope and Charity." In *Christian Belief*, translated by B. Harbert, edited by B. Ramsey, 273–343. New York: New City Press, 2005. E. Evans, *Corpus Christianorum Series Latina*. Vol. 46. Turnholt: 1969, 49–114.

Augustine. "Free Choice of the Will." In *Teacher; The Free Choice of the Will; Grace and Free Will*, translated by R. Russell, 72–242. Vol. 59 of *The Fathers of the Church*. Washington, DC: Catholic University of America Press, 1968. W. Green, *Corpus scriptorium ecclesiasticorum latinorum*. Vol. 74. Vienna: 1956.

Augustine. *Letters*. Part II, Vol. 1, *Letters 1–99*. *The Works of Saint Augustine*. Translated by R. Teske. Edited by J. Rotelle. New York: New City Press, 2001. *Letters*. Part II, Vol. 2, *Letters 100–155*. Translated by R. Teske. Edited by B. Ramsey. New York: New City Press, 2003. *Letters*. Part II, Vol. 3, *Letters 156–210*. Translated by R. Teske. Edited by B. Ramsey. New York: New City Press, 2004. *Letters*. Part II, Vol. 4, *Letters 211–270, 1*–29**. Translated by R. Teske. Edited by B. Ramsey. New York: New City Press, 2005. D. Dekkers and J. Fraipont, *Corpus Christianorum Series Latina*. Vol. 38–40. Turnholt: 1946, 1–2196.

Augustine. *On Genesis*. Translated by R. Teske. Vol. 84 of *The Fathers of the Church*. Washington, DC: Catholic University of America Press, 1990. J. Zycha, *Corpus scriptorium ecclesiasticorum latinorum*. Vol. 28. Vienna: 1894.

Augustine. "The Punishment and Forgiveness of Sins and the Baptism of Little Ones." In *Selected Writings on Grace and Pelagianism*, translated by R. Teske, edited by B. Ramsey, 91–214. New York: New City Press, 2011. C. F. Urba and J. Zycha, *Corpus scriptorium ecclesiasticorum latinorum*. Vol. 60. Vienna: 1913, 3–151.

Augustine. *Revisions*. Translated by B. Ramsey. Edited by R. Teske. New York: New City Press, 2010. P. Knöll, *Corpus scriptorium ecclesiasticorum latinorum*. Vol. 36. Vienna: 1902.

Augustine. *Sermons 1–19*. Translated by E. Hill. New York: New City Press, 1990.

Augustine. "The Spirit and the Letter." In *Selected Writings on Grace and Pelagianism*, translated by R. Teske, edited by B. Ramsey, 229–92. New York: New City Press, 2011. C. F. Urba and J. Zycha, *Corpus scriptorium ecclesiasticorum latinorum*. Vol. 60. Vienna: 1913, 155–229.

Augustine. *The Trinity*. Translated by E. Hill. New York: New City Press, 2012. J. G.Ph Borleffs, *Corpus Christianorum Series Latina*. Vols. 50 and 50A. Turnhout: 1968, 1–380, 381–535.

Augustine. "Questions on the Heptateuch." *In Writings on the Old Testament. The Works of St. Augustine: A Translation for the 21st Century*, translated by J. Lienhard, 3–445. New York: New City Press, 2016. I. Fraipont, Corpus Christianorum Series Latina. Vol. 33. Vienna: 1958, 1–337.

Basil. *Letters*. Vol. 1, *1–185*. Vol. 13 of *The Fathers of the Church*. Translated by A. Way. Vol. 2, *186–368*. Vol. 28 of *The Fathers of the Church*. Translated by A. Way. Washington, DC: Catholic University of America Press, 1951 and 1955. J. P. Migne, *Patrologiae cursus completus: Series graeca*. Vol. 32. Paris: 1857, 219–1112.

Basil. "On the Hexaemeron." In *Exegetic Homilies*. Vol. 46 of *The Fathers of the Church*, translated by A. C. Way. Washington, DC: Catholic University of America Press, 1963. J. P. Migne, *Patrologiae cursus completus: Series graeca*. Vol. 29. Paris: 1857, 4–208.

Basil. "On the Holy Spirit." In *Basil: Letters and Select Works*, edited by P. Schaff and H. Wace. Series II, Vol. VIII of *Nicene and Post Nicene Fathers*. Grand Rapids, MI: Eerdmans, 1968.

Basil. "On Psalm 32." In *Basil: Letters and Select Works*, edited by P. Schaff and H. Wace. Series II, Vol. VIII of *Nicene and Post Nicene Fathers*. Grand Rapids, MI: Eerdmans, 1968. J. P. Migne, *Patrologiae cursus completus: Series graeca*. Vol. 29. Paris: 1857, 323–50.

Boethius. "A Treatise against Eutyches and Nestorius." In *Tractates: The Consolation of Philosophy*, translated by H. F. Stewart, E. K. Rand, and S. J. Tester. Loeb Classical Library 74. Cambridge, MA: Harvard University Press, 1973.

Boethius. "De Trinitate." In *Tractates: The Consolation of Philosophy*, translated by H. F. Stewart, E. K. Rand, and S. J. Tester. Loeb Classical Library 74. Cambridge, MA: Harvard University Press, 1973.

Caelestius. "Fragment." In *Faith of the Early Fathers*. Vol. 2, edited by W. Jurgens. Collegeville, MN: Liturgical Press, 1979.

Cicero. *De Officiis*. Book I. Constitution Society, accessed August 11, 2019. http://www.constitution.org/rom/de_officiis.htm.

Clement of Alexandria. *Christ the Educator*. Translated by S. Wood. Vol. 23 of *The Fathers of the Church*. Washington, DC: Catholic University of America Press, 1954. Otto Stahlin, *Die griechischen christlichen Schriftsteller der ersten Jahrhunderte*. Vol. 12. Leipzig: 1936, 87–340.

Clement of Alexandria. "Exhortation to the Heathen." In *Fathers of the Second Century*, edited by A. Roberts and J. Donaldson. Vol. II of *The Ante-Nicene Fathers*. Grand Rapids, MI: Eerdmans, 1983. Otto Stahlin, *Die griechischen christlichen Schriftsteller der ersten Jahrhunderte*. Vol. 12. Leipzig: 1936, 3–86.

Clement of Alexandria. "*Stromata*." In *Fathers of the Second Century*, edited by A. Roberts and J. Donaldson. Vol. II of *The Ante-Nicene Fathers*. Grand Rapids, MI: Eerdmans, 1983. Otto Stahlin, *Die griechischen christlichen Schriftsteller der ersten Jahrhunderte*. Vol. 15 (Books 1–6). Leipzig: 1906 [reprinted in 1939 and 1960], 3–102. Vol. 17 (Books 7–8). Leipzig: 1909 [reprinted in 1970].

Constantine. "Letter to Alexander and Arius." In *A New Eusebius: Documents Illustrating the History of the Church to AD 337*, edited by J. Stevenson, 350–51. London: SPCK, 1995.

Cyril of Alexandria. "Against Diodore of Tarsus and Theodore of Mopsuestia." In *St Cyril Archbishop of Alexandria: Five Tomes against Nestorius; Scholia on the Incarnation; Christ Is One; Fragments against Diodore of Tarsus and Theodore of*

Mopsuestia, the Synousiasts, translated by P. E. Pusey. Vol. 47 of *Library of Fathers of the Holy Catholic Church*. Oxford: James Parker, 1881.

Cyril of Alexandria. *Commentary on John*. Vol. 1. Translated by D. Maxwell and J. Elowsky. Downers Grove, IL: Intervarsity Press, 2013. P. E. Pusey, *Sancti patris nostri Cyrilli archiepiscopi Alexandrini in Divi Johannis evangelium*. Oxford: 1872.

Cyril of Alexandria. *On the Unity of Christ*. Translated by J. McGuckin. New York: St. Vladimir's Seminary Press, 1995. J. P. Migne, *Patrologiae cursus completus: Series graeca*. Vol. 75. Paris: 1863, 1254–362.

Cyril of Alexandria. "Scholia on the Incarnation." In *St Cyril Archbishop of Alexandria: Five Tomes against Nestorius; Scholia on the Incarnation; Christ Is One; Fragments against Diodore of Tarsus and Theodore of Mopsuestia, the Synousiasts*, translated by P. E. Pusey. Vol. 47 of *Library of Fathers of the Holy Catholic Church*. Oxford: James Parker, 1881.

Cyril of Alexandria. *St. Cyril of Alexandria, Letters 1–50*. Translated by J. McEnerney. Vol. 76 of *The Fathers of the Church*. Washington, DC: Catholic University of America Press, 1987. E. Schwartz, *Acta Conciliorum Oecumenicorum*. Berlin: De Gruyter, 1914.

Cyril of Jerusalem. "Catechetical Lectures." In *Nicene and Post Nicene Fathers*. Second Series, Vol. 7, edited by P. Schaff and H. Wace, Grand Rapids, MI: Eerdmans, 1996. J. P. Migne, *Patrologiae cursus completus: Series graeca*. Vol. 33. Paris: 1857, 331–1128.

"Didache." In *Apostolic Fathers*, translated by F. Glimm. Vol. 1 of *The Fathers of the Church*. Washington, DC: Catholic University of America Press, 2008. Funk-Bihlmeyer-Schneemelcher, *Die apostolischen Väter*. Vol. 1. Tübingen: 1947, 1–9.

Dionysius. "Letter against the Sabellians." In *A New Eusebius*, edited by J. Stevenson, 252–53. London: SPCK, 1987.

Dionysius of Rome. "Letter of Dionysius of Rome to Dionysius of Alexandria." In *The Faith of the Early Fathers*. Vol. 1, edited by W. A. Jurgens, 248–49. Collegeville, MN: Liturgical Press, 1970.

Epiphanius. *The Panarion of Epiphanius of Salamis*. Translated by F. Williams. Leiden: Brill, Book I, 1997; Books II and III, 1994. K. Holl, *Die griechischen christlichen Schriftsteller der ersten Jahrhunderte*. Vols. 25, 31, 37. Leipzig: 1915, 1922, 1933.

Ephraim the Syrian. "Homily on Our Lord." In *Gregory the Great II, Ephriam Syrus, Aphrahat*, edited by Philip Schaff and Henry Wace, 33. Series II, Vol. XIII of *Nicene and Post Nicene Fathers*. Grand Rapids, MI: Eerdmans, 1898. T. J. Lamy, *S. Ephraem Syri hymni et sermons*. Mechlin: 1882–1902.

Eunomius. *The Extant Works*. Translated by R. P. Vaggione. Oxford: Clarendon Press, 1987.

Eusebius Pamphili. *Ecclesiastical History, Books 1–5*. Translated by R. Deferrari. Vol. 19 of *The Fathers of the Church*. Washington, DC: Catholic University of America Press, 1953. E. Klostermann, *Die griechischen christlichen Schriftsteller der ersten Jahrhunderte*. Vol. 14. Leipzig: 1906, 59–182.

Eusebius of Caesarea. "Letter to His Church on the Creed of Nicaea." In *A New Eusebius: Documents Illustrating the History of the Church to AD 337*, edited by J. Stevenson, 344–47. London: SPCK, 1995.

Eutyches. "Admission of Eutyches." In *Creeds, Councils and Controversies*, edited by J. Stevenson, 335–36. London: SPCK, 1989.

Gaius. *The Institutes of Gaius*. Translated by W. M. Gordon and O. F. Robinson. London: Duckworth, 1988.

Gregory of Nazianzus. "Against the Arians." In *Cyril of Jerusalem, Gregory Nazianzen*, edited by P. Schaff and H. Wace. Series II, Vol. VII of *Nicene and Post Nicene Fathers*. Grand Rapids, MI: Eerdmans, 1996.

Gregory of Nazianzus. "Epistle 101." In *Cyril of Jerusalem, Gregory Nazianzen*, edited by P. Schaff and H. Wace. Series II, Vol. VII of *Nicene and Post Nicene Fathers*. Grand Rapids, MI: Eerdmans, 1996. J. P. Migne. *Patrologiae cursus completus: Series graeca*. Vol. 37. Paris: 1857, 20–396.

Gregory of Nazianzus. "Fifth Theological Oration (Oration 31)." In *Cyril of Jerusalem, Gregory Nazianzen*, edited by P. Schaff and H. Wace. Series II, Vol. VII of *Nicene and Post Nicene Fathers*. Grand Rapids, MI: Eerdmans, 1996. J. P. Migne, *Patrologiae cursus completus: Series graeca*. Vol. 36. Paris: 1857. A. J. Mason, *The Five Theological Orations of Gregory of Nazianz. Cambridge Patristic Texts*. Cambridge: 1899.

Gregory of Nazianzus. "Orations." In *Cyril of Jerusalem, Gregory Nazianzen*, edited by P. Schaff and H. Wace. Series II, Vol. VII of *Nicene and Post Nicene Fathers*. Grand Rapids, MI: Eerdmans, 1996. J. P. Migne, *Patrologiae cursus completus: Series graeca*. Vol. 36. Paris: 1857. A. J. Mason, *The Five Theological Orations of Gregory of Nazianz*. Cambridge Patristic Texts. Cambridge: 1899.

Gregory of Nyssa. "Against Eunomius." In *Gregory of Nyssa: Dogmatic Treatises; Select Writings and Letters*, edited by P. Schaff and H. Wace. Series II, Vol. V of *Nicene and Post Nicene Fathers*. Grand Rapids, MI: Eerdmans, 1972. J. P. Migne, *Patrologiae cursus completus: Series graeca*. Vol. 45. Paris: 1863, 24–118.

Gregory of Nyssa. "Answer to Eunomius." In *Gregory of Nyssa: Dogmatic Treatises; Select Writings and Letters*, edited by P. Schaff and H. Wace. Series II, Vol. V of *Nicene and Post Nicene Fathers*. Grand Rapids, MI: Eerdmans, 1972. J. P. Migne, *Patrologiae cursus completus: Series graeca*. Vol. 45. Paris: 1863, 237–1122.

Gregory of Nyssa. "*Antirrheticus*." In *St. Gregory of Nyssa: Anti-Apollinarian Writings*, translated by R. Orton, 41–58. Vol. 131 of *The Fathers of the Church*. Washington, DC: Catholic University of America Press, 2015. T. J. Carter, "Commentary upon the Fragments of Apollinarius' Apodeixis." In *Apollinarian Christologies: A Study of the Writings of Apollinarius of Laodicea*, 339–84. London: Hamley King, 2011. H. Lietzmann, *Apollinaris von Laodicea und seine Schule, Texte und Untersuchungen*. Tubingen: 1904.

Gregory of Nyssa. "The Great Catechism." In *Gregory of Nyssa: Dogmatic Treatises; Select Writings and Letters*, edited by P. Schaff and H. Wace. Series II, Vol. V of *Nicene and Post Nicene Fathers*. Grand Rapids, MI: Eerdmans, 1972. J. P. Migne, *Patrologiae cursus completus: Series graeca*. Vol. 45. Paris: 1863, 9–106.

Gregory of Nyssa. *Homilies on the Song of Songs*. Translated by R. Norris. Atlanta: Society of Biblical Literature, 2012, Homily 15. J. P. Migne, *Patrologiae cursus completus: Series graeca*. Vol. 44. Paris: 1863, 755–1120.

Gregory of Nyssa. "On the Holy Trinity." In *Gregory of Nyssa: Dogmatic Treatises;*

Select Writings and Letters, edited by P. Schaff and H. Wace. Series II, Vol. V of *Nicene and Post Nicene Fathers*. Grand Rapids, MI: Eerdmans, 1972. J. P. Migne, *Patrologiae cursus completus: Series graeca*. Vol. 44. Paris: 1863.

Gregory of Nyssa. "On Infants' Early Deaths." In *Gregory of Nyssa: Dogmatic Treatises; Select Writings and Letters*, edited by P. Schaff and H. Wace. Series II, Vol. V of *Nicene and Post Nicene Fathers*. Grand Rapids, MI: Eerdmans, 1972. J. P. Migne, *Patrologiae cursus completus: Series graeca*. Vol. 46. Paris: 1863, 161–92.

Gregory of Nyssa. "On the Making of Man." In *Gregory of Nyssa: Dogmatic Treatises; Select Writings and Letters*, edited by P. Schaff and H. Wace. Series II, Vol. V of *Nicene and Post Nicene Fathers*. Grand Rapids, MI: Eerdmans, 1972. J. P. Migne, *Patrologiae cursus completus: Series graeca*. Vol. 44. Paris: 1863, 123–256.

Gregory of Nyssa. "On Not Three Gods." In *Gregory of Nyssa: Dogmatic Treatises; Select Writings and Letters*, edited by P. Schaff and H. Wace. Series II, Vol. V of *Nicene and Post Nicene Fathers*. Grand Rapids, MI: Eerdmans, 1972. J. P. Migne, *Patrologiae cursus completus: Series graeca*. Vol. 45. Paris: 1863, 115–36.

Hilary. *The Trinity*. Translated by S. McKenna. Vol. 25 of *The Fathers of the Church*. Washington, DC: Catholic University of America Press, 1954. J. P. Migne, *Patrologiae cursus completus: Series latina*. Vol. 10. Paris: 1845, 23–472.

Hippolytus. *Contra Noetum*. Translated by R. Butterworth. London: Heythrop Monographs, 1977. P. Nautin, *Hippolyte: Contre les heresies, fragment, etude et edition critique*. Paris: 1949.

Horsiesios. "Instructions." In *Pachomian Koinonia*. Vol. 3, translated by A. Veilleux. Michigan: Cistercian, 1982.

Ignatius of Antioch. "Letters." In *Apostolic Fathers*, translated by F. Glimm. Vol. 1 of *The Fathers of the Church*. Washington, DC: Catholic University of America Press, 2008. J. P. Migne, *Patrologiae cursus completus: Series graeca*. Vol. 5. Paris: 1857.

Irenaeus. "Against Heresies." In *Apostolic Fathers with Justin Martyr and Irenaeus Ante-Nicene Fathers*. Vol. 1, edited by A. Roberts and J. Donaldson. Grand Rapids, MI: Eerdmans, 1985. J .P. Migne, *Patrologiae cursus completus: Series graeca*. Vol. 7. Paris: 1857, 433–1224.

Irenaeus. *Demonstration of the Apostolic Preaching*. Translation and commentary by I. MacKenzie. Aldershot: Ashgate, 2002. *Texte und Untersuchungen* 31.1. Leipzig: 1907.

Julian of Eclanum. "To Florus." In Augustine, *Answer to the Pelagians, III* [Unfinished work in answer to Julian], translated by R. Teske, edited by J. Rotelle. New York: New City Press, 1999. E. Kalinka, *Corpus scriptorium ecclesiasticorum latinorum*. Vol. 85, Part 1. Vienna: Hoelder Pichler Tempsky, 1974.

Justin Martyr. *The First Apology, The Second Apology, Dialogue with Trypho, Exhortation to the Greeks, Discourse to the Greeks, The Monarchy of the Rule of God*. Translated by T. Falls. Vol. 6 of *The Fathers of the Church*. Washington, DC: Catholic University of America Press, 1948. J. P. Migne, *Patrologiae cursus completus: Series graeca*. Vol. 6. Paris: 1857, 327–471 (First and Second Apology); 471–800; 241–312.

Justin Martyr. "Fragments on the Resurrection." In *Apostolic Fathers with Justin Martyr and Irenaeus Ante-Nicene Fathers*. Vol. 1, edited by A. Roberts and J. Donaldson. Grand Rapids, MI: Eerdmans, 2001. J. C. T. von Otto, *Corpus apologetarum christianorum saeculi secundi*. Vol. III. Ienae: 1879, 211–49.

Lactantius. "On the Workmanship of God." In *Fathers of the Third and Fourth Centuries Ante-Nicene Fathers*. Vol. VII, edited by A. Roberts and J. Donaldson. Grand Rapids, MI: Eerdmans, 1979. S. Brandt, *Corpus scriptorium ecclesiasticorum latinorum*. Vol. 27. Vienna: 1897, 3–64.

Leo I (pope). *Pope Leo I, Letters*, translated by E. Hunt. Vol. 34 of *The Fathers of the Church*. Washington, DC: Catholic University of America Press, 1957. J. P. Migne, *Patrologiae cursus completus: Series latina*. Vol. 54. Paris: 1846, 581–1218.

Leo I (pope). *Sermons*. Translated by J. Freeland and A. Conway. Vol. 93 of *The Fathers of the Church*. Washington, DC: Catholic University of America Press, 1996. J. P. Migne, *Patrologiae cursus completus: Series latina*. Vol. 54. Paris: 1846, 137–468.

Leporius. "Libellus emendationis." In *Faith of the Early Fathers*. Vol. 3, edited by W. Jurgens. Collegeville, MN: Liturgical Press, 1979.

Marcus Aurelius. *Meditations*. Translated by M. Staniforth. London: Penguin, 2003.

"[The] Martyrdom of Saint Polycarp." In *Apostolic Fathers*, translated by F. Glimm. Vol. 1 of *The Fathers of the Church*. Washington, DC: Catholic University of America Press, 1947. Funk-Bihlmeyer-Schneemelcher, *Die apostolischen Väter*. Vol. 1. Tübingen: 1956, 120–32.

Methodius. "From the Discourse on the Resurrection." In *Fathers of the Third Century Ante-Nicene Fathers*. Vol. VI, edited by A. Roberts and J. Donaldson. Grand Rapids, MI: Eerdmans, 1971. J. P. Migne, *Patrologiae cursus completus: Series graeca*. Vol. 18. Paris: 1857.

Nemesius of Emesa. "A Treatise on the Nature of Man." In *Cyril of Jerusalem and Nemesius of Emesa*, translated by W. Telfer. Vol. IV of *Library of Christian Classics*. London: SCM Press, 1955. *Nemesii Episcopi Premnon Physicon: Sive Peri physeos anthropou liber a N. Alfano*, K. Burkhard, Leipzig: Tuebner, 1917.

Nestorius. *The Bazaar of Heracleides*. Translated by G. R. Driver and L. Hodgson. Oxford: Clarendon Press, 1925. P. Bedjan, *Nestorius: Le Livre d'Héraclide de Damas*. Paris: 1910.

Nestorius. "Fragment." In *Faith of the Early Fathers*. Vol. 3, edited by W. Jurgens. Collegeville, MN: Liturgical Press, 1979. F. Loof, *Nestoriana: Die Fragmente des Nestorius, gesammelt, untersucht und herausgeben, mit Beiträgen von S.A. Cook und G. Kampffmeyer*. Halle: 1905.

Nestorius. "Letter 5, Second Letter to Cyril." In *St. Cyril of Alexandria, Letters 1–50*, translated by J. McEnerney, 43–48. Vol. 76 of *The Fathers of the Church*. Washington, DC: Catholic University of America Press, 1987.

Origen. "Against Celsus." In *Fathers of the Third Century*, edited by A. Roberts and J. Donaldson. Vol. IV of *The Ante-Nicene Fathers*. Grand Rapids, MI: Eerdmans, 1982. P. Koetschau, *Die griechischen christlichen Schriftsteller der ersten Jahrhunderte*. Vols. 2 and 3. Leipzig: 1899.

Origen. *Commentary on the Gospel According to John, Books 1–10*. Translated by R. Heine. Vol. 80 of *The Fathers of the Church*. Washington, DC: Catholic University of America Press, 1989. E. Preuschen *Die griechischen christlichen Schriftsteller der ersten Jahrhunderte*. Vol. 10. Leipzig: 1903, 1–574.

Origen. "*De Principiis, First Principles.*" In *Fathers of the Third Century*, edited by A. Roberts and J. Donaldson. Vol. IV of *The Ante-Nicene Fathers*. Grand Rapids, MI: Eerdmans, 1982. P. Koetschau, *Die griechischen christilichen Schriftsteller der ersten Jahrhunderte*. Vol. 22. Leipzig: 1913.

Origen. "Dialogue with Heracleides." In *Treatise on the Passover and Dialogue with Heracleides*, translated by R. Daly. Mahwah, NJ: Paulist Press, 1992.

Origen. *An Exhortation to Martyrdom, Prayer and Selected Works*. Edited and translated by Rowan Greer. Mahwah, NJ: Paulist Press, 1979.

Origen. *Homilies on Genesis and Exodus*. Translated by R. Heine. Vol. 71 of *The Fathers of the Church*. Washington, DC: Catholic University of America Press, 1982. ("On Genesis," 47–224; "On Exodus," 227, 387–96.) J. P. Migne, *Patrologiae cursus completus: Series graeca*. Vol. 12. Paris: 1862.

Origen. *Homilies on Luke*. Translated by J. Leinhard. Vol. 94 of *The Fathers of the Church*. Washington, DC: Catholic University of America Press, 1996. J. P. Migne, *Patrologiae cursus completus: Series graeca*. Vol. 13. Paris: 1862, 1801–908.

Pamphilus. "Apology for Origen." In *St Pamphilus Apology for Origen and Rufinus on the Falsification of the Books of Origen*, translated by T. Scheck. Vol. 120 of *The Fathers of the Church*. Washington, DC: Catholic University of America Press, 2010.

Paul of Samosata. "Fragments." In *A New Eusebius: Documents Illustrating the History of the Church to AD 337*, edited by J. Stevenson. London: SPCK, 1995.

Pelagius. "Letter to Demetrias." In *Pelagius: Life and Letters*, translated by B. R. Rees, 35–70. Vol. II of *The Letters of Pelagius and His Followers*. Woodbridge: Boydell, 1998. J. P. Migne, *Patrologiae cursus completus: Series latina*. Vol. 30. Paris: 1846, 15–45.

Philo. "Allegorical Interpretation 1, 2 and 3." In *Works of Philo*, translated by C. Yonge. Peabody, MA: Hendrickson, 1993.

Philo. *On the Creation of the Cosmos According to Moses*. Translated and commentary by D. Runia. Leiden: Brill, 2001.

Plato. *Phaedo*. Edited by C. J. Rowe. Cambridge Greek and Latin Classics. Cambridge: Cambridge University Press, 2001.

Tertullian. "Against Marcion." In *Latin Christianity: Its Founder, Tertullian*, edited by A. Roberts and J. Donaldson. Vol. III of *Ante-Nicene Fathers*. Peabody, MA: Hendrickson, 1995. J. G.Ph Borleffs, *Corpus Christianorum*. Vol. 2. Turnhout: 1954, 441–726.

Tertullian. "Against Praxeas." In *Latin Christianity: Its Founder, Tertullian*, edited by A. Roberts and J. Donaldson. Vol. III of *Ante-Nicene Fathers*. Peabody, MA: Hendrickson, 1995. Kroymann-Evans text, *Corpus Christianorum*. Vol. 2. Turnhout: 1954, 1159–205.

Tertullian. "Apology 1." In *Tertullian Apologetical Works; Octavius*, translated by R. Arbesmann. Vol. 10 of *The Fathers of the Church*. Washington, DC: Catholic University of America Press, 1950. E. Dekkers, *Corpus Christianorum*. Vol. 1. Turnhout: 1954. 85–171.

Tertullian. "On Baptism." In *Latin Christianity: Its Founder, Tertullian*, edited by A. Roberts and J. Donaldson. Vol. III of *Ante-Nicene Fathers*. Peabody, MA: Hendrickson, 1995. J. G.Ph Borleffs, *Corpus Christianorum*. Vol. 1. Turnhout: 1954, 277–95.

Tertullian. "On the Flesh of Christ." In *Latin Christianity: Its Founder, Tertullian*, edited by A. Roberts and J. Donaldson. Vol. III of *Ante-Nicene Fathers*. MA: Hendrickson, 1995. Kroymann, *Corpus Christianorum*. Vol. 2. Turnhout: 1954, 873–917.

Tertullian. "On the Resurrection of the Flesh." In *Latin Christianity: Its Founder*, edited by A. Roberts and J. Donaldson. Vol. III of *Ante-Nicene Fathers*. Peabody, MA: Hendrickson, 1995. J. G.Ph Borleffs, *Corpus Christianorum*. Vol. 2. Turnhout: 1954, 921–1012.

Tertullian. "The Chaplet." In *Latin Christianity: Its Founder*, edited by A. Roberts and J. Donaldson. Vol. III of *Ante-Nicene Fathers*. Peabody, MA: Hendrickson, 1995. J. G.Ph Borleffs, *Corpus Christianorum*. Vol. 2. Turnhout: 1954, 1039–65.

Tertullian. "On the Soul." In *Tertullian Apologetical Works; Octavius*, translated by R. Arbesmann. Vol. 10 of *The Fathers of the Church*. Washington, DC: Catholic University of America Press, 1950. J. G.Ph Borleffs, *Corpus Christianorum*. Vol. 2. Turnhout: 1954, 781–869.

Theodore of Mopsuestia. "Commentary on Haggai." In *Theodore of Mopsuestia Commentary on the Twelve Prophets*, translated by R. Hill. Vol. 108 of *The Fathers of the Church*. Washington, DC: Catholic University of America Press, 2004.

Theodore of Mopsuestia. *Commentary of Theodore of Mopsuestia on the Nicene Creed*. Translated by A. Mingana. Vol. V of *Woodbrooke Studies*. Piscataway, NJ: Gorgias, 2009. [First published by Woodbrooke, 1932.]

Theodore of Mopsuestia. "Fragment of a Letter to Domnus." In *Faith of the Early Fathers*, edited by W. Jurgens. Vol. 2. Collegeville, MN: Liturgical Press, 1979.

Theodore of Mopsuestia. "On the Incarnation"; "Catechetical Homilies"; "In Opposition to Apollinaris." In *Theodore of Mopsuestia*, edited by F. McLeod. New York: Routledge, 2009.

Florigelium

Bardy, G. *Recherches sur Saint Lucien d'Antioche et son école*. Paris: 1936.

Bettenson, H. *The Later Christian Fathers*. London: Oxford University Press, 1974.

Harmless, W., ed. *Augustine in His Own Words*. Washington, DC: Catholic University of America Press, 2010.

Jurgens, W. A. *The Faith of the Early Fathers*. Vols. 1–3. Collegeville, MN: Liturgical Press, 1970, 1979, 1979.

Kelly, J. N. D. *Early Christian Creeds*. New York: Routledge, 2014. [First published 1950.]

Stevenson, J. *A New Eusebius. Documents Illustrating the History of the Church to AD 337*. London: SPCK, 1995.

Stevenson, J. *Creeds, Councils and Controversies: Documents Illustrating the History of the Church, AD 337–461*. London: SPCK, 1989.

Modern Sources

Ad Hoc Committee of the Harvard Medical School. "A Definition of Irreversible Coma." *Journal of the American Medical Association* 205, no. 6 (1968): 337–40.

Albrecht, G., ed. *Encyclopedia of Disability*. London: Sage, 2006.
Anatolios, K. *Athanasius*. London: Routledge, 2004.
Annas, J. *Hellenistic Philosophy of Mind*. Los Angeles: University of California Press, 1994.
Annas, J. *Platonic Ethics Old and New*. Ithaca, NY: Cornell University Press, 1999.
Anscombe, G. E. M. "Murder and the Morality of Euthanasia." In *Human Life, Action and Ethics: Essays by G. E. M. Anscombe*, edited by M. Geach and L. Gormally. Exeter: Imprint Academic, 2005.
Ashley, B. "The Anthropological Foundations of the Natural Law." In *St. Thomas Aquinas and the Natural Law Tradition: Contemporary Perspectives*, edited by J. Goyette, M. Latkovic, and R. Myers, 3–16. Washington, DC: Catholic University of America Press, 2004.
Ayres, L. *Augustine and the Trinity*. Cambridge: Cambridge University Press, 2010.
Ayres, L. "Not Three People: The Fundamental Themes of Gregory of Nyssa's Trinitarian Theology as Seen in 'To Ablabius: On Not Three Gods.'" *Modern Theology* 18, no. 4 (2002): 450.
Ayres, L. *Nicaea and Its Legacy*. Oxford: Oxford University Press, 2006.
Ayres, L., and A. Radd-Gallwitz. "Doctrine of God." In *The Oxford Handbook of Early Christian Studies*, edited by Susan Harvey and David Hunter, 864–85. Oxford: Oxford University Press, 2008.
Bammel, C. "The State of Play with Regard to Hippolytus and the Contra Noetum." *Heythrop Journal* 31, no. 2 (1990): 197.
Barnes, M. "Anti-Arian Works." In *Augustine through the Ages*, edited by A. Fitzgerald. Grand Rapids, MI: Eerdmans, 1999.
Barnes, M. "Augustine in Contemporary Theology." *Theological Studies* 56, no. 2 (1995): 237–38.
Barnes, M. *The Power of God: Δύναμις in Gregory of Nyssa's Trinitarian Theology*. Washington, DC: Catholic University of America Press, 2001.
Barnes, M. "Contra Eunomium III.6." In *Gregory of Nyssa: Contra Eunomium*, edited by J. Leemans and M. Cassin, 369–82. Leiden: Brill, 2014.
Barnes, T. *Tertullian*. Oxford: Oxford University Press, 1985.
Barnhart, R. *Chambers Dictionary of Etymology*. New York: Chambers Harrap, 1988.
Barth, K. *Church Dogmatics*. Vol. 1, Part I. Edinburgh: T & T Clark, 1975.
Baskin, J., ed. *The Cambridge Dictionary of Judaism and Jewish Culture*. Cambridge: Cambridge University Press, 2011.
Battin, M. *Ending Life: Ethics and the Way We Die*. Oxford: Oxford University Press, 2005.
Battin, M., and T. Quill, eds. *Physician-Assisted Dying: The Case for Palliative Care and Patient Choice*. Baltimore: Johns Hopkins University Press, 2004.
Bauckham, R. "The Origin of the Ebionites." In *The Image of the Judeo-Christians in Ancient Jewish and Christian Literature*, edited by P. Tomson and D. Lambers-Petry. Tubingen: Mohr Siebeck, 2003.
Beatrice, P. F. "The Word '*Homoousios*' from Hellenism to Christianity." *Church History* 71 (2002): 269–70.
Beauchamp, T. "The Failure of Theories of Personhood." In *Personhood and Health-*

care, edited by D. Thomasma, D. Weisstub, and S. Herve. Dordrecht: Kluwer, 2001.

Beauchamp, T. "The Right to Die as the Triumph of Autonomy." *Journal of Medicine and Philosophy* 31, no. 6 (2006): 643–44.

Beauchamp, T. *Standing on Principles: Collected Essays*. Oxford: Oxford University Press, 2010.

Beauchamp, T., and J. Childress. *The Principles of Biomedical Ethics*. Oxford: Oxford University Press, 1979. [2nd ed., 1983; 3rd ed., 1989; 6th ed., 2009; 7th ed., 2013.]

Beeley, C. *Gregory of Nazianzus on the Trinity and the Knowledge of God*. Oxford: Oxford University Press, 2008.

Behr, J. *Formation of Christian Theology*. Vol. 1 of *The Way to Nicaea*. Crestwood, NY: St. Vladimir's Seminary Press, 2001.

"*Belmont Report*: Ethical Principles and Guidelines for the Protection of Human Subjects of Research." In *Source Book in Bioethics: A Documentary History*, edited by A. Jonsen, R. Veatch, and L .R. Walters, 22–28. Washington, DC: Georgetown University Press, 1998.

Benedict XVI (pope). *Fathers of the Church from St Clement of Rome to St Augustine of Hippo*. Edited by J. Leinhard. Grand Rapids, MI: Eerdmans, 2009.

Bennett, S. "Chimera and the Continuum of Humanity: Erasing the Line of Constitutional Personhood." *Emory Law Journal* 55, no. 2 (2006): 347–87.

Berkman, J. "From Theological Speciesism to a Theological Ethology." *Journal of Moral Theology* 3, no. 2 (2014): 11–34.

Berlin, A., et al. *Jewish Study Bible*. Oxford: Oxford University Press, 2004.

Bernat, J. *Ethical Issues in Neurology*. Philadelphia: Kluwer, 2008.

Betcher, S. *Spirit and the Politics of Disablement*. Minneapolis: Fortress Press, 2007.

Bianchi, U. "The Religio-Historical Relevance of Lk 20:34–36." In *Studies in Gnosticism and Hellenistic Religions*, edited by R. Van Den Broek and M. J. Vermaseren. Leiden: Brill, 1981.

Biggar, N. *Aiming to Kill: The Ethics of Suicide and Euthanasia*. Cleveland: Pilgrim Press, 2004.

Bindley, T. H., and F. W. Green. *The Oecumenical Documents of the Faith*. London: Methuen, 1950.

Black, K. *A Healing Homiletic: Preaching and Disability*. Nashville: Abingdon Press, 1996.

Blosser, B. *Become Like the Angels: Origen's Doctrine of the Soul*. Washington, DC: Catholic University of America Press, 2012.

Blowers, P. *Drama of the Divine Economy: Creator and Creation in Early Christian Theology and Piety*. Oxford: Oxford University Press, 2012.

Boersma, H. *Embodiment and Virtue in Gregory of Nyssa: An Anagogical Approach*. Oxford: Oxford University Press, 2013.

Bonfante, G., and L. Bonfante. *The Etruscan Language: An Introduction*. Manchester: Manchester University Press, 2002.

Borkowski, A. *Textbook on Roman Law*. London: Blackstone, 1997.

Bortolotti, L., and J. Harris. "Disability, Enhancement and Harm Benefit Continuum."

In *Freedom and Responsibility in Reproductive Choice*, edited by J. Spencer and A. Du Bois-Pedain. Oxford: Hart, 2006.

Bouteneff, P. "Essential or Existential: The Problem of the Body in the Anthropology of St Gregory of Nyssa." In *Gregory of Nyssa: Homilies on the Beatitudes*, edited by H. Drobner and A. Viciano. Leiden: Brill, 2000.

Bowery, A. M. "Boethius." In *Augustine through the Ages: An Encyclopedia*, edited by A. Fitzgerald. Grand Rapids, MI: Eerdmans, 1999.

Bradshaw, D. "The *Opuscula Sacra*: Boethius and Theology," In *The Cambridge Companion to Boethius*, edited by John Marenbon, 105–28. Cambridge: Cambridge University Press, 2009.

Branson, J., and D. Miller. *Damned for Their Difference*. Washington, DC: Gallaudet University Press, 2002.

Briggman, A. *Irenaeus of Lyons and the Theology of the Holy Spirit*. Oxford: Oxford University Press, 2012.

British Council of Churches. *The Forgotten Trinity: Report of the BCC Study Commission on Trinitarian Doctrine Today*. Vol. 1. London: BCC Inter-Church House, 1989.

Brock, B. "Augustine's Hierarchies of Human Wholeness and Their Healing." In *Disability in the Christian Tradition: A Reader*, edited by B. Brock and J. Swinton. Grand Rapids, MI: Eerdmans, 2012.

Brock, D. *Life and Death: Philosophical Essays in Biomedical Ethics*. Cambridge: Cambridge University Press, 1993.

Brown, D. *The Divine Trinity*. London: Duckworth, 1985.

Brown, P. *Augustine of Hippo*. London: Faber and Faber, 2000.

Brown, P. *The Body and Society*. London: Faber and Faber, 1990.

Brown, R. *The Community of the Beloved Disciple*. Mahwah, NJ: Paulist Press, 1979.

Brown, R., et al., eds. *New Jerome Biblical Commentary*. London: Geoffrey Chapman, 2000.

Buckland, W. *A Textbook of Roman Law from Augustus to Justinian*. Cambridge: Cambridge University Press, 1963.

Burns, P., ed. *Butler's Lives of the Saints: January*. Collegeville, MN: Liturgical Press, 1995.

Burns, S. "Cappadocian Encratism and the Macarian Community." In *Studia Patristica*. Vol. XXXVII 1999, edited by M. E. Wiles et al. Leuven: Peeters, 2001.

Calame, C. *The Craft of Poetic Speech in Ancient Greece*. Ithaca, NY: Cornell University Press, 1995.

Calhoun, D. "Prospects for Human Dignity after Darwin." In *Human Dignity in Bioethics from Worldviews to the Public Square*, edited by S. Dilley and N. Palpant. New York: Routledge, 2013.

Camosy, C. *Beyond the Abortion Wars*. Grand Rapids, MI: Eerdmans, 2015.

Camosy, C. *For Love of Animals*. Cincinnati: Franciscan Media, 2013.

Camosy, C. "Other Animals as Persons? A Roman Catholic Inquiry." In Animals as Religious Subjects, Transdisciplinary Perspectives, edited by C. Deane-Drummond, R. Artinian-Kaiser, and D. Clough. London: Bloomsbury, 2013.

Camosy, C. *Peter Singer and Christian Ethics: Beyond Polarization*. Cambridge: Cambridge University Press, 2012.

Carlson, L. *The Faces of Intellectual Disability: Philosophical Reflections*. Bloomington: Indiana University Press, 2010.

Carter, T. *The Apollinarian Christologies: A Study of the Writings of Apollinarius of Laodicea*. London: Hamley King, 2011.

Catechism of the Catholic Church. Dublin: Veritas, 1994

Cavalieri, P., and P. Singer. "The Great Ape Project." In *Peter Singer: Unsanctifying Human Life*, edited by H. Kuhse. Oxford: Blackwell, 2002.

Chadwick, H. *The Early Church*. Middlesex: Penguin, 1974.

Chestnut, R. "The Two *Prosopa* in Nestorius' *Bazaar of Heraclides*." *Journal of Theological Studies* 29 (1978).

Clayton, P. *The Christology of Theodoret of Cyrus*. Oxford: Oxford University Press, 2007.

Clifford, R., and R. Murphy. "Genesis." In *The New Jerome Biblical Commentary*, edited by R. Brown et al., 8–43. London: Geoffrey Chapman, 2000.

Clough, D. "Not a Not-Animal: The Vocation to be a Human Animal Creature." *Studies in Christian Ethics* 26, no. 1 (2013): 4–17.

Coakley, S. "Does Kenosis Rest on a Mistake? Three Kenotic Models in Patristic Exegesis." In *Exploring Kenotic Christology*, edited by C. S. Evans. Oxford: Oxford University Press, 2006.

Colish, M. *The Stoic Tradition from Antiquity to the Early Middle Ages: Stoicism in Classical Latin Literature*. Vol. 1. Leiden: Brill, 1990.

Congregation for the Doctrine of the Faith. *Dignitas Personae*. Rome: Congregation for the Doctrine of the Faith, 2008.

Conradie, E. *Christianity and Earthkeeping: In Search of an Inspiring Vision*. Stellenbosch: African Sun Media, 2011.

Coope, C. *Worth and Welfare in the Controversy over Abortion*. Basingstoke: Palgrave Macmillan, 2006.

Corrigan, K. *Evagrius and Gregory: Mind, Soul and Body in the 4th Century*. Farnham: Ashgate, 2009.

Cranford, R. "The Case of Mr. Stevens." *Issues in Law and Medicine* 97, no. 2 (1991): 199–211.

Cranford, R., and D. Smith. "Consciousness: The Most Critical Moral (Constitutional) Standard for Human Personhood." *American Journal of Law and Medicine* 13, no. 2–3 (1987): 242.

Creamer, D. "Embracing Limits: Queering Embodiment: Creating/Creative Possibilities for Disability Theology." *Journal of Feminist Studies in Religion* 26, no. 2 (2010): 109.

Crosby, J. *The Selfhood of the Human Person*. Washington, DC: Catholic University of America Press, 1996.

Cross, R. "Form and Universal in Boethius." *British Journal for the History of Philosophy* 20, no. 3 (2012): 439–58.

Daley, B. "Divine Transcendence and Human Transformation: Gregory of Nyssa's Anti-Apollinarian Christology." *Modern Theology* 18, no.4 (2002): 502.

Daley, B. *The Hope of the Early Church: A Handbook of Patristic Eschatology*. Cambridge: Cambridge University Press, 1991.
Davies, B. *The Reality of God and the Problem of Evil*. London: Continuum, 2006.
Davis, L. *The First Seven Ecumenical Councils*. Collegeville, MN: Liturgical Press, 1990.
Dawson, K. "Introduction: An Outline of Scientific Aspects of Human Embryo Research." In *Embryo Experimentation: Ethical, Legal and Social Issues*, edited by P. Singer et al. Cambridge: Cambridge University Press, 1993.
DeGrazia, D. "Genetic Enhancement, Post-Persons and Moral Status: A Reply to Buchanan." *Journal of Medical Ethics* 38 (2012): 135–39.
DeGrazia, D. *Human Identity and Bioethics*. Cambridge: Cambridge University Press, 2005.
DeGrazia, D. "On the Question of Personhood beyond Homo Sapiens." In *In Defense of Animals*, edited by P. Singer, 40–53. Oxford: Blackwell, 2006.
DeGrazia, D. *Taking Animals Seriously*. Cambridge: Cambridge University Press, 1996.
Dennett, D. "Conditions of Personhood." In *The Identities of Persons*, edited by A. Oksenberg Rorty, 175–96. Berkeley: University of California Press, 1976.
Descartes, R. *Descartes Philosophical Essays and Correspondence*, edited by R. Ariew. Indianapolis: Hackett, 2000.
DeWolf Bosek, M., and T. Savage. *The Ethical Component of Nursing Education: Integrating Ethics into Clinical Experience*. Philadelphia: Lippincott, Williams and Wilkins, 2007.
De Young, R., C. McCluskey, and C. Van Dyke. *Aquinas's Ethics: Metaphysical Foundations, Moral Theory and Theological Context*. Notre Dame, IN: University of Notre Dame Press, 2009.
Doran, R. *The Birth of a Worldview*. Lanham, MD: Rowman and Littlefield, 1999.
Dunn, G. *Tertullian*. London: Routledge, 2005.
Dunn, J. *The Theology of Paul the Apostle*. Grand Rapids, MI: Eerdmans, 1998.
Dupuis, J., and J. Neuner, eds. *The Christian Faith in the Doctrinal Documents of the Catholic Church*. New York: Alba House, 1996.
Dworkin, R. *Life's Dominion*. New York: Vintage, 1994.
Edwards, M. "Constructions of Physical Disability in the Ancient Greek World: The Community Concept." In *The Body and Physical Difference: Discourses of Disability*, edited by D. Mitchell and S. Snyder. Ann Arbor: University of Michigan Press, 1997.
Edwards, R. "Ethics and Embryology: The Case for Experimentation." In *Experiments on Embryos*, edited by A. Dyson and J. Harris. London: Routledge, 1991.
Eiesland, N. *The Disabled God: Toward a Liberatory Theology of Disability*. Nashville: Abingdon Press, 1994.
Elford, R. J. *The Pastoral Nature of Theology: An Upholding Presence*. New York: Cassell, 1999.
Engberg-Pedersen, T. "Setting the Scene: Stoicism and Platonism in the Transitional Period in Ancient Philosophy." In *Stoicism in Early Christianity*, edited by T. Rasimus, T. Engberg-Pedersen, and I. Dunderberg, 1–14. Grand Rapids, MI: Baker, 2010.

Engelhardt, H. T. "Infanticide in a Post-Christian Age." In *Euthanasia and the Newborn*, edited by R. McMillan, H. T. Engelhardt, and S. Spiker. Boston: D. Reidel, 1987.

Engelhardt, H. T. "Moral Pluralism, the Crisis of Secular Bioethics, and the Divisive Character of Christian Bioethics: Taking the Culture Wars Seriously." *Christian Bioethics* 15, no. 3 (2009): 234–53.

Engelhardt, H. T. "A Skeptical Reassessment of Bioethics." In *Bioethics Critically Reconsidered: Having Second Thoughts*, edited by H. T. Engelhardt, 1–28. New York: Springer, 2012.

Evans, J. *The History and Future of Bioethics: A Sociological View*. New York: Oxford University Press, 2012.

Evans, J. *Playing God: Human Genetic Engineering and the Rationalization of Public Bioethical Debate*. Chicago: University of Chicago Press, 2002.

Fackre, G. *The Christian Story*. Grand Rapids, MI: Eerdmans, 1996.

Fairbairn, D. *Grace and Christology in the Early Church*. Oxford: Oxford University Press, 2003.

Fitzmyer, J. "Introduction to the New Testament Epistles." In *The New Jerome Biblical Commentary*, edited by R. Brown et al., 768–71. London: Geoffrey Chapman, 2000.

Fitzmyer, J. "Pauline Theology." In *The New Jerome Biblical Commentary*, edited by R. Brown et al., 1390–93. London: Geoffrey Chapman, 2000.

Fletcher, J. *The Ethics of Genetic Control*. Buffalo: Prometheus, 1988.

Fletcher, J. "Four Indicators of Humanhood: The Enquiry Matures." In *On Moral Medicine: Theological Perspectives in Medical Ethics*, edited by S. Lammers and A. Verhey. Grand Rapids, MI: Eerdmans, 1998.

Fletcher, J. *Humanhood: Essays in Biomedical Ethics*. Buffalo: Prometheus, 1979.

Fletcher, J. *Morals and Medicine*. Boston: Beacon, 1954.

Fletcher, J. *Situation Ethics: The New Morality*. London: Westminster John Knox Press, 1997. [1st ed., 1966.]

Fotion, N., and J. C. Heller, eds. *Contingent Future Persons: On the Ethics of Deciding Who Will Live, or Not, in the Future*. Dordrecht: Kluwer, 1997.

Fox, P. *God as Communion: John Zizioulas, Elizabeth Johnson and the Retrieval of the Symbol of the Triune God*. Collegeville, MN: Liturgical Press, 2001.

Frampton, M. *Embodiments of Will: Anatomical and Physiological Theories of Voluntary Animal Motion from Greek Antiquity to the Latin Middle Ages, 400 B.C.–A.D. 1300*. Berlin: Verlag Dr Muller, 2008.

Francis (pope). *Laudato Si*. London: Catholic Truth Society, 2015.

Frede, M., and G. Striker, eds. *Rationality in Greek Thought*. Oxford: Oxford University Press, 1996.

Frier, B., and T. McGinn. *A Casebook on Roman Family Law*. Oxford: Oxford University Press, 2004.

Gaine, S. *Will There Be Free Will in Heaven? Freedom, Impeccability and Beatitude*. London: T & T Clark, 2003.

Garland, R. *The Eye of the Beholder: Deformity and Disability in the Graeco-Roman World*. London: Bristol Classical Press, 1995.

Garr, W. R. *In His Own Image and Likeness: Humanity, Divinity and Monotheism.* Leiden: Brill, 2003.
Gavrilyuk, P. *The Suffering of the Impassible God: The Dialectics of Patristic Thought.* Oxford: Oxford University Press, 2004.
Gavrilyuk, P. "Theopatheia: Nestorius's Main Charge against Cyril of Alexandria." *Scottish Journal of Theology* 56, no. 2 (2003): 190–207.
George, R., and P. Lee. "Acorns and Embryos." *New Atlantis* 7 (2004/2005): 90–100.
Gill, C. "Personhood and Personality: The Four Personae Theory." In Cicero, *De Officiis I,* edited by J. Annas, 169–99. Vol. VI of *Oxford Studies in Ancient Philosophy.* Oxford: Oxford University Press, 1988.
Gillon, R. "Human Reproductive Cloning." In *The Cloning Sourcebook*, edited by A. Klotzko. Oxford: Oxford University Press, 2003.
Glover, J. *Causing Death and Saving Lives.* London: Penguin, 1977.
Goodley, C., and M. Lynn-Rose. "Mental States, Bodily Dispositions and Table Manners: A Guide to Reading 'Intellectual' Disability from Homer to Late Antiquity." In *Disabilities in Roman Antiquity: Disparate Bodies A Capite Ad Calcem*, edited by C. Laes et al., 17–43. Leiden: Brill, 2013.
Goodley, D. *Disability Studies: An Interdisciplinary Introduction.* London: Sage, 2011.
Goodley, D. *Dis/Ability Studies: Theorising Disability and Ableism.* Oxford: Routledge, 2014.
Gordijn, B. "The Troublesome Concept of the Person." *Theoretical Medicine and Bioethics* 20, no. 4 (1999): 347–59.
Goulder, M. "Ignatius' Docetists." *Vigiliae Christianae* 53, no. 1 (1999): 16–30.
Green, M., and D. Winkler. "Brain Death and Personal Identity." *Philosophy and Public Affairs* 9, no. 2 (1980): 105–33.
Grenz, S. *The Social God and the Relational Self.* Louisville, KY: Westminster John Knox Press, 1991.
Grenz, S. *Theology for the Community of God.* Grand Rapids, MI: Eerdmans, 1994.
Grillmeier, A. *Christ in Christian Tradition: From the Apostolic Age to Chalcedon.* Translated by J. S. Bowden. London: Mowbray, 1965.
Gunton, C. *The Promise of Trinitarian Theology.* London.... Clark, 1997.
Gunton, C. "Trinity, Ontology and Anthropology: Towards a Renewal of the Doctrine of the Imago Dei." In *Persons, Divine and Human*, edited by C. Schwobel and C. Gunton. Edinburgh.... Clark, 1991.
Gwynn, D. *Athanasius of Alexandria, Bishop, Theologian, Ascetic, Father.* Oxford: Oxford University Press, 2012.
Hall, D. *The Trinity: An Analysis of Thomas Aquinas' Exposito of the De Trinitate of Boethius.* Leiden: Brill, 1992.
Hall, S. *Doctrine and Practice in the Early Church.* London: SPCK, 1995.
Hannah, D. *Michael and Christ: Michael Traditions and Angel Christology in Early Christianity.* Tubingen: Mohr Siebeck, 1999.
Hanson, R. P. C. *The Search for the Christian Doctrine of God: The Arian Controversy, 318–381.* Edinburgh.... Clark, 1988.
Harris, J. "The Concept of the Person and the Value of Life." In *Personhood and Health*

Care, edited by D. Thomasma, D. Weisstub, and C. Hervé, 99–111. Dordrecht: Kluwer, 2001.

Harris, J. "Embryos and Hedgehogs: On the Moral Status of the Embryo." In *Experiments on Embryos*, edited by A. Dyson and J. Harris, 69–70. London: Routledge, 1990.

Harris, J. *Enhancing Evolution: The Ethical Case for Making Better People*. Princeton, NJ: Princeton University Press, 2007.

Harris, J. "Euthanasia and the Value of Life." In *Euthanasia Examined*, edited by J. Keown. Cambridge: Cambridge University Press, 1995.

Harris, J. *The Value of Life: An Introduction to Medical Ethics*. Oxford: Routledge, 1985.

Harris, J. *Wonderwoman and Superman: The Ethics of Human Biotechnology*. Oxford: Oxford University Press, 1992.

Harrison, C. *Augustine: Christian Faith and Fractured Humanity*. Oxford: Oxford University Press, 2000.

Harrison, P. "Subduing the Earth: Genesis 1, Early Modern Science, and the Exploitation of Nature." *Journal of Religion* 79, no. 1 (1999): 86–109.

Herring, G. *An Introduction to the History of Christianity*. London: Continuum, 2001.

Hildebrand, S. *The Trinitarian Theology of Basil of Caesarea: A Synthesis of Greek Thought and Biblical Truth*. Washington, DC: Catholic University of America Press, 2007.

Hill, E. "Response: St Augustine and R.R.R. on Women." *New Blackfriars* 66, no. 785 (1985): 503–4.

Hobbes, T. *Leviathan with Selected Variants from the Latin Edition of 1668*. Edited by E. Curley. Indianapolis: Hackett, 1994.

Hoekema, A. *Created in God's Image*. Grand Rapids, MI: Eerdmans, 1994.

Hofer, A. *Christ in the Life and Teaching of Gregory of Nazianzus*. Oxford: Oxford University Press, 2013.

Holmes, A. *Building the Christian Academy*. Grand Rapids, MI: Eerdmans, 2001.

Horgan, M. "The Letter to the Colossians." In *The New Jerome Biblical Commentary*, edited by R. Brown et al., 876–82. London: Geoffrey Chapman, 2000.

House of Lords Select Committee on Stem Cell Research. *Stem Cell Research*. London: House of Lords, 2001. https://publications.parliament.uk/pa/ld200102/ldselect/ldstem/83/8301.htm.

Hull, J. "Blindness and the Face of God: Toward a Theology of Disability." In *The Human Image of God*, edited by H. Zeibertz et al. Leiden: Brill, 2001.

Hunter, D. *Marriage, Celibacy, and Heresy in Ancient Christianity: The Jovinianist Controversy*. Oxford: Oxford University Press, 2007.

Iltis, A. "The Failed Search for the Neutral in the Secular: Public Bioethics in the Face of the Culture Wars." *Christian Bioethics* 15, no. 3 (2009): 220–33.

International Theological Commission. "The Hope of Salvation for Infants Who Die without Being Baptised (2007)." In *Texts and Documents, 1969–1985*, Vol. 1, 353–400. San Francisco: Ignatius Press, 2009.

Jagersma, H. *A History of Israel to Bar Kochba*. London: SCM Press, 1994.

Jennett, B. *The Vegetative State: Medical Facts, Ethical and Legal Dilemmas*. Cambridge: Cambridge University Press, 2002.

Jensen, S., ed. *The Ethics of Organ Transplantation*. Washington, DC: Catholic University of America Press, 2011.
Johnson, H. M. "Unspeakable Conversations." *New York Times Magazine*. February 16, 2003. http://www.nytimes.com/2003/02/16/magazine/unspeakable-conversations.html.
John Paul II (pope). *Evangelium Vitae*. Website of the Holy See, March 25, 1995. http://w2.vatican.va/content/john-paul-ii/en/encyclicals/documents/hf_jp-ii_enc_25031995_evangelium-vitae.html.
John Paul II (pope). *Fides et Ratio*. Website of the Holy See, September 14, 1998. http://w2.vatican.va/content/john-paul-ii/en/encyclicals/documents/hf_jp-ii_enc_14091998_fides-et-ratio.html.
John Paul II (pope). *General Audience: Marriage in the Integral Vision of Man*. Website of the Holy See, April 2, 1980. http://w2.vatican.va/content/john-paul-ii/en/audiences/1980/documents/hf_jp-ii_aud_19800402.html.
John Paul II (pope). *General Audience (Psalm 150)*. Website of the Holy See, February 26, 2003. http://w2.vatican.va/content/john-paul-ii/en/audiences/2003/documents/hf_jp-ii_aud_20030226.html.
John Paul II (pope). "Mentally Ill Are Also Made in God's Image." *L'Osservatore Romano*. December 11, 1996.
John Paul II (pope). *Redemptor Hominis*. Website of the Holy See, March 4, 1979. http://w2.vatican.va/content/john-paul-ii/en/encyclicals/documents/hf_jp-ii_enc_04031979_redemptor-hominis.html.
John Paul II (pope). *Salvifici Doloris*. Website of the Holy See, February 11, 1984. http://w2.vatican.va/content/john-paul-ii/en/apost_letters/1984/documents/hf_jp-ii_apl_11021984_salvifici-doloris.html.
John Paul II (pope). *Sollicitudo Rei Socialis*. Website of the Holy See, December 30, 1987. http://w2.vatican.va/content/john-paul-ii/en/encyclicals/documents/hf_jp-ii_enc_30121987_sollicitudo-rei-socialis.html.
John Paul II (pope). *Veritatis Splendour*. Website of the Holy See, August 6, 1993. http://w2.vatican.va/content/john-paul-ii/en/encyclicals/documents/hf_jp-ii_enc_06081993_veritatis-splendor.html.
Jolowicz, H. F., and B. Nicholas. *Historical Introduction to the Study of Roman Law*. Cambridge: Cambridge University Press, 1972.
Jonas, H. "Against the Stream: Comments on the Definition and Redefinition of Death." In *Philosophical Essays: From Ancient Creeds to Technological Man*, edited by L. E. Long. Chicago: University of Chicago Press, 1974.
Jones, D. *The Soul of the Embryo*. London: Continuum, 2004.
Kannengeisser, C. "Origen's Doctrine Transmitted by Antony the Hermit and Athanasius of Alexandria." In *Origeniana Octava*, Vol. II, edited by Lorenzo Perrone. Louvain: Leuven University Press, 2003.
Karras, V. "Science and the Cappadocians: Orthodoxy and Science in the Fourth Century." In *Science and the Eastern Orthodox Church*, edited by D. Buxhoeveden and G. Woloschak. Farnham: Ashgate, 2011.
Kasper, W. *The God of Jesus Christ*. London: SCM Press, 1983.
Kasper, W. *Jesus the Christ*. Mahwah, NJ: Paulist Press, 1977.

Kearney, M. *Mortally Wounded*. New York: Touchstone, 1997.
Keating, J. F., and T. J. White, eds. *Divine Impassibility and the Mystery of Human Suffering*. Grand Rapids, MI: Eerdmans, 2009.
Kelly, D. *Medical Care at the End of Life: A Catholic Perspective*. Washington, DC: Georgetown University Press, 2006.
Kelly, J. N. D. *Early Christian Creeds*. New York: Routledge, 2014. [First published 1950.]
Kelly, J. N. D. *Early Christian Doctrines*. London: Continuum, 2006.
Kennedy, I. *Treat Me Right*. Oxford: Oxford University Press, 2001.
Keown, J. *Euthanasia, Ethics and Public Policy*. Cambridge: Cambridge University Press, 2002.
Keown, J. *The Law and Ethics of Medicine*. Oxford: Oxford University Press, 2012.
Keown, J., and D. Jones, "Surveying the Foundations of Medical Law: A Reassessment of Glanville Williams's the Sanctity of Life and the Criminal Law." *Medical Law Review* 16, no. 1 (2008): 85–126.
Kitwood, T. *Dementia Reconsidered: The Person Comes First*. Berkshire: Open University Press, 1997.
Kitwood, T. *On Dementia: A Reader and Critical Commentary*, edited by C. Baldwin and A. Capstick. Berkshire: Open University Press, 2007.
Knight, K. *Aristotelian Philosophy: Ethics and Politics from Aristotle to MacIntyre*. Cambridge: Polity Press, 2007.
Knuuttila, S. *Emotions in Ancient and Medieval Philosophy*. Oxford: Oxford University Press, 2006.
Koosed, J., and D. Schumm, "Out of the Darkness: Examining the Rhetoric of Blindness in the Gospel of John." In *Disability in Judaism, Christianity, and Islam: Sacred Texts, Historical Traditions, and Social Analysis*, edited by D. Schumm and M. Stoltzfus, 77–92. New York: Palgrave Macmillan, 2011.
Kuhse, H., and P. Singer, eds. *Bioethics: An Anthology*. Oxford: Blackwell, 2006.
Kuhse, H., and P. Singer, eds. *A Companion to Bioethics*. Oxford: Wiley-Blackwell, 2009.
Küng, H., and W. Jens, eds. *A Dignified Dying*. London: SCM Press, 1995.
Laes, C. *Disability in Antiquity*. London: Routledge, 2017.
Lamberigts, M. "Caelestius." In *Augustine through the Ages: An Encyclopedia*, edited by G. W. H. Lampe. Oxford: Clarendon Press, 1961.
Lampe, G. W. H., ed., *A Patristic Lexicon*. Oxford: Clarendon Press, 1961.
Lancel, S. *St Augustine*. London: SCM Press, 2002.
Laurie, G. *Introducing Early Christianity*. New York: Intervarsity Press, 2004.
Leader, Z. *Revision and Romantic Authorship*. Oxford: Oxford University Press, 2002.
Leinhard, J. *Orthodox Readings of Augustine*. Edited by G. Demacopoulos and A. Papanikolaou. Crestwood, NY: St. Vladimir's Seminary Press, 2008.
Leithart, P. *Athanasius*. Grand Rapids, MI: Baker, 2011.
Lesky, A. *Greek Tragedy*. London: Ernest Benn, 1967.
Levinas, E. *Totality and Infinity: An Essay on Exteriority*. London: Kluwer Academic, 1991. [First published in French 1961.]
Lewis, H. *Deaf Liberation Theology*. Aldershot: Ashgate, 2007.
Liddell, H. G., and R. Scott. *Greek English Lexicon*. Oxford: Clarendon Press, 1940.

Linzey, A. *Animal Theology*. London: SCM Press, 1994.
Lizza, J. "Persons at the Beginning and End of Life." In *Bioethics in India: Proceedings of the International Bioethics Workshop in Madras, Biomanagement of Biogeoresources 16–19 January*, edited by J. Azariah, H. Azariah, and D. Macer. Chennai: University of Madras, 1997.
Locke, J. *An Essay Concerning Human Understanding*. Edited by K. Winkler. Cambridge: Hackett, 1996. [First published 1689.]
Lockwood, M. "The Moral Status of the Embryo: Implications for IVF." *Reproductive BioMedicine Online* 10, no. 1 (2005): 17–20.
Logan, A. *Gnostic Truth and Christian Heresy*. Edinburgh.... Clark, 1996.
Long, A. A. *From Epicurus to Epictetus: Studies in Hellenistic and Roman Philosophy*. Oxford: Oxford University Press, 2006.
Louth, A. "The Place of Theosis in Orthodox Tradition." In *Partakers of the Divine Nature*, edited by M. Christensen and J. Wittung. Cranbury, NJ: Associated University Presses, 2007.
MacDonald, P. *History of the Concept of the Mind*. Aldershot: Ashgate, 2003.
Machery, E. "Apeism and Racism, Reasons and Remedies." In *The Politics of Species, Reshaping Our Relationships with Other Animals*, edited by R. Corbey and A. Lanjouw. Cambridge: Cambridge University Press, 2013.
MacKellar, C., and D. Jones. *Chimera's Children: Ethical, Philosophical and Religious Perspectives on Human-Nonhuman Experimentation*. London: Continuum Press, 2012.
Macquarrie, J. *Christology Revisited*. London: SCM Press, 1998.
Manninen, B. "Revisiting the Argument from Fetal Potential." *Philosophy, Ethics and Humanities in Medicine* 2 (2007).
Marenbon, J. *Boethius*. Oxford: Oxford University Press, 2003.
Matthews, P. "Communication Strategies and Intensive Interaction Therapy Meet the Theology of the Body: Bioethics in Dialogue with People with Profound Disabilities." *New Bioethics* 19, no. 2 (2013): 97–110.
Matthews, P. "Human Dignity and the Profoundly Disabled: A Theological Perspective." *Human Reproduction and Genetic Ethics* 17, no. 2 (2011).
Matthews, P. "Participation and the Profoundly Disabled: 'Being' Engaged—A Theological Approach." *Journal of Religion, Disability and Health* 17 (2013): 431–32.
Matthews, P. *Pope John Paul II and the "Apparently" Non-Acting Person*. Leominster: Gracewing, 2013.
Matthews, P. "Right Rights, Authentic Autonomy: Disability as a Human Rights Issue." *Catholic Medical Quarterly* 63, no. 4 (2013).
Mauss, M. "A Category of the Human Mind: The Notion of Person; the Notion of Self." In *The Category of the Person*, edited by M. Carrithers, S. Collins, and S. Lukes. Cambridge: Cambridge University Press, 1985.
McCabe, H. *God Matters*. London: Continuum, 1987.
McCarthy Spoerl, K. "Apollinarius on the Holy Spirit." In *Studia Patristica*. Vol. XXXVII of *Papers Presented at the 13th International Conference on Patristic Studies*, edited by M. F. Wiles and E. J. Yarnold. Louvain: Peeters, 2001.

McCruden, K. "Monarchy and Economy in Tertullian's *Adversus Praxeam. Scottish Journal of Theology* 55, no. 3 (2002): 332.
McGowan, A. "Tertullian and the 'Heretical' Origins of the 'Orthodox' Trinity." *Journal of Early Christian Studies* 14, no. 4 (2006): 437–57.
McGrath, A. *Christian Theology: An Introduction*. Oxford: Wiley-Blackwell, 2011.
McGrath, A. *Historical Theology*. Oxford: Blackwell, 1998.
McGuckin, J. "Did Augustine's Christology Depend on Theodore of Mopsuestia?" *Heythrop Journal* 31, no. 1 (1990): 39–52.
McGuckin, J. *St Cyril of Alexandria: The Christological Controversy*. Crestwood: St. Vladimir's Seminary Press, 2004.
McGuckin, J. *St Gregory of Nazianzus*. Crestwood: St. Vladimir's Seminary Press, 2001.
McKim, D. *Theological Turning Points*. Louisville, KY: Westminster John Knox Press, 1988.
McLaughlin, B. "Vitalism and Emergence." In *The Cambridge History of Philosophy, 1870–1945*, edited by T. Baldwin. Cambridge: Cambridge University Press, 2003.
McLeod, F. *The Image of God in the Antiochene Tradition*. Washington, DC: Catholic University of America Press, 1999.
McLeod, F. *The Roles of Christ's Humanity in Salvation: Insights from Theodore of Mopsuestia*. Washington, DC: Catholic University of America Press, 2005.
McLeod, F. *Theodore of Mopsuestia*. New York: Routledge, 2009.
McLeod, F. "Theodore of Mopsuestia Revisited." *Theological Studies* 61, no. 3 (2000): 447–80.
McMahan, J. *The Ethics of Killing: Problems at the Margins of Life*. Oxford: Oxford University Press, 2002.
McMahan, J. "Infanticide." *Utilitas* 19, no. 2 (2007): 131–59.
McWilliam, J. "Augustine at Ephesus?" In *One Lord, One Faith, One Baptism*, edited by M. Dutton and P. T. Gray. Grand Rapids, MI: Eerdmans, 2006.
Meilaender, G. *Neither Beast nor God: The Dignity of the Human Person*. New York: Encounter Books, 2009.
Merrill, S. B. *Defining Personhood: Toward the Ethics of Quality in Clinical Care*. Amsterdam: Rodopi, 1998.
Messer, N. "Human Genome Project, Health and the Tyranny of Normality." In *Brave New World?*, edited by C. Deanne-Drummond. London: Continuum, 2003.
Middleton, R. *The Liberating Image*. Grand Rapids, MI: Brazos Press, 2005.
Migliore, D. *Faith Seeking Understanding*. Grand Rapids, MI: Eerdmans, 2004.
Miller, P., S. Parker, and S. Gillinson. *Disablism: How to Tackle the Last Prejudice*. London: Demos, 2004.
Mingana, A. *Catechetical Homilies: Commentary of Theodore of Mopsuestia on the Nicene Creed*. Vol. 5 of *Woodbrooke Studies*. Cambridge: Cambridge University Press, 1932. [Reprint, Gorgias, 2009.]
Moll, S. *The Arch-Heretic Marcion*. Tubingen: Mohr Siebeck, 2010.
Mori, M. "Is the Human Embryo a Person? No." In *Conceiving the Embryo: Ethics, Law and practice in Human Embryology*, edited by D. Evans, 151–63. London: Martinus Nijhoff, 1996.

Moss, C. "Heavenly Healing: Eschatological Cleansing and the Resurrection of the Dead in the Early Church." *Journal of the American Academy of Religion* 79, no. 4 (2011): 991–1017.
Muller, R. "The Role of Church History in the Study of Systematic Theology." In *Doing Theology in Today's World*, edited by J. Woodbridge and T. McComiskey. Grand Rapids, MI: Zondervan, 1991.
Murphy, T. "In Defence of Irreligious Bioethics." *American Journal of Bioethics* 12, no. 12 (2012): 3–10.
Neil, B. *Leo the Great*. London: Routledge, 2009.
Neil, B., and P. Allen. *Crisis Management in Late Antiquity (410–590 CE): A Survey of the Evidence from Episcopal Letters*. Leiden: Brill, 2013.
Ngaire Williams, A. *The Divine Sense*. Cambridge: Cambridge University Press, 2007.
Nicholas, B. *An Introduction to Roman Law*. Oxford: Oxford University Press, 2008.
O'Collins, G. *The Tripersonal God*. Mahwah, NJ: Paulist Press, 1999.
O'Connor, J. M. "The First Letter to the Corinthians." In *The New Jerome Biblical Commentary*, edited by R. Brown et al., 798–815. London: Geoffrey Chapman, 2000.
O'Donovan, O. "Again: Who Is a Person?" In *On Moral Medicine, Theological Perspectives in Medical Ethics*, edited by S. Lammers and A. Verhey. Grand Rapids, MI: Eerdmans, 1998.
O'Donovan, O. *Begotten or Made?* Oxford: Oxford University Press, 1984.
O'Keefe, J. "Impassible Suffering? Divine Passion and Fifth Century Christology." *Theological Studies* 58 (1997): 39–60.
Olson, R. *The Mosaic of Christian Belief*. Downers Grove, IL: Intervarsity Press, 2002.
Olson, R. *The Story of Christian Theology*. Downers Grove, IL: Intervarsity Press, 1999.
O'Rourke, K. "Reflections on the Papal Allocution Concerning Care for Persistent Vegetative State Patients." *Christian Bioethics* 12, no. 1 (2006): 93.
O'Rourke, K., and P. Norris. "Care of the PVS Patient: Catholic Opinion in the US." *Linacre Quarterly* 68, no. 3 (2001): 207–17.
O'Rourke Boyle, M. *Senses of Touch: Human Dignity and Deformity from Michelangelo to Calvin*. Leiden: Brill, 1998.
Osborn, E. *Clement of Alexandria*. Cambridge: Cambridge University Press, 2005.
Osborn, E. *Irenaeus of Lyons*. Cambridge: Cambridge University Press, 2004.
Osborn, E. *Tertullian, First Theologian of the West*. Cambridge: Cambridge University Press, 2003.
Parfit, D. *Reasons and Persons*. Oxford: Clarendon Press, 1984.
Pasnau, R. *Thomas Aquinas on Human Nature*. Cambridge: Cambridge University Press, 2002.
Patterson, B. "Redeemed Bodies: Fullness of Life." In *Human Disability and the Service of God: Reassessing Religious Practice*, edited by N. Eiesland and D. Saliers. Nashville, TN: Abingdon Press, 1998.
Persson, I., and J. Savulescu. *Unfit for the Future: The Need for Moral Enhancement*. Oxford: Oxford University Press, 2012.
Peterson, J. *Genetic Turning Points: The Ethics of Human Genetic Intervention*. Grand Rapids, MI: Eerdmans, 2001.

Pius XII (pope). "Address to an International Congress of Anesthesiologists." *L'Osservatore Romano*. November 25–26, 1957.
Placher, W. *Narratives of a Vulnerable God*. Louisville, KY: Westminster John Knox Press, 1994.
Pollard, T. E. *Johannine Christology and the Early Church*. Cambridge: Cambridge University Press, 1970.
Pollock, D. "Masks and the Semiotics of Identity." *Journal of the Royal Anthropological Institute* 1, no. 3 (1995): 582.
Pontifical Council for Justice and Peace. *Compendium of the Social Doctrine of the Church*. Washington, DC: Libreria Editrice Vaticana, 2004.
President's Commission for the Study of Ethical Problems in Medicine and Biomedical and Behavioural Research. *Defining Death: Medical, Legal and Ethical Issues in the Definition of Death*. Washington, DC: Government Printing Office, 1981.
Prestige, G. L. *God in Patristic Thought*. London: SPCK, 1975.
Pritchard, A. M. *Leage's Roman Private Law*. London: MacMillan, 1961.
Purcell, E. "Narrative Ethics and Vulnerability: Kristeva and Ricoeur on Interdependence." *Journal of French and Francophone Philosophy* 21, no. 1 (2013): 43–59.
Quasten, J. *Patrology*. Vol. III. Utrecht: Spectrum, 1960.
Quin, P. "Disputing the Augustinian Legacy: John Locke and Jonathan Edwards on *Romans 5:12–19*." In *The Augustinian Tradition*, edited by G. Matthews, 238–42. Berkeley: University of California Press, 1999.
Quispel, G. *Gnostica, Judaica, Catholica. Collected Essays of Gilles Quispel*, edited by J. Van Oort. Leiden: Brill, 2008.
Rachels, J. *Can Ethics Provide Answers? And Other Essays in Moral Philosophy*. Lanham, MD: Rowman and Littlefield, 1997.
Rachels, J. *Created from Animals: The Moral Implications of Darwinism*. Oxford: Oxford University Press, 1990.
Rachels, J. *The End of Life: Euthanasia and Morality*. Oxford: Oxford University Press, 1986.
Rachels, J., and W. Ruddick. "Lives and Liberty." In *The Legacy of Socrates Essays in Moral Philosophy*, edited by S. Rachels. New York: Columbia Press, 2007.
Rahner, K. *Theological Investigations*. Vol. IV. Translated by K. Smyth. London: Darton, Longman and Todd, 1974.
Rakestraw, R. "The Persistent Vegetative State and the Withdrawal of Nutrition and Hydration." In *Readings in Christian Ethics*. Vol. 2, edited by D. Clark and R. Rakestraw, 126–27. Grand Rapids, MI: Baker, 2008.
Ramsey, P. *The Patient as Person*. New Haven, CT: Yale University Press, 1970.
Raven, C. *Apollinarianism: An Essay on the Christology of the Early Church*. Eugene, OR: Wipf and Stock, 2004. [Originally published by Cambridge University Press, 1923.]
Rees, B. R. *Pelagius: Life and Letters*. Vol. I, *Pelagius: A Reluctant Heretic*. Woodbridge: Boydell, 1998.
Rehm, R. *Greek Tragic Theatre*. London: Routledge, 1994.
Reinders, H. *Receiving the Gift of Friendship*. Grand Rapids, MI: Eerdmans, 2008.

Reist, M. T., ed. *Defiant Birth: Women Who Resist Medical Eugenics*. North Melbourne, VIC: Spinifex, 2009.
Reynolds, T. *Vulnerable Communion: A Theology of Disability and Hospitality*. Grand Rapids, MI: Brazos Press, 2008.
Ricoeur, P. *Oneself as Another*. Translated by K. Blamey. Chicago: Chicago University Press, 1994.
Rist, J. *Human Value: A Study in Ancient Philosophical Ethics*. Leiden: Brill, 1982.
Rodriguez-Arias, D., M. Smith, and N. Lazar. "Donation after Circulatory Death: Burying the Dead Donor Rule." *American Journal of Bioethics* 11, no. 8 (2011): 36–43.
Rollin, B. "The Moral Status of Animals and Their Use as Experimental Subjects." In *A Companion to Bioethics*, edited by H. Kuhse and P. Singer, 497–98. Oxford: Wiley-Blackwell, 2009.
Rolnick, P. *Person, Grace and God*. Grand Rapids, MI: Eerdmans, 2007.
Romero, M. "Aquinas on the *Corporis Infirmitas*: Broken Flesh and the Grammar of Grace." In *Disability in the Christian Tradition: A Reader*, edited by B. Brock and J. Swinton, 101–51. Grand Rapids, MI: Eerdmans, 2012.
Rondet, H. *Original Sin: The Patristic and Theological Background*. Florence, AZ: Ecclesia Press, 1972.
Rosen, M. *Dignity: Its History and Meaning*. Cambridge, MA: Harvard University Press, 2012.
Ruddick, W. " 'Biographical Lives' Revisited and Extended." *Journal of Ethics* 9 (2005): 502.
Ruether, R. R. "The Liberation of Christianity from Patriarchy." *New Blackfriars* 66, no. 781/782 (1985), 325–26.
Runia, D. *Philo of Alexandria and the Timaeus of Plato*. Leiden: Brill, 1986.
Runia, D. *Philo in Early Christian Literature: A Survey*. Assen: Van Gorcum Fortress Press, 1993.
Russell, N. *Cyril of Alexandria*. London: Routledge, 2000.
Russell, N. *The Doctrine of Deification in the Greek Patristic Tradition*. Oxford: Oxford University Press, 2006.
Ruston, R. *Human Rights and the Image of God*. London: SCM Press, 2004.
Ryder, R. *The Political Animal: The Conquest of Speciesism*. Jefferson, NC: McFarland, 1998.
Ryder, R. "Speciesism Revisited." *Think* 2, no. 6 (2004): 89–90.
Sanders, E. P. "Paul between Judaism and Hellenism." In *St. Paul among the Philosophers*, edited by J. Caputo and L. Alcoff. Bloomington: Indiana University Press, 2009.
Savulescu, J., and G. Kahane. "The Moral Obligation to Create Children with the Best Chance of the Best Life." *Bioethics* 23, no. 5 (2009): 274–90.
Saxton, M. "Disability Rights and Selective Abortion." In *The Disability Studies Reader*, edited by L. Davis. New York: Routledge, 2006.
Schaefer, J. "Appreciating the Beauty of the Earth." *Theological Studies* 62, no. 1 (2001): 23–52.
Schaefer, J. *Theological Foundations for Environmental Ethics: Reconstructing Medieval*

and Patristic Concepts. Washington, DC: Georgetown University Press, 2009.
Scope. *Getting Away with Murder: Disabled People's Experience of Hate Crime in the UK* London: SCOPE, 2008.
Scope. "Memorandum from Scope to the House of Lords, House of Commons Joint Committee on Human Rights." In *A Life Like Any Other? Human Rights of Adults with Learning Disabilities. Seventh Report of Session 2007–08*. Vol. II of *Oral and Written Evidence*, 79–80. London: Parliamentary Bookshop, 2008.
Second Vatican Council. *Dei Verbum*. Website of the Holy See, November 18, 1965. http://www.vatican.va/archive/hist_councils/ii_vatican_council/documents/vat-ii_const_19651118_dei-verbum_en.html.
Second Vatican Council. *Gaudium et Spes*. Website of the Holy See, December 7, 1965. *http://www.vatican.va/archive/hist_councils/ii_vatican_council/documents/vat-ii_const_19651207_gaudium-et-spes_en.html.*
Select Committee on Science and Technology. "Memorandum 21: Submission from Christian Action Research and Education (CARE)." UK Parliament website, accessed April 11, 2012. http://www.publications.parliament.uk/pa/cm200607/cmselect/cmsctech/272/272we23.htm.
Shannon, T. "Grounding Human Dignity." *Dialog: A Journal of Theology* 43, no. 2 (2004): 114.
Shults, L. R. *Christology and Science*. Aldershot: Ashgate, 2008.
Silvas, A. *Gregory of Nyssa: The Letters, Introduction, Translation and Commentary*. Leiden: Brill, 2007.
Simpson, D. P. *Cassell's Latin Dictionary*. London: Cassell, 2007.
Singer, G. "People with Mental Retardation and the Developmental Disabilities Philosophy." In *Handbook of Human Development for Health Care Professionals*, edited by K. Thies and J. Travers, 267–86. London: Jones and Bartlett, 2006.
Singer, P. "All Animals Are Equal." In *Bioethics: An Anthology*, edited by H. Kuhse and P. Singer, 568–77. Oxford: Blackwell, 2006.
Singer, P. *Animal Liberation*. New York: HarperCollins, 1975.
Singer, P. "An Intellectual Autobiography." In *Peter Singer under Fire: The Moral Iconoclast Faces His Critics*, edited by J. Schaler. Peru, IL: Open Court, 2009.
Singer, P. "Killing Humans and Killing Animals." In *Peter Singer: Unsanctifying Human Life*, edited by H. Kuhse, 112–22. Oxford: Blackwell, 2002.
Singer, P. *Practical Ethics*. 2nd ed. Cambridge: Cambridge University Press, 1993. [3rd ed., Cambridge University Press, 2011.]
Singer, P. "Reply to Stephen Drake." In *Peter Singer under Fire: The Moral Iconoclast Faces His Critics*, edited by J. Schaler. Peru, IL: Open Court, 2009.
Singer, P. *Rethinking Life and Death*. Oxford: Oxford University Press, 1994.
Singer, P. "Speciesism and Moral Status." *Metaphilosophy* 40, no. 3–4 (2009): 567–81.
Singer, P. *Writings on an Ethical Life*. London: Fourth Estate, 2002.
Smith, C. U. M. "Beginnings: Ventricular Psychology." In *Brain, Mind and Consciousness in the History of Neuroscience*, edited by C. U. M. Smith and Harry Whitaker. Dordrecht: Springer, 2014.
Sorabji, R. *The Philosophy of the Commentators, 200–600 AD: A Sourcebook*. Vol. 2, *Physics*. Ithaca, NY: Cornell University Press, 2005.

Spaemann, R. *Persons: The Difference between "Someone" and "Something."* Oxford: Oxford University Press, 2006.

Stammers, T., and S. Bullivant. "Secularism." In *Oxford Textbook of Spirituality in Healthcare*, edited by M. Cobb, C. Pcualski, and B. Rumbold, 83–88. Oxford: Oxford University Press, 2012.

Stevenson, James. *A New Eusebius: Documents Illustrating the History of the Church to AD 337*. London: SPCK, 1987.

Stiver, D. *The Philosophy of Religious Language*. Oxford: Blackwell, 1996.

Strawson, G. *Locke on Personal Identity: Consciousness and Concernment*. Princeton, NJ: Princeton University Press, 2011.

Strecker, G. *Theology of the New Testament*. New York: Westminster John Knox Press, 2000.

Sulmasy, D. "End-of-Life Care Revisited." In *Artificial Nutrition and Hydration and the Permanently Unconscious Patient: The Catholic Debate*, edited by R. Hamel and J. Walter. Washington, DC: Georgetown University Press, 2007.

Swinburne, R. *The Christian God*. Oxford: Oxford University Press, 1994.

Swinburne, R. *The Coherence of Theism*. Oxford: Oxford University Press, 1993.

Swinburne, R. *The Existence of God*. Oxford: Oxford University Press, 2004.

Swinburne, R. *Is There a God?* Oxford: Oxford University Press, 1996.

Takala, T. "Genetic Knowledge and Our Conception of Ourselves as Persons." In *Personhood and Healthcare*, edited by D. Thomasma, D. Weisstub, and C. Hervé, 91–97. Dordrecht: Kluwer, 2001.

Tallis, R. *In Defence of Wonder and Other Philosophical Reflections*. London: Routledge, 2014.

Tanner, J. "Eugenics before 1945." *Journal of Modern European History* 10, no. 4 (2012): 458–79.

Taylor, C. *Sources of the Self: The Making of Modern Identity*. Cambridge: Cambridge University Press, 1989.

Tellbe, M. *Christ-Believers in Ephesus*. Tubingen: Mohr Siebeck, 2009.

ter Haar Romney, R. B. "Eusebius of Emessa's Commentary on Genesis and the Origins of the Antiochene School." In *The Book of Genesis in Jewish and Oriental Christian Interpretation*, edited by J. Frishman and L. Van Rompay. Louvain: Peeters, 1997.

Teske, R. *To Know God and the Soul: Essays on the Thought of St. Augustine*. Washington, DC: Catholic University of America Press, 2008.

Thiel, U. *The Early Modern Subject: Self-Consciousness and Personal Identity from Descartes to Hume*. Oxford: Oxford University Press, 2011.

Thunberg, L. "The Human Person as Image of God." In *Christian Spirituality: Origins to the 12th Century*, edited by B. McGinn et al. London: Routledge, 1986.

Tooley, M. *Abortion and Infanticide*. Oxford: Oxford University Press, 1983.

Tooley, M. "Personhood." In *A Companion to Bioethics*, edited by H. Kuhse and P. Singer. Oxford: Wiley Blackwell, 2009.

Toom, T. "The Potential of a Condemned Analogy: Augustine." *Heythrop Journal* 48, no. 2 (2007): 205–6.

Torchia, J. *Exploring Personhood*. New York: Rowman & Littlefield, 2008.

Torrance, I. "Chemists or Terminologists? The Christological Debate from Apollinaris to Severus of Antioch." In *Jesus Christ Today: Studies of Christology in Various Contexts*, edited by S. Hall. Berlin: De Gruyter, 2009.

Torrance, T. *The Christian Doctrine of God*. Edinburgh.... Clark, 1996.

Trigg, J. *Origen*. London: SCM Press, 1983.

Truog, R., and F. Miller. "The Dead Donor Rule and Organ Transplantation." *New England Journal of Medicine* 359, no. 7 (2008): 674–75.

Turcescu, L. *Gregory of Nyssa and the Concept of Divine Persons*. Oxford: Oxford University Press, 2005.

Turcescu, L. "Soteriological Issues on the 1999 Lutheran-Catholic Joint Declaration on Justification: An Orthodox Perspective." *Journal of Ecumenical Studies* 28, no. 1 (2001): 64–72.

Turner, J. *Sethian Gnosticism and the Platonic Tradition*. Paris: Peeters, 2001.

Tutu, D. *No Future without Forgiveness*. London: Random House, 1999.

Upson-Saia, K. "Resurrecting Deformity: Augustine on Wounded and Scarred Bodies in the Heavenly Realm." In *Disability in Judaism, Christianity, and Islam: Sacred Texts, Historical Traditions, and Social Analysis*, edited by D. Schumm and M. Stoltzfus. New York: Palgrave Macmillan, 2011.

van Kooten, G. "Image, Form and Transformation: A Semantic Taxonomy of Paul's 'Morphic' Language." In *Jesus, Paul, and Early Christianity*, edited by R. Buitenwerf et al. Leiden: Brill, 2008.

van Kooten, G. *Paul's Anthropology in Context*. Tübingen: Mohr Siebeck, 2008.

van Loon, H. *The Dyophysite Christology of Cyril of Alexandria*. Leiden: Brill, 2009.

Veatch, R. "The Dead Donor Rule: True by Definition." *American Journal of Bioethics* 3, no. 1 (2003): 10–11.

Veatch, R. "The Death of Whole-Brain Death: The Plague of the Disaggregators, Somaticists and Mentalists." *Journal of Medicine and Philosophy* 30 (2005): 353–78.

Veatch, R. "The Impending Collapse of the Whole-Brain Definition of Death." *Hastings Center Report* 23, no. 4 (1993): 18–24.

Vine, W. E. *Vine's Complete Expository Dictionary of Old and New Testament Words*, edited by M. Ungar and W. White. Nashville, TN: Thomas Nelson, 1984.

Wallace-Hadrill, D. *Christian Antioch*. Cambridge: Cambridge University Press, 1982.

Ware, K. *The Orthodox Church*. London: Penguin, 1997.

Ware, T. "The Human Person as an Icon of the Trinity." Sobornost 18, no. 2 (1986): http://trinityinyou.com/pdfs/the_Human_Person_as_an_Icon_of_the_Trinity.pdf.

Warnock, M. "Do Human Cells Have Rights?" *Bioethics* 1 (1987): 2.

Warnock, M. "In Vitro Fertilisation: The Ethical Issue." *Philosophical Quarterly* 33, no. 132 (1983): 239.

Warnock, M. *The Warnock Report on Human Fertilisation and Embryology*. Oxford: Blackwell, 1984.

Watermeyer, B. *Towards a Contextual Psychology of Disability*. Oxford: Routledge, 2013.

Weinandy, T. *Athanasius*. Aldershot: Ashgate, 2007.

Weinandy, T. "Cyril and the Mystery of the Incarnation." In *The Theology of St Cyril*

of Alexandria: A Critical Appreciation, edited by T. Weinandy and D. Keating, 23–54. London.... Clark, 2003.
Weinandy, T. *Does God Change?* Still River, MA: St. Bede's, 1984.
Weinandy, T. *Does God Suffer?* Notre Dame, IN: University of Notre Dame Press, 2000.
Weinandy, T. "Zizioulas: The Trinity and Ecumenism." *New Blackfriars* 83 (2002): 411.
Weiss Block, J. *Copious Healing: A Theology of Access for People with Disabilities*. New York: Continuum International, 2002.
Wessel, S. *Leo the Great and the Spiritual Rebuilding of a Universal Rome*. Leiden: Brill, 2008.
Westermann, C. *Genesis 1–11*. London: SPCK, 1984.
Wickham, L. "Pelagianism in the East." In *The Making of Orthodoxy: Essays in Honour of Henry Chadwick*, edited by R. Williams. Cambridge: Cambridge University Press, 2002.
Wikler, D. "Can We Learn from Eugenics?" *Journal of Medical Ethics* 25 (1999): 183–94.
Wildes, K. "Religion in Bioethics: A Rebirth." *Christian Bioethics* 8, no. 2 (2002): 163–74.
Wilkinson, D. *Death or Disability? The "Carmentis Machine" and Decision-Making for Critically Ill Children*. Oxford: Oxford University Press, 2013.
Williams, F., ed. *The Panarion of Epiphanius of Salamis, Books II and II. De Fide*. Leiden: Brill, 2013.
Williams, R. *Arius: Heresy and Tradition*. London: Darton, Longman and Todd, 1987.
Williams, R. "Origen." In *The First Christian Theologians*, edited by G. R. Evans. Oxford: Blackwell, 2004.
Winterbottom, M. *Roman Declamation*. London: Bristol Classical Press, 1980.
Wirzba, N. *The Paradise of God: Renewing Religion in an Ecological Age*. Oxford: Oxford University Press, 2003.
Wojtyła, K. *Love and Responsibility*. London: Fount, 1982.
Wojtyła, K. *Sign of Contradiction*. San Francisco: HarperCollins, 1979.
Young, F. "Alexandrian and Antiochene Exegesis." In *A History of Biblical Interpretation: The Ancient Period*, edited by A. Hauser and D. Watson. Grand Rapids, MI: Eerdmans, 2003.
Young, F. *Biblical Exegesis and the Formation of Christian Culture*. Cambridge: Cambridge University Press, 1997.
Young, F. *God's Presence: A Contemporary Recapitulation of Early Christianity*. Cambridge: Cambridge University Press, 2013.
Young, F. "*Theotokos:* Mary and the Pattern of Fall and Redemption in the Theology of Cyril of Alexandria." In *The Theology of St Cyril of Alexandria: A Critical Appreciation*, edited by T. Weinandy and D. Keating. London.... Clark, 2003.
Zimmermann, J. *Humanism and Religion: A Call for the Renewal of Western Culture*. Oxford: Oxford University Press, 2012.
Zimmermann, J. *Incarnational Humanism: A Philosophy of Culture for the Church in the World*. Downers Grove, IL: Intervarsity Press, 2012.
Zimmermann, N. *Levinas and Theology*. London: Bloomsbury, 2013.
Zizioulas, J. *Being as Communion*. New York: St. Vladimir's Seminary Press, 1985.

Index

Scripture Index

Subject Index